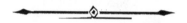

ISBN 978-0-266-56155-2
PIBN 10257591

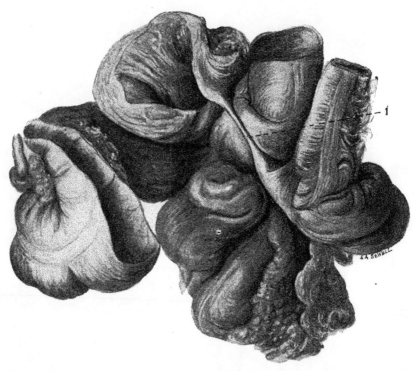

FIG. 1.—Strangulation of Intestine by Fibrous Band (1): 379, St. Thomas's
Hospital Museum.

THE ACUTE ABDOMEN

BY

WILLIAM HENRY BATTLE,

Senior Surgeon to St. Thomas's Hospital.

Formerly Joint Lecturer on Systematic Surgery, and on Practical Surgery to St. Thomas's Hospital Medical School ; Surgeon to the Royal Free Hospital ; Assistant Surgeon to the East London Hospital for Children ; Hunterian Professor, Royal College of Surgeons ; Orator to the Medical Society of London, etc. ; Joint Author (with Mr. Corner) of the Surgical Diseases of the Vermiform Appendix and their Complications (2nd ed), etc.

SECOND EDITION. ENLARGED AND ILLUSTRATED

THE MACMILLAN COMPANY OF CANADA, LTD.,
TORONTO

PREFACE

THE first edition of Lectures on "The Acute Abdomen" having become exhausted some months ago, I was requested by the publishers to write a second edition, with such alterations and additions as might seem advisable. The continued advance of our knowledge of the acute conditions which may arise in the abdomen has necessitated an increase in size of the volume, whilst it has appeared desirable to add the accounts of many cases and illustrations with the view of more thoroughly elucidating the subject. So many acute abdominal diseases have proved curable by operation, when it is performed early, that I hope my readers will not consider the subject unduly magnified considering its importance in modern practice. The treatment of the acute abdomen (including that of lesions the result of traumatism) demands an acquaintance with the surgical part of the subject which cannot always be obtained in text-books on surgery. In addition, it may be added that in order to be of general application the methods described should be as simple as possible, so that no practitioner need fear to make an attempt to save a threatened life because he has not some particular clamp, bobbin or brand of catgut in his possession. Silk is still recommended, because it is strong and can be trusted. Moreover, it is easily sterilised by boiling, even in a cottage.

The principal additions to the present volume, which is divided into sections, are those on the planning of abdominal incisions and injuries to the abdomen, external and internal, including most of the subject-matter of the Oration given before the Medical Society of London in 1910. There is a special section on the after effects of abdominal injuries. An endeavour has been made to differentiate clinically some of the varieties of peritonitis dependent on infection of the peritoneum through the blood stream ; whilst in addition there are sections on perforations of tuberculous ulceration of the intestine ; perforations of diverticula of the large bowel ; intraperitoneal abscesses ; concealed abscesses ; sigmoiditis ; important changes complicating tumours of the uterus and tumours of the ovaries ; and torsion of the omentum. In Part VII. an account is given of diverticulum of the cystic duct of congenital origin. Since I commenced my task a book has appeared by my colleagues, Messrs. Adams and Cassidy, which covers the same field to a great extent. It is an excellent one, and will meet with a wide acceptance. As this book is written from a different standpoint, I hope it will also prove useful and fulfil a want. The subject-matter has been mostly given in the form of lectures to students, and the personal form of address has been retained, as it seems to present advantages from the teaching point of view.

With the approval of my colleague, Dr. Hector Mackenzie, the plan of placing a mark ✳ when the patient was admitted into St. Thomas's Hospital under his care has been adopted in order to economise space and prevent repetition. It is hardly possible to speak too highly of the help which he has afforded during the years that we have been colleagues, but the reader of the following pages will be able to appreciate some of the debt which I owe him, and will understand that I am not ungrateful.

I have much pleasure in acknowledging the great assistance which Dr. John Harold has given me in passing the book through the press. Mr. Stewart Rouquette has been very helpful in the preparation of some of the subject-matter and statistics, whilst I am indebted to him (and to Mr. W. K. Bigger) for some photographs.

Most of the illustrations have been made for this edition by Mr. Sewell, whose excellent work is in such request by medical authors.

WILLIAM HENRY BATTLE.

HARLEY STREET,
LONDON, W.
September, 1914.

CONTENTS

CONTENTS

PART II.

PART III.

PART IV.

A.A.   *b*

LIST OF ILLUSTRATIONS

THE ACUTE ABDOMEN

INTRODUCTION

THE PLANNING OF ABDOMINAL INCISIONS

OWING to the frequency with which incisional hernia follows the making of an abdominal wound, it would be well that any one engaged, or hoping to be engaged, in the practice of abdominal surgery should have clearly in mind the anatomical structure of the parts through which he will have to pass in order to treat lesions of the viscera whether acute or not. It must be fully recognised, however, that in some acute abdominal conditions it is not always possible, or perhaps wise, to elaborate an incision ; the quickest and most direct route must be followed at any cost. Professor F. G. Parsons has kindly made a dissection which he has permitted me to show in this illustration. It gives clearly the relationship of the parts. The rectus muscle appears, however, as usual in the dead subject, more narrow than it is in the living. It then covers two thirds instead of half of the distance betwcen the anterior superior spine and the umbilicus, as shown. This is important, as will be seen later on.

There are certain lines and arrangements of muscular fibres which must be remembered, and of the former the most important is the linea alba, the second in importance the linea semilunaris.

It was once the rule to do all abdominal operations through one of these lines, and most commonly the linea alba was selected. For this there were many reasons :—

1. Such an incision gave direct access to the diseased parts, could be easily extended upwards or downwards, and permitted

the operator to secure the pedicle of an ovarian tumour with equal facility on either side.   Operation was mostly required for disease in the lower abdomen or pelvis, and not for acute conditions, or for diseases of the stomach, gall-bladder, or appendix.

2. The wall was at its thinnest in this line ; therefore it took little time to get through it, and a comparatively short time to close it when the surgeon had finished.

3. There was hardly any hæmorrhage to embarrass the operator, and in the days when Spencer Well's artery forceps were unknown this was of great importance.

Once it appeared to be the aim of an operator to extract an ovarian tumour from the abdomen through an incision as minute as possible.   In a short correspondence in the *Lancet* on this question I ventured to protest against the principle of such an incision.   The immediate danger of suppuration was considerable, and fear of peritonitis great, in those days. Experience had not shown the danger of subsequent yielding of the scar.   The dislike of making a large opening only departed when our methods of wound treatment rendered any cut in the abdominal wall made by a surgeon practically safe.   The injury inflicted on the edges of a small wound by the surgeon's hands and retractors increased the danger of the suppuration which it was intended to minimise, whilst it limited the area which it was possible to adequately explore.

We have for a long time reached a stage when we not only plan a particular operation but try to do it in such a manner that the abdominal wall at the site selected for the necessary incision shall afterwards be as strong as it was before the operation was commenced.   We want, in other words, an incision which will give adequate access to the disease but leave behind no weakness which can give uneasiness in the future. An accurate knowledge of the anatomical structure of the abdominal wall is therefore of the utmost importance.   You must appreciate the peculiar arrangement of the rectus muscle as regards its sheath, also the extent of the wall which this muscle covers.   The part which the lateral muscles play in rendering the abdomen secure must also be remembered, for neglect to do so may lead to trouble, in consequence of a badly-planned incision.

For practical purposes there are two muscular groups, the anterior and the lateral : of the former, we need only mention the recti-abdominis, running from above downwards ; in the

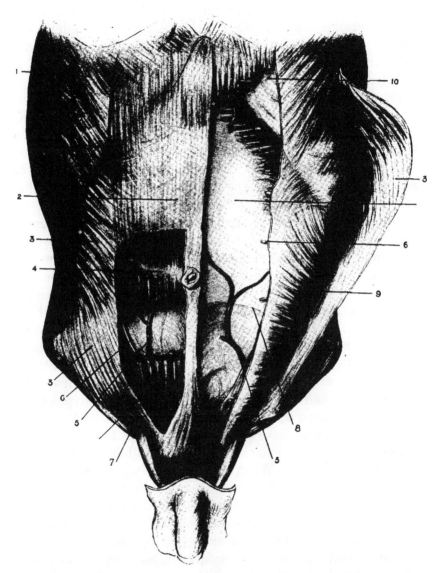

FIG. 2.—From a Dissection of the Muscles of the Abdominal Wall by Professor F. G. Parsons :—1. Serratus magnus. 2. Sheath of the rectus. 3. External oblique.   4. Rectus muscle.   5. Deep epigastric artery.   6. Dorsal nerves. 7. Cord and cremaster muscle. 8. Semilunar line of transversalis fascia. 9. Internal oblique. 10. Costal cartilages.

latter, the external and internal obliques and the transversalis, running in different directions but united in action. The recti-abdominis hold the front of the abdomen, extending laterally towards the iliac spines over a space greater than is usually allotted to them, for they reach to within 2 inches of the anterior superior spine of the ilium on each side in the adult, being thus spread over a great part of the anterior abdominal wall. Each muscle is unusual, inasmuch as it is mostly contained in a sheath, is broad, long, flattened and very strong. The sheath, although of great strength, is loosely attached to the muscle which it encloses, excepting at the lineæ transversæ, and permits of no outward deviation in the line of pull, so long as the two are attached together by an uninjured linea alba. The tendinous intersections of the recti possess value from the surgical as well as from other points of view.

There is no difference of opinion on one point, for all surgeons are agreed that suppuration within the abdomen which requires the employment of drainage after incision through the abdominal wall is likely to be followed by weakness later on ; they are apt to differ in their replies when asked their experience concerning incisions which have not been complicated by suppuration either before or after operation. Some do not admit that hernia occurs in their practice, others perhaps confess that operation is followed by weakness of the incision in a small percentage of clean cases. It is of course very annoying to find that a patient for whom an exploratory operation has been done, or perhaps one for the rectification of a painless disease, has developed a ventral hernia which is causing more inconvenience than the trouble for which the incision was made. When the original operation was for something which required a long and difficult manipulation, or the patient knows that life was saved by it, there is less disposition to gird at the operator should a hernia afterwards develop, and less surprise is expressed by the surgeon when it is met with. It must be recognised, however, that even at the present day, with our greatly improved technique, it is impossible to guarantee absolutely that an incision in the linea alba, whether made above or below the umbilicus, will not yield during after-life. (Convalescence may have been quite perfect, no cough troubled the patient, nor did the anæs-thetic cause undue strain or vomiting, yet the unpleasant fact remains and has to be faced, a hernia may form in spite of all our care.) All scar tissue has a tendency to contract, but this may be overcome, and there are special reasons why a cicatrix should stretch when it enters into the formation of the abdominal wall. In every part of this it is subjected to the action of two forces—(a) intra-abdominal tension, which varies considerably at different times of the day, and tends to a more permanent increase as we get older and more sedentary in our habits ; and (b) the action of the muscles of the abdomen, which again is of varying power, and sometimes indeed violent and irregular, in consequence of disease. The intra-abdominal pressure is fairly evenly distributed over the whole of the anterior part of the abdomen, but in addition, over the lower part especially, there is the added weight of the abdominal contents when the patient is either sitting or in the erect position.

It may be asked what kind of incision should be substituted for those through the linea alba and the linea semilunaris. It is obvious that if the rectus muscle can be temporarily displaced to one side during an operation, and put back uninjured in its normal bed after the operation has been finished, there will be no possibility of the development of a hernia at the site of the incision. In the operation for the removal of the appendix which I suggested many years ago, and have practised regularly since, advantage is taken of the anatomical arrangement of the rectus. An opening is made to the inner side of the linea semilunaris through the anterior sheath of the muscle, the muscle itself is drawn inwards with a retractor, the posterior sheath incised, the appendix removed, and the incision sutured. This operation possesses many advantages, not the least important of which is the possibility of extending it to any reasonable distance. Modifications of this method have since been adopted for other operations, the advantages of it being so obvious.

At an appendix operation, if the right ovary or tube be found diseased and requires removal, this can be done through the same incision. Should the left ovary or tube require removal, it can be excised through a similar incision on the other side at the same sitting, and a perfect wall will be left.

Displacement of the rectus outwards after incision of the sheath should be substituted in the early stage of many operations for those which were formerly carried out entirely through the middle line, e.g., the removal of fibroids, ovariotomy, tubal disease, etc. ; exploratory operations generally, and operations on the stomach.

It is occasionally advisable to go through the substance of the rectus muscle in some operations, such as gastrostomy by the method of Senn, operations on the gall-bladder and bile-ducts, and for the treatment of acute suppurative peritonitis in children and young adults, for although such an incision may be followed by hernia, it is not so in every case, and there is less danger of its giving way during the immediate after-treatment than if it is made through the linea semilunaris.

If the anterior sheath of the rectus is not restored after these incisions going directly through the muscle, then there will be some bulging of the muscle with consequent weakness of the abdominal wall. It is sometimes mistaken for a paralysis, but the rectus cannot fulfil its functions properly without a sheath, and will act perfectly again when the defect is remedied.

In the majority of patients benefit is gained by a careful and regulated course of exercises after all abdominal operations ; the danger is still that of keeping them recumbent or fettered by bandages and belts for too long a time. Abdominal hernia may be prevented by appropriate exercises, but it is not of much use prescribing a " course of Sandow " for an irreducible ventral hernia!

During an abdominal operation in which the linea semilunaris is exposed it is easy to observe the action of the external oblique, for should the patient make any effort to cough or vomit, tendinous fibres forming its insertion are pulled upwards and outwards, frequently forming parallel folds which are continuous with the anterior sheath of the rectus. The continued pull of the muscles in the lateral group is strongly backwards away from the middle line, and if an incision has left any weakness either at the linea alba or linea semilunaris the weak incision will be stretched, as these lines are really insertions of the lateral muscles. It is not necessary for the weak spot to be a large one in the first instance, for the omentum seems to have the power of finding the most minute and of dilating it. We owe much to the omentum for the use of its defensive powers against intra-abdominal disease, and perhaps its pushing character and insinuating qualities in cases of a defective abdominal wall are only an effort of Nature to give the individual early notice of his danger, so that he may remedy the defect in his armour as soon as possible. Be that as it may, such warnings should not be so frequently neglected.

Not only, then, are incisions in the median line very liable to be followed by hernial protrusion possibly years later, but also those which have been placed in the linea semilunaris, and for a similar reason the lateral pull of the muscles, which is so difficult to regulate and control. In both these situations there are practically only three layers which prevent a protrusion from forming, and an incision through the middle layer places a weak line between peritoneum and skin, for in the prevention of abdominal hernia the resistance of the skin, and indeed of the peritoneum, may be regarded as non-existent ; they are both of them too elastic and easily stretched, even when uninjured, to afford any permanent protection. The aponeurotic structures constitute our main reliance, their value after division again depending almost entirely on the accuracy of apposition secured by the method of suturing adopted. If the line of suture is not accurate but irregular, the edges not meeting well, then we must expect to have a weak scar—indeed the wonder is, not that we occasionally get one, but that we do not get one more often. The edges to be joined are commonly so narrow that they can rarely be in perfect apposition over the whole length of the incision. Both this layer and the peritoneum must be sutured with the greatest care, for although we may hold it as a fact that if the aponeurotic layer becomes perfectly united no hernia will develop, should there be any depression in the peritoneal line of suture you may be sure that a piece of omentum will find and insinuate itself into it. By this means, and also as a possible result of the inclusion of a piece of omentum during the process of the insertion of sutures, a great pressure may be exerted on the aponeurotic union at one or more points, one of which may yield. The tendency to-day, therefore, should be to avoid the linea alba and the linea semilunaris as much as possible, and, if it is necessary to open the abdomen in these lines, to plan an incision which shall not divide more than is absolutely necessary, since weak points in the semilunar line, the line formerly chosen for Langenbüch's incision, will not prove to be easily managed if of old standing with contracted muscles posteriorly. A strong aponeurotic layer is most useful, but the transversalis fascia is also of service, and its accurate union will assist in keeping the contents of the abdomen in their proper place. It is sutured with the peritoneum as the innermost layer, and as a reinforcement to it its value is great, especially in men, in whom the peritoneum is often less elastic than in women, and does not stretch or hold sutures with satisfaction. But I do not think that the most accurate apposition of this layer by any method of suturing is calculated to prevent a protrusion taking place unless the line of incision is reinforced externally by other structures. If it is possible to place the lines of reunion of the divided tissues so that these lines are not exactly superimposed, the result may sometimes be better.

As regards the other positions in which incisions may be made, we cannot over-estimate the great importance of the rectus abdominis, and we should endeavour to preserve it from injury as much as possible. If its fibres have been separated by a blunt instrument instead of having been cut by a knife, the resulting union may be less secure, for the parallel bundles of fibres when rolled apart may not unite when placed side by side. Wire sutures have been tried, and when their presence was not resented it was hoped they would ensure that security for all time which is obtained whilst the patient is in bed and his wound kept free from any possible strain or adverse influence. I do not myself use any other material than silk (mostly No. 1) for the suturing of wounds of the abdominal wall ; all the buried sutures are of this material, and it is reliable : you can always trust it, and the interrupted silk suture gives me a sense of security which catgut never affords. The only cases in which I have known a bursting open of an abdominal wound after operation, during the course of my personal experience, have been when I have employed catgut, or silk of less strength than that of No. 1. Perhaps I am prejudiced, but I am not alone in my preference for silk, for Sir Alfred Pearce Gould, whose experience is large, also advocates its use for the deep sutures. As some of you may know, I have advised silk for the routine sutures in these cases for many years in the lecture-room, and used it in the operating theatre. Kocher asks : " How can people go on using catgut for suturing the wall of the abdomen, when Madelung has recorded over a hundred cases where the wound has burst open because of it ? "

If the surgeon has to operate quickly because of the urgency of the case, then he must insert strong sutures which will include all the layers on both sides of the wound, and there are none better for this purpose than the larger-sized fishgut, which is readily sterilised, makes a good knot, and will resist any strain. This necessity for rapid operating is found in cases of the " acute abdomen " in stout adults, when the operation must be rapid to be successful ; there is another point in the urgent operations for this class of case, and that is the incision through the semilunaris should be chosen deliberately, as this gives much the least difficulty when it comes to closing the wound and the surgeon is short-handed. The possibility of a hernia after recovery is not worth a moment's consideration in such cases ; it can be easily put right by a second operation. In the ordinary operation where the surgeon is not hurried, the abdominal wall should be closed in layers : forty-four out of the fifty-five German and Austrian surgeons quoted by Dr. Swaffield were in favour of this procedure, and it agrees with the experience of most British surgeons. The importance of operating early when a wound shows signs of yielding later on, because of the greater benefit to be derived from the operation when practised on a small hernia, must be self-evident ; there is also the smaller risk of an operation of short duration in a bad type of patient to be considered, for shock is absent, and the administration of an anæsthetic need not be prolonged, or one may be employed locally. In bad cases we can use the intra-venous infusion of a solution of hedonal.

It must not be forgotten that muscles that have been contracted undergo change, so that after a long interval of time it may be impossible to stretch them to their former length sufficiently to cover the weak place in the abdominal wall. I think this statement particularly applies to the lateral muscles on the spinal side of a hernia following an incision through the upper right rectus in an operation for treatment of some hepatic disease.

The herniæ which occupy the middle line below the umbilicus sometimes assume rather startling proportions, falling down between the thighs and causing distress both from the dragging of their contents and their occasional disturbance or inflammation. Their formation is therefore a real danger to be guarded against.

In the herniæ which follow incisions for the relief of appendix abscesses, although much may be done to prevent them by the gridiron method, the skin and peritoneum become joined together in a thin cicatricial layer to which the omentum is often adherent. This covering may be dangerously thin, for sometimes it does not much exceed the thickness of paper. Hernia is rare after operations on the kidney by the lumbar route, if the incision is made obliquely from above downwards and the fascial planes are sutured after the operation.

Never cut across muscular fibres unless it is absolutely necessary from the particular needs of the case ; muscular fibres must always be separated, not cut, and as the aponeurosis of the external oblique forms the strongest layer in the lateral wall, incisions should follow the direction of that muscle. There are nerves likewise to be considered, and often a little care in the arrangement of a wound will result in the avoidance of any injury to them. In some instances when the fibres of the rectus have been split in the performance of cholecystotomy or gastro-enterostomy, without reference to the position of the nerves, that part of the muscle to the inner side of the incision has undergone atrophy and a hernia has consequently developed. At Czerny's instance Assmy investigated the after-results of cases in which a wide vertical splitting of the rectus fibres had been performed, and he showed that an atrophy of that part of the muscle dissociated from its nerve supply always followed.[1]

---

[1] Moynihan, "Abdominal Operations," p. 91.

THE ADMINISTRATION OF ANÆSTHESIA IN ACUTE CONDITIONS OF THE ABDOMEN.

Dr. Z. Mennell, who has most ably administered anæsthetics for me for some years, advises as follows :—

" For the successful performance of an operation for acute abdominal disease, the method of anæsthesia and choice of one to be used must be carefully considered.

" In the first place the patients are generally suffering from more or less severe toxæmia due to absorption from the abdominal condition, and· secondly, it is rarely possible to prepare them for operation on account of urgency.

" Generally speaking, ether should be selected and chloroform avoided, and in the less severe cases the ordinary nitrous oxide ether sequence may be used : the number of cases in which a perfectly satisfactory anæsthesia can be obtained by this means varies directly with the skill of the anæsthetist in the use of this method.

" When morphine has been given before the operation it is usually possible to obtain anæsthesia by means of open ether, that is ether dropped on to a Skinners or Schimmelbusch mask : there are, however, many cases in which a preliminary narcotic (morphine, scopolamine) is inadmissible.

" In cases where there is already severe shock the responsibility of the anæsthetist is great ; the condition may appear to be desperate, but usually the anæsthetic is taken better than would appear to be likely. Here the minimum of the anæsthetic must be used which is compatible with the necessary surgical manipulations, and the less anæsthetic used the less addition there is to the pre-existing shock. Oxygen must be used freely to counteract any cyanosis, and saline infusion subcutaneously, or if necessary intravenously, should be resorted to at the commencement of the operation. The use of strychnine and other cardiac stimulants is to be deprecated. The body warmth must be maintained ; the room should be kept at a temperature of 70° F.; the body must not be unnecessarily exposed, and the legs and arms may be bandaged and covered with cotton wool ; any saline or lotions used must be slightly above the body temperature.

" Children take ether well, but are specially liable to the

condition known as acidosis ; when this is present the dangers of a general anæsthetic are greatly increased—when the breath of a patient smells of acetone or when there is the acetone reaction in the urine, ether, and especially chloroform, are contra-indicated, and it is in such cases that intra-spinal anæsthesia is specially useful.

" For some years in America, and more recently in this country, a mixture of nitrous oxide and oxygen in definite percentages has been used for prolonged operations.　In severe abdominal conditions it may be used with advantage, either with or without nerve blocking by means of novocaine sub-cutaneously.　This without doubt diminishes shock, but the method is difficult and has its limitations.

" At St. Thomas's Hospital hedonal, and elsewhere ether, has been used intravenously.

" The most dangerous perhaps of cases met with under the heading of the Acute Abdomen are those of acute intestinal obstruction with consequent severe vomiting. When an anæsthetic is given in such cases, great care must be taken of the position in which the patient is placed : the head must be on a level or little below that of the body and turned to one side with a gag in the mouth, the danger being that of inhaling the vomit into the air passages.　Here again intra-spinal anæsthesia is indicated, and more recently we have been using intratracheal ether ; with this method, as soon as the catheter has been passed into the trachea, all danger of inhalation of vomit ceases."

PART I·

INJURIES OF THE ABDOMEN

CONTUSIONS

For purposes of clearness it will be best to divide these injuries into two groups :—

A. *Contusions without Rupture of the Abdominal Contents.*

B. *Contusions in which there is Evidence of Internal Injury.*

A. These contusions are of varying degrees of gravity, according to the severity of the injury, the region of the abdomen struck, the physical condition of the individual, his preparedness for the blow, the time which has elapsed since the last meal, etc. Any contusion of the abdomen may be serious, and it must be remembered that a patient without symptoms of importance, when seen soon after an injury, may be suffering from a rupture of the intestine or other internal organ, which will prove fatal if not recognised in time. Such cases have been only too frequent in the history of surgery, and whenever the cause of the injury has been "possibly" sufficient to produce internal damage, however slight, the case should be taken under observation and carefully watched. There may be no bruising of the skin and yet there may be a rupture of the intestine. In these days, when football is so popular, it is hardly necessary to say that a contusion of the abdomen is frequently followed by severe pain, shock and vomiting, yet the effects pass off in a short time. There are not many cases recorded in which the shock of a contusion without internal injury has proved fatal, but at least one is known about which there can be no doubt. On the other hand, the absence of an unusual amount of initial shock has been frequently observed when an injury has been inflicted which has caused death in a few hours.

The amount of extravasation of blood following a contusion of this part of the body varies much, according to the nature of

the injury, but beyond stiffness and pain on movement, swelling
and the usual discoloration of skin, does not as a rule produce
continued inconvenience unless there is associated with it a
rupture of some muscular tissue.   In a case under the care of
Mr. C. A. Ballance in which extravasation of blood had taken
place in the subperitoneal tissue, there was a large area of
dulness over the front of the abdomen not attended with
evidence of free fluid in the peritoneal cavity.   If the blood is
not absorbed, a fluid swelling may be found long afterwards ;
in one case I opened such a swelling the contents of which were
serous, which persisted five years after an injury.   Suppuration may follow but is not common, yet in the aged it may·
cause anxiety, and an early incision is indicated should there
be evidence that it has commenced.

Rupture of part of an abdominal muscle is not unusual as a
result of a direct injury, especially if the condition of the
muscle has deteriorated from some illness.   The patient will
complain of local pain on movement, and tenderness of the
part, whilst a defect may be felt on examination when the muscle
is put into action.   Such an injury, if involving a complete
rupture of the rectus muscle, will give rise to much discomfort
but not to a hernia.   In rupture of the muscles, on the lateral
aspect of the abdominal wall, a protrusion may be found as a
temporary condition forming at the site of the laceration, or
as a permanent one from yielding of the scar tissue formed in
the process of healing.

An operation for the closure of such a weak spot is indicated,
because, although the danger of strangulation may appear
remote, a truss is inconvenient, is not always easily kept in
position, and does not prevent an increase in size.

Rupture of the recti muscles is sometimes seen as a result of
intense strain, during parturition, vomiting, tetanic spasms,
and gymnastic feats.   Professor Alexis Thomson says that it has
been chiefly observed in cavalry recruits, through attempting
to mount a horse without placing the foot in the stirrup.

These ruptures always occur in the lower part of the rectus
muscle, because of the absence of the posterior layer of its
sheath in that situation.   There is violent pain at the site of
the rupture, with inability to straighten the body, which is
kept flexed to prevent traction on the part.   There is found a

very tender swelling to one side of the middle line ; this swelling is chiefly produced by extravasation between the ruptured ends which are concealed by it.

In cases where operation can be performed the sheath of the muscle should be opened and the ends sutured ; in this way the patient will obtain a stronger union and recover most quickly. Should his condition not permit of the operation, he should be placed on his back in bed, in such a position that the abdominal wall is fully relaxed. On account of the strength of the anterior sheath of the muscle it is unnecessary to make the patient wear a truss afterwards.

The ruptures of the diaphragm which occur independently of gunshot wounds, stabs, etc., are usually found on the left side, and are produced by a sudden and great increase of intra-abdominal pressure. Severe muscular efforts, as in vomiting and parturition, have caused this lesion, but there may be a less evident cause, as in the patient whose case is recorded in the *British Medical Journal* of 1858.

Here a man of 20 was admitted to St. Mary's Hospital "suffering from pneumothorax and diaphragmatic hernia," from which he died thirty-two hours after admission. He had slipped while walking in his own house, and in trying to save himself from falling given himself a severe twist, when he felt something snap at the lower ribs on the left side, followed by great pain, to such an extent that he could hardly breathe for some minutes.

B. When complicated with injury to the viscera there has been some severe violence inflicted, such as a crush between buffers in shunting, or the subject has been run over.

In Holmes's " System of Surgery," Vol. IL, the case of a man aged 24 who had fallen from a scaffold is given. He lived for eleven weeks, and at the *post-mortem* examination the inferior surface of the diaphragm was lacerated from the median line to the extent of 6 inches to the left side. The spleen had been separated into two pieces ; there were the remains of an extensive extravasation of blood and much suppuration both below and above the diaphragm in the region of the rupture.

A wound of the diaphragm may be very readily produced. A stab from a knife in civil brawls or a lunge from a bayonet in warfare may produce it, either from the front or the side. It is then likely to be seriously complicated with injury to one of the viscera and dangerous hæmorrhage. If the patient recovers from the immediate dangers incidental to such wounds he will very probably develop a hernia into the pleural cavity at a later date.

A good example of the course of such cases will be found on p. 236.

A case in which a rupture of the diaphragm was associated with escape of viscera into the chest was operated on by Mr. Berry in the Royal Free Hospital.

Male, aged 19, buffer accident. Admitted November 11, 1898, in a state of collapse, with superficial evidence of injury over the upper part of the abdomen, in the loin, and over the lower ribs. No air could be heard in the chest below the third rib on the left side, and the left side was dull behind the mid-axillary line. Very marked pallor was a prominent sign. There was much sickness (beginning on the third day), the vomit being coffee-coloured, great thirst, and not much pain. On November 15 the heart was evidently displaced to the right and a tympanic resonance extended over the front of the left chest almost to the clavicle, and blended below with the abdominal resonance. A "bruit d'airain" was heard over the tympanitic area. The breath sounds were normal over the right lung. The diagnosis lay between pneumothorax and gastric hernia. Operation, midnight of 16th. A large hole was felt in the diaphragm, through which about half the stomach, the transverse colon, the duodenum, half the spleen, and the upper half of the left kidney had passed into the thorax. The hole was as large as a man's fist, situated between the diaphragm and the last rib. Two stitches secured the liver over the opening after reduction of the protrusion. The patient died at the close of the operation.

It is possible in performing an operation for empyema in a child to pass through the diaphragm when making the incision, if the lower part of the pleural cavity is obliterated by adhesions. Such an opening should be carefully sutured and the pleura drained at a higher point.

In gunshot injuries the diaphragm is frequently traversed by a ball, but the injury to this muscle need not be specially considered, as it is probably unimportant compared with that inflicted on the other structures.

From the great danger of diaphragmatic hernia which almost invariably follows rupture or wound of the diaphragm, such injuries should be repaired as much as possible by means of direct interrupted sutures when the condition of the patient permits. The transpleural route will be the better one to use.

I cannot too strongly impress upon those responsible for any patient suffering from an abdominal injury the importance of watching the pulse. It is necessary to insist upon a careful examination from hour to hour ; it is now many years since I tried to impress the importance of this careful observation upon my juniors, and I still strongly urge it. The small pulse of the patient with shock should not increase in frequency in cases of simple contusion, when the shock is passing away.   If it does so, and the temperature is falling, you have a danger signal which may mean much.   Other signs of importance, to which reference will be made later, are severe local pain, rigidity of the abdominal wall, alteration in the percussion note, continued vomiting, and an anxious and distressed appearance.   A rise in temperature may indicate the need for exploration, but less importance may be attached to the onset of distension unless other symptoms show it to be the result of an inflammation of the peritoneum.

Meteorism without any lesion that can be found on abdominal exploration may result from a simple contusion of the abdomen.

Some years ago a boy of 12 was admitted to St. Thomas's Hospital under my care, and a somewhat rapid distension of the abdomen with rise of temperature ensued.   There was, however, no rigidity, special complaint of pain, or vomiting. The resident assistant-surgeon explored the abdomen at my request, but could find nothing abnormal.   The distension subsided after operation and the boy made a good recovery. It was very much on a par with the excessive meteorism which is some- times seen after surgical interference with the peritoneum, for instance in the performance of a radical cure of hernia.

A far more important condition as indicative of internal injury is a rigid abdomen without any distension.   Absence of liver dulness will be referred to later ; it is not a sign to which any importance should be attached.   In no case should a surgeon wait for its development, or refuse to operate because it is not demonstrable.

When the shock has passed off, there is usually no difficulty in coming to a conclusion, but in many cases, especially the more severe injuries, it is the wisest plan to interfere before the patient is further exhausted by loss of blood.   The damage must be treated in the same way as a wounded artery is attacked in more accessible parts of the body.

Statistical tables show how very important it is to operate early both in these cases of hæmorrhage and in those in which an infection of the peritoneum may follow.   There are, how-ever, many instances in which it may be necessary to consider the question of operation in apparently hopeless and neglected cases ; here the verdict in favour of operation should not be put aside too readily. The many ways now available of pro-ducing anæsthesia and treating collapse, with the evidences given of recovery under the most desperate circumstances which published cases afford, justify and often compel an attempt, however hazardous it may appear.

WOUNDS OF THE ABDOMEN.

I remember very well when we were taught that it was a wrong practice to interfere with wounds of the abdomen ; appropriate dressings were to be applied and we were to wait for symptoms. The important thing in all these injuries is to ascertain whether there is penetration of the peritoneum, and a careful examination of the part should be made under anæsthesia. Let the region be painted with iodine as soon as the wound can be exposed, and do not complicate matters by doing an imperfect examination either with probe or finger. Cover it with a sterilised or antiseptic dressing, and bandage this into position. In cases where there is hæmorrhage from the parietes this must be arrested in the usual manner. When the bleeding point is not easily found, it may be advisable to place a temporary plug in the wound. Explore as soon as possible, and so make certain of the extent of the wound ; if the peritoneum has not been penetrated, the bleeding is arrested, the wound cleaned, and cut muscles sutured. The most dangerous cases are not necessarily those in which the escape of abdominal contents proves the fact that the peritoneum has been invaded ; they are subjected to operation without loss of time. Do not wait for symptoms ; it is bad surgery. If at the operation the wound is found to extend into the peritoneal cavity, then a most careful examination of the parts within should be made through an incision of adequate size. Should the patient not apply for treatment until some days have elapsed, you must be guided by the symptoms which are present, paying special attention to the condition of the pulse and signs of local inflammation. It may still be necessary to explore. If there are no symptoms it would be best to keep the patient under observation—for serious symptoms have developed after some days in cases of stab wounds.

In making these exploratory incisions through the abdominal wall, it is usually possible to extend them in such a direction that the anatomical arrangement of the muscles is taken into consideration, as already advised in the planning and making of abdominal incisions. Avoid the middle line if possible. The after-development of a ventral hernia may make the life of a man miserable and his support a burden to the community, still the first consideration is the making of an adequate opening for the examination.

If the wound is of considerable size and permits of the protrusion of intestine, omentum, etc., the parts protruded must be carefully washed with warm sterilised saline solution, boracic acid solution, or even boiled water before they are returned to the abdomen. The question of treatment of the wounds inflicted on these parts will be considered later. General principles must guide you in the first place. The herniated contents will be reduced after repair of wounded parts and enlargement of the opening. Reduction should then be no more difficult than it is after examination during an operation, where it has been necessary to bring much bowel outside in exploring for the cause of an obstruction. If the bowel has not been compressed by the small opening for any great length of time, there should be no distension of it. The protruded parts must be most carefully cleansed, let it be repeated, for if there is any contamination of the peritoneum later it will be most commonly caused by septic material carried in when the herniated part is reduced. Drainage is seldom required, and should be avoided if possible. The wound should be carefully sutured in layers, as after the making of irregular wounds by the surgeon. If the state of the patient does not permit of careful suturing in layers, use strong interrupted sutures of salmon gut, passing through all the layers.

When the wounds are of longer standing, and the protrusion is adherent to the lips of the wound, it must be cleansed and returned if its structure is not injured beyond repair. When there is a septic wound with possibly gangrenous protrusion, in some instances little can be done beyond cleansing the part and making provision for relief of any constriction. The question of excision of the whole protrusion will have to be considered ; in some this would be the best treatment, if the condition of the patient is hopeful and the surroundings permit of it.   Drainage is usually necessary in all late cases.

There may be occasions when attempts at reduction of a protrusion would be bad surgery.   I remember when the subject of internal injuries was under discussion at the Portsmouth meeting of the British Medical Association an officer in the R.A.M.C. gave an account of a case of protrusion of the omentum, which followed a bullet wound, when the patient was on active service in the Hills.   The enemy was sniping the retreating force, and the wound was an oblique one of the abdominal wall.   The circumstances were against successful operation, therefore it was postponed.   After removal of the omentum a few days later the soldier made a good recovery.

Even large intestinal protrusions have been safely reduced without surgical help when the opening has not been too constricted and the usual septic inflammation has not super-vened.   Some of these accounts appear almost incredible.

It may be well to mention here the protrusions which follow spontaneous rupture of the coverings of large herniæ.   These accidents may occur when the skin and other tissues have become very thin from stretching, but are more likely to happen when there is weakness in the parts due to scar tissue resulting from a former operation.

In one case in which the coverings of a femoral hernia had ruptured, Mr. Bernard Pitts, who treated the case, found a woman applying for admission " because something had given way."   When her clothing was lifted, almost the whole of her small intestine was found to be out-side, covered more or less with a towel.   She recovered after cleansing, reduction, and suturing of the parts.   Here a former operation for strangulation had left a large femoral ring from too free division of Gimbernat's ligament.

It is easy to make the section of Gimbernat's ligament too freely during an operation for strangulated femoral hernia.

There are two cases included amongst the ventral and umbilical herniæ in the St. Thomas's Hospital records in which a similar accident occurred ; one of these died.   The sloughing of skin which sometimes follows fæcal abscess in gangrenous hernia is quite a different thing, and is far more frequent.   The mortality is very high.

Gunshot wounds of the abdomen in civil life should be subjected to immediate exploration, or to an operation at the earliest possible moment.   I do not recollect a single case in which the patient recovered where operation was declined or not advised when there was reason to suspect from the direction

of the bullet that the intestine had been injured.   There may be
many wounds in the bowel, the operation will be not only prolonged but difficult, wound after wound may present itself, each
succeeding one proving more certainly the need for the operation.   There must be no waiting for symptoms.   The surgeon
has more reason for urging operation than in cases of suspected
subcutaneous rupture of the gut.   It is true that there may be
doubt as to a wound of intestine in the latter injury, but in the
former there can be none.   The incision should extend through
the track of the bullet down to the peritoneum, any foreign
substance that may be found being removed and kept.   The
edges of this wound should be excised, especially in wounds
which have been inflicted for some time.   An opening large
enough to admit of thorough inspection of the abdominal
contents underlying should be made through the peritoneum,
and after packing off the area of probable injury with sterilised
gauze any blood or escaped fluid should be wiped away and the
track of the bullet followed further.   Wounded gut should be
drawn outside and immediately sutured.   As there may be
many openings in opposed loops, no abdomen should be closed
until actual inspection has proved that none have been overlooked.   Cleanse the intestine and parts involved in the
examination with sterilised saline.   Do not hesitate to bring
all the intestine outside the wound inch by inch if necessary,
beginning at the cæcum and working from that as a fixed point.
If the operation has been done early, there will be no distension
of the intestine, and manipulation of the parts will be comparatively easy and quickly performed.   When there is commencing
infection and distension of the intestine, it will be best to empty,
possibly through a puncture, one or more of the most distended coils, and the need for drainage will be evident.

Although it will be advisable to follow the track of the
wound down to the peritoneum in all cases, this incision may
require to be supplemented by another nearer the middle line
to enable you to deal adequately with the injured bowel.
In most cases, however, the linea alba can and should be
avoided, on account of the danger of later development of a
hernia ;   but rapidity of operating is important, and for the
surgeon who has not had a great deal of practice the less
complicated incision may be best.

Some American surgeons, pioneers in this branch of surgery, have successfully dealt with multiple bullet wounds of the intestine which have been inflicted with a revolver. In these they have boldly brought the whole of the small intestine outside through a long incision and sutured the wounds. Hamilton not only sutured eleven wounds of the small intestine, but two of the large, and ligatured a bleeding mesenteric artery. The amount of shock must be proportionally greater, but there is no doubt that this method of total evisceration has a great advantage over the more careful method of exploration, for it enables a more thorough examination to be made of parts which might other, wise escape attention. In addition, the surgeon knows quickly the amount of damage which has been inflicted, and can arrange either to suture perforations singly, or to resect when there are several closely situated, and perform an anastomosis.

As regards the treatment of bullet wounds of the abdomen on active service, the opinion of my senior colleague, Mr. G. H. Makins, as expressed after his experiences in the South African war, is valuable. He writes :—

"A careful consideration of the whole of the cases that I saw leaves me with the firm impression that perforating wounds of the small intestine differ in no way in their results and consequences when produced by small-calibre bullets from those of every-day experience, although when there is reason merely to suspect their presence an exploration is not indicated under circumstances that may add a fresh danger to the patient." [1]

He gives general rules regarding the treatment of injuries to the intestine,[2] which we also venture to quote because of their importance, coming as they do from such an eminent authority.

"First the patients must be removed with as little disturbance as possible, and absolute starvation must be insisted on. If the patients be suffering from severe shock, hypodermic injections of strychnine should be administered, or possibly some stimulant by the rectum."

He advises that all abdominal injuries should be placed in the same marquee, and kept absolutely quiet until they are evidently out of danger.

"When feeding is commenced at the end of twenty-four or thirty-six hours, it must be in the form at first of warm water, then milk adminis. tered in teaspoonfuls only. In doubtful cases morphine must be avoided. Operative treatment is required in a certain number of cases, but in the

[1] "Surgical Experiences in South Africa," p. 457.
[2] Ibid., p. 452.

majority we are met with the extreme difficulty that in a very large proportion of the occasions. on which these wounds are received an abdominal section is not warranted in consequence of the conditions under which it would have to be performed."

It is necessary to emphasise the fact that bullet wounds of the intestine are often widely separated, and a search limited to the parts underlying the surface wound may be inadequate to reveal their number.

Gunshot wounds of the stomach vary very considerably according to the nature of the weapon, the size of the bullet, its shape, the distance from which it was fired, etc. The state of the organs as to distension or emptiness must be taken into consideration. The bullet may contuse the anterior wall, pass into the cavity of the stomach and remain there, or more probably penetrate the posterior wall also. The angle at which it entered must also be taken into consideration, as the probability of damage to other parts will much depend upon this.

Early operation in these as in other injuries penetrating, or possibly penetrating, the intestinal tract is very important. Forgue and Jeanbrau[1] give a series of 112 cases, in which the stomach was wounded by bullets, and the results of operation are shown as follows :—

When the stomach only was wounded—

	Recovered.	Died.
Operations within six hours . .	9	4
„ after this period . .	2	4
Wounds of stomach and other parts—		
Operations within six hours . .	13	16
„ „ six to twelve hours .	2	11
„ after twelve hours . .	2	11
„ time not stated . .	3	5

In these cases the opening should be a median one, made quickly and freely, so that the stomach may be easily seen and manipulated. If escape of the contents of the stomach has taken place, the peritoneum underlying the wound must be cleansed, the stomach wound located and sutured, a double row of sutures being used. The gastro-colic omentum should then be freely opened below the greater curvature of the stomach and its main vessel and search made for a posterior opening. This will probably afford evidence of its existence

[1] *Revue de Chirurgie*, 1903.

by the blood and stomach contents present in the lesser sac. The opening in the omentum must be of adequate size and the wound in the posterior surface sutured in a similar manner to the anterior wound. Search may be made for the bullet and any other injury which it may have caused in its progress. Omission to make an examination of the other structures possibly involved may render useless all your efforts.

Sir Berkeley Moynihan[1] writes :—

"It is remarkable how often they are overlooked. Forgue and Jeanbrau quote many cases where at the *post-mortem* examination gross damages, overlooked at the operation, were laid bare. Bertram records a case where the spleen and left kidney were found injured ;

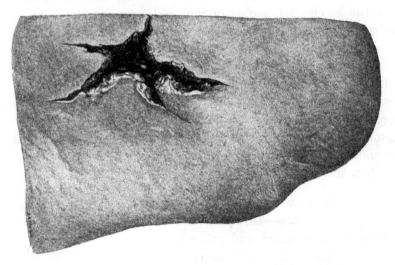

FIG. 3.—Bayonet Wound of Liver: 432, St. Thomas's Hospital Museum.

Briddon, one where four perforations of the small intestine were found ; Gabzewicz, one where an injury to the colon was seen ; and Poucet and others, examples of injury to the liver. The minutest search must be made, despite the fact that, because of the patient's collapse from shock or hæmorrhage, a prolongation of the operation is not without its own danger."

The treatment of the stomach wounds and the general peritoneal conditions does not differ very much from that required after perforation of a gastric ulcer, and will vary according to the position of the wound as regards the pylorus and the time that has elapsed since the escape of the stomach

---

[1] "Abdominal Operations," p. 321.

contents began. Gastro-enterostomy is rarely required, but in a large number, however careful the peritoneal toilet may have been, drainage will be necessary.

In gunshot wounds and stabs of the liver it is best to open up and cleanse the wounds, although more serious signs of internal hæmorrhage may be absent. Attention must again be drawn to the fact that a case which may be quite without symptoms at first may become alarming in a few hours as a result of internal hæmorrhage. Later there may be infection of effused blood or bile-stained fluid which has become localised.

When the injury has been inflicted below the ribs, it will be necessary to conduct the operation as in explorations for the treatment of biliary calculus in the bileducts. The important thing is to get an opening of adequate size through which full exploration and, if necessary, suturing can be done.

In wounds penetrating the pleura and the diaphragm, it has been found necessary to enlarge the opening and follow the track, resecting ribs to give more room. A further incision of the diaphragm may be required. A combination of the thoracic and abdominal routes has been very successfully employed by Professor M. Ferrier and Professor Lejars.

The actual wound in the liver must be treated by suture or by gauze packing, as described in subcutaneous ruptures of this organ. The thermocautery is very unreliable, and should be avoided in abdominal surgery.

In bullet wounds of the liver both surfaces must be examined, for if the wound of exit is overlooked, hæmorrhage may continue from that and cause a fatal ending. As a rule, it is not possible (even in civil life) to localise the bullet before these operations ; and no prolonged search should be made for it. If easily found and accessible it should be removed, and search should also be made for any portion of clothing which may have been carried in with it. The danger to the patient is not the presence of a bullet in the liver, it is the internal hæmorrhage from the wound.

Wounds of the portal vessels usually prove rapidly fatal and seldom present much chance of surgical aid. When the gall-bladder has been wounded, its greater accessibility permits of rapid suture of the lesion. If bile is found in the peritoneum mixed with the blood, a most careful search should be made for the opening from which it has escaped. No abdomen should be closed without drainage if a definite opening cannot be found. Wounds of the gall-bladder may be treated in one of three ways :—(1) Suture, as in the operation of. cholecystotomy, sometimes after excision of the edges of the wound. (2) Suture of the opening to the wound in the parietes, as in cholecystostomy. (3) Excision of the whole of the gall-bladder, with drainage of the part.

In wounds of the splenic region a possibly penetrating wound makes exploration imperative. This should be carried out through an incision to the left of the abdomen. An incision through the median line will not give adequate approach to it, yet such an incision may be advisable for exploration in the first place. In very few instances has it been of any use to apply sutures to wounds of this organ, but in some slight lacerations and one or two cases of gunshot it has proved successful. As a rule it is necessary to excise it quickly, on account of the amount of bleeding which is taking place (see p. 61). Packing may be successful when it is evident that excision would be unusually difficult and dangerous on account of the added shock. It may enable the patient to tide over the shock which results from the serious nature of such an injury.

In cases of protrusion of the spleen (recent protrusion) when there is no wound of that organ, cleansing and replacement should be carried out. The danger of replacing a septic spleen is so great that the wound should be enlarged, the intra-abdominal part of the pedicle ligatured, and such a spleen cut away ; this should be followed by repair of the abdominal wall. It is not satisfactory to leave a weak spot by suturing the pedicle in the parietal incision.

The possibility of a wound of other parts by the weapon or missile must be remembered and the kidney examined ; the diaphragm also requires to be searched.

Wounds in the epigastric region may also injure the pancreas, but such are commonly complicated by damage to other organs near.

In a case treated by Ninni[1] a revolver bullet had entered quite close to the second lumbar vertebra, traversed the first lumbar vertebra, produced six perforations in the small gut and another in the colon near the hepatic flexure, and finally emerged on the right of the epigastrium.

[1] Lejars, p. 380.

Laparotomy was performed, the seven intestinal perforations were found and sutured, and then, as blood was seen to be escaping from between the stomach and transverse colon, the gastro-colic omentum was opened, and a wound of the pancreas at the junction of the head and body was discovered; two deep sutures were introduced and stopped the bleeding, and drainage was provided. The patient was cured in five weeks.

The use of thick catgut sutures will be required to close these wounds and arrest hæmorrhage, and as far as possible the peritoneum should be closed over the wounded spot. In all instances the wound should be drained, the line selected being that through the gastro-colic omentum, another opening being made there, even if the gastro-hepatic omentum has been chosen to give access to the wound.[1]

Wounds of the kidney are indicated by hæmaturia, escape of urine from the wound, symptoms of internal hæmorrhage, pain in the loin, possible renal colic, and the formation of a swelling in the region of the kidney. The prognosis will be much worse—it is already serious—if there is any intraperitoneal complication. It follows, therefore, that wounds inflicted from the front are the more dangerous. In any case, if there is reason to think that a wound of this organ is bleeding, it will be best to explore through a lumbar incision, clear away extravasated blood, and pack with gauze. Any wound involving the renal pelvis and permitting of escape of urine may require secondary interference on account of septic infection; free drainage will then be necessary. Should it be evident that an important vessel has been divided, or that it is unsafe to trust to plugging, then a primary resection is required. Nephrectomy may be necessary if secondary hæmorrhage occurs during the after-treatment. Removal through a lumbar incision is to be done when there is no strong indication in favour of the abdominal route.

Hernia of the kidney through a wound in the loin is a rare effect of injury, and is rarely complete. Nephrectomy is most commonly required, but if the injury to the kidney is limited to the body of the organ and does not involve the vessels of the hilum, much can be done by cleansing, drainage, and appropriate suturing of the wound after it has been returned to its bed.

[1] See "Rupture of Pancreas," p. 52.

Wounds of the renal pelvis are usually inflicted by the surgeon in removal of calculi. It is not infrequently possible to take away a calculus by a posterior incision and close the opening with fine catgut ; in some instances, however, the main vessels will be in danger from the needle, and safety will be gained by approximating the edges of the wounds with forceps and passing a ligature round two opposed points. This will also save time. In accidental stab wounds it is not often that the wound is limited to the pelvis ; other parts are frequently involved, so that a removal of the whole organ is necessary.

Wounds of the ureter are almost entirely complications of a surgical operation, and require to be repaired at the time. When the wound is an incised lateral one, suturing may be done as after ureterotomy for removal of calculus, the opening being closed with lateral catgut sutures of small size not involving the mucous lining.

In complete transverse section without loss of substance there are three methods which may be employed :—(1) Lateral anastomosis, as in lateral anastomosis of the small intestine, the two ends being closed with ligatures. The difficulties of this method will be apparent when it is remembered that the suturing has to be done at a considerable distance from the surface and within the abdomen. (2) The upper end of the ureter is implanted in the lower through an opening in the side. The end of the lower is ligatured, and a lateral incision made about one-tenth of an inch below this. The upper end is incised and then implanted in the lower by means of a suture (passed like a mattress suture) from within outwards, opposite to the slit. It is then carried into the lower tube, and from within outwards at a distance which will permit of the complete invagination of the upper end. It is then tied, and the insertion of about four stitches, uniting the superficial parts, completes the junction. (3) Implantation of the upper end into the lower is effected by making a slit in the latter and drawing the former into position by means of special sutures passed like the one de-scribed in the last method. This slit is closed after the other sutures have been tied and the upper part held in its place.

Sometimes it is not possible to unite the separated ends— there has been loss of substance. Under these circumstances there are three courses open to the surgeon :—(1) implantation of the upper end in the bladder ; (2) implantation in the wall of the large bowel, cæcum or sigmoid ; (3) nephrectomy.

In (1) and (2) the operations are similar in technique. The lower end must be closed with a ligature. The upper end is slit so that it may not contract too much afterwards. The position of the opening must be such that no tension will be left after the sutures have been put in. In the bowel the retroperitoneal surface nearest to the ureter will be selected. Two rows of fine sutures will be necessary, the inner row taking the submucous tissues and the outer row the muscular and cellular coverings. It has been recommended that the bladder wall should be lifted up and fixed to the pelvic peritoneum with a catgut suture, so as to prevent anything like dragging on the line of incision.

Excision of the kidney can be easily performed, and may be the only possible method to employ on some occasions.

Wounds of the bladder are the result of gunshot injuries, punctured wounds inflicted by pointed instruments, or wounds inflicted by a surgeon during some abdominal operation. Gunshot wounds inflicted in warfare are most serious, because of the difficulty in obtaining adequate treatment soon after the wound has been received. They resemble in this respect the intestinal injuries. Mr. Makins, in his " Experiences," p. 457, found that " an uncomplicated perforation in the intraperitoneal portion of the viscus was frequently recovered from. When the perforation was at the base of the bladder, however, the prognosis was very bad, and, as far as I know, not a single patient escaped death. The increase of risk in an extraperitoneal wound of this viscus is indeed very great, while an intraperitoneal perforation may be considered an injury of lesser severity, provided the urine be of normal character." " Drainage by a catheter tied in proved worse than useless." He considers that a suprapubic opening might be better, but is not hopeful under the conditions which obtain in war time.

There can be no doubt that in ordinary life exploration with the provision of drainage will prove the most successful.

The accidental wounds are most commonly the result of falls on some pointed instrument, such as a spike in a railing, the broken leg of a chair, a stake, etc., when the injury is inflicted below the pubes, through the rectum, vagina, or perineum. A stab may reach the bladder above the pubes.

I have no doubt about the treatment that should be employed here ; the wound of entry should be explored for foreign bodies, and cleansed as far as possible. A suprapubic opening should be made and the peritoneal aspect of the bladder exposed. If this is not injured, the peritoneum should be sutured and the anterior aspect of the bladder examined. If there is a wound which cannot be brought to the surface or sutured *in situ*, free drainage must be provided. Should no wound be found, it would be better to open the bladder and clear it of clots and foreign substances through a suprapubic opening, the edges of the bladder being attached to the skin. It is a mistake to confine your attention to the wound of entry only, when this is below the pubes ; these wounds are dangerous from their liability to septic infection, and the prognosis will depend on the perfection of the drainage provided.

Surgical wounds of the bladder are less commonly seen at the present day than they were when laparotomy was an infrequent operation. The beginner is warned so often about the danger of opening a bladder which has been drawn up in front of a tumour or pelvic inflammatory mass that he does not attempt to open the peritoneum in the danger zone. It may, however, be injured during the separation of adhesions, and in doubtful cases the injection of saline solution into the bladder before the abdomen is closed will afford evidence as to whether this has occurred or not. The frequency with which the bladder is present in hernia varies a good deal ; it is most commonly found in the inguinal variety, and is then opened during the separation of the sac, or after the application of a ligature to the neck of the sac. In the majority there has been no evidence that it was accompanying the protrusion before operation, and therefore it has been opened before its presence was suspected. Occasionally, especially in femoral hernia, it is included with the sac ligature ; this accident produces much pain, and blood in the urine, with frequent micturition. This mistake is very fatal.

The appearance of an unusual amount of clear fluid in the wound during the separation of an inguinal sac should lead to careful search. In doubtful cases the injection of saline solution into the bladder will be of use in determining the injury. A probe passed into a doubtful pouch can (if it is a part of the bladder) be made to touch a silver catheter introduced in the usual manner. I have met with this complication in four out of one thousand cases of radical cure of inguinal hernia.

If the wound is an irregular one, it should be trimmed up and the edges brought together with a row of sutures not invading the mucous membrane. As these herniæ are often not covered by peritoneum, they are difficult to differentiate from the cellular tissue in which they lie, and nothing like a defined margin may be felt to enable you to recognise it. They are also, at times, very thin, and must be carefully sutured. After the bladder has been sutured, it should be reduced with the neck of the sac and the operation completed by the particular method favoured.

The uterus is rarely ruptured by any form of external violence, even when pregnancy is far advanced, but when it is, a very serious problem is presented. The danger is great from internal hæmorrhage, which can only be checked by early operation. This is true also of a wound, and in both there must be no delay. When a pregnant woman has received a kick over the abdomen, the amount of damage to the uterine wall will vary considerably ; sometimes it is very extensive, and there is no chance of saving the patient unless the uterus is emptied and afterwards removed. In the case of ruptures of limited extent, where there has been but slight escape of amniotic fluid (as also in wounds of similar importance), strong silk sutures or catgut should be passed through the full thickness of the wall down to the lining and tied, others being introduced between them to close the peritoneum. The blood-clots and fluid should be cleared away and the external wound closed without drainage.

If the fœtus or membranes are prolapsed, then it is advisable to place these within the uterus and if the wound is not a large one suture it, leaving the fœtus to come away *per vias naturales.*

In later stages of pregnancy when there is prolapse of the fœtus, or the wound is large, rendering suturing unsafe, it will be best to empty the uterus in the manner employed during Cæsarian section. Occasionally after extraction of uterine contents, when there has been prolapse of much or all of the fœtus and membranes, it may be possible to repair the opening ; but the bleeding may prove difficult to arrest, whilst the condition of·the patient is bad.   Here and in other cases where the damage is extensive a safer treatment will be hysterectomy.

A most important and encouraging case is one described by Albarran [1] :—

" . . . A young woman came under his care, who was about four and a half months pregnant, for a self-inflicted revolver wound of the umbilical region.   She was almost unconscious, cold and with a temperature of 95° F.   The abdomen was slightly distended.   Operation five hours after infliction of the wound.   About four pints of fluid mixed with blood was found, and five wounds were discovered in the small intestine, four in the upper third of the ileum, and one in the jejunum about 16 inches below duodeno-jejunal junction.   About 8 inches of intestine which contained four of these was excised and end-to-end anastomosis performed ; the wound higher in the intestine was sutured.   A long loop of the umbilical cord protruded through a wound in the fundus uteri, and low down in the posterior wall the wound of exit was found.   Albarran resected the loop of prolapsed cord, reduced the stump into the uterus, and sutured the bullet openings with silk.   The peritoneum was cleansed, a gauze drain placed in Douglas's pouch, and the wound closed up to it.   The patient miscarried next day, but made a perfect recovery."

In many cases removal of the uterus will be required if the rupture is large enough to permit of the escape of the fœtus, or any considerable portion of it.

Rupture of the uterus during parturition is a most serious accident, and is most frequently fatal as a result of the hæmor-rhage.   Blood may flow *per vaginam*, but more often escapes into the peritoneal cavity, producing the symptoms which follow extensive bleeding from one of the solid viscera without external wound.   If extensive external hæmorrhage occurs, with cessation of the labour pains, etc., the vagina must be plugged whilst preparations are made for operation.   There must be no attempt at delivery in the usual way.   When the rupture is solely into the peritoneum, the danger is that it may be quite overlooked until the occurrence of a secondary collapse due to renewed hæmorrhage.

Nothing less than hysterectomy will be of any avail, and the sooner this is recognised and the operation performed the better chance will the patient have of recovery.   A total removal of the uterus above the vagina is not really difficult

[1] Bull. de la Société de Chir., 1895, p. 243.

when the operator has had experience, but more lives will be saved by removal of the uterus and extra-abdominal treatment of the stump, because less time is occupied in carrying it out.

In the extra abdominal treatment of the stump (Porro's operation) the abdominal incision is made with due regard to the position of the bladder, presenting clots cleared away, and a rubber tube passed over the fundus and adjusted as low down as possible. It is drawn tight and clamped or tied. The uterus is then opened at one point and the incision enlarged or the rupture extended by quick tearing with the fingers. The child is rapidly extracted through the opening by pulling on the feet. The uterus is brought outside, the rubber tube tightened, and the intestine packed off. "Two knitting needles are passed through the flattened rubber tube and the cervix and the uterus cut off about $\frac{3}{4}$ inch above the needles." [1] The peritoneum is cleansed and the external wound closed, the lowest suture being passed through the stump also. When time and surroundings are favourable, a supravaginal amputation, with intraperitoneal treatment of the stump, is the better treatment.

In this operation after the uterus has been emptied the following procedures should be carried out, provision having been made for the temporary arrest of hæmorrhage, either by pressure by the hands of an assistant or by placing a rubber band as low as possible :—(1) Clamp the upper two-thirds of the left broad ligament, and cut between the clamps. (2) Search for the uterine vessels, which will be felt by the side of the cervix. Secure them with a large clamp and divide near uterus. (3) Make an anterior peritoneal flap and carry it downwards ; do the same posteriorly ; see that the bladder is taken down with the anterior flap. (4) Open vagina on left side near attachment, and cut in front and behind the cervix. (5) Take the cervix strongly in a pair of vulsellum forceps and carry it forward ; by this means the right border of the uterus comes well up. (6) Clamp the uterine vessels on the right side, and divide them near the uterus. (7) Clamp and divide the upper part of the broad ligament. (8) Examine for any bleeding vessels that may have escaped the clamps. (9) Apply strong ligatures beyond the clamps and not too near them.

[1] Jacobson, Vol. II., p. 869; Herman, "Difficult Labour."

(10) Close the vaginal vault if the conditions are favourable (no suspicion of possible sepsis), otherwise put a gauze drain in the vagina. Search for any extension of wound beyond the area which has been specially involved in the main laceration.

Mr. Grimsdale,[1] in relating a case of recovery after abdominal hysterectomy with removal of tubes and ovaries for rupture which occurred at the fourth confinement in a woman of 27, gives the average occurrence as 1 in 2,433. He gives also the average mortality in 1874 (Hugenberger) as 95 per cent. and in 1892 (Schultz) 55 per cent., and says the lowest mortality is obtained when prompt abdominal operation can be performed. He adds : " I feel confident that the safest treatment in the long run will be found in the boldest measures. It is impossible to know how much damage has been done and how much the peritoneum has been soiled until the abdomen has been opened," etc.

TRAUMATIC RUPTURE OF THE VISCERA WITHOUT EXTERNAL WOUND.

In the group of injuries of the abdominal organs the result of violence not associated with wound of the abdominal wall are comprised those cases which within my recollection were admitted to our hospitals only to die, lulled to their last sleep by the administration of sufficient opium to procure physiological rest. That a person who had received a ruptured viscus would die was almost universally accepted as a matter of course, and it was only the increased boldness that came to surgeons as a consequence of improved wound treatment that enabled a different practice to be followed and many lives saved. The presence of a wound of the abdominal wall was considered by some an indication for surgical interference, but not by all. None were sufficiently bold to operate when there was no wound, although a diagnosis was correctly made. The frequency with which peritonitis followed opening of the peritoneum and killed the patient after abdominal section made the suggestion of interference appear overbold. The knowledge that death, which would probably follow, would be ascribed to the operation and not to the injury, made surgeons unwilling to face the result. To the surgeons of St. Thomas's Hospital is due much of the credit for an improved prospect in this branch of surgery. About 1886 Mr. John Croft, surgeon to the hospital, performed an operation for ruptured small intestine.

[1] *Journal of Obstetrics and Gynæcology*, 1903, p. 558.

in a patient without external wound (Fig. 4).   An artificial anus was established, and the patient survived for a month ; in fact he did well until resection of this artificial anus and end - to - end enterorraphy was done, but the second operation was not survived. It was not long, however, before a similar case came into the hospital ; this time Croft sutured the rent in the gut and closed the external wound.   This patient made a perfect recovery.   The   same surgeon was the first to operate for a rupture of the spleen, and Mr. A. O. Mackellar did a similar operation for a like injury in a second case.   Sir W.

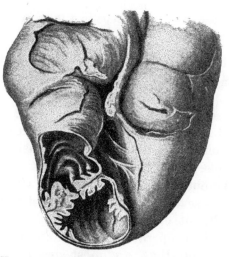

FIG. 4.—The portion of intestine excised by John Croft in the first successful case of operation for traumatic rupture (St. Thomas's Hospital Museum).

MacCormac operated for intraperitoneal rupture of the urinary bladder, and repeated his success in another case two months later. These were the first of their kind in which success was obtained, and naturally made a deep impression on the profession.

A table of abdominal injuries admitted to all the London hospitals which publish statistical reports is perhaps of some interest and is as follows :—

St. Bartholomew's (1873–1906), St. Thomas's (1866–1907), Middlesex (1873–1904), University College (1879–1904), Westminster (1880–1903) :—

	Per cent.
Simple contusion of the abdomen	64
With injury to kidney	7·7
,, alimentary canal	4·7
liver	4·5
spleen	2·6
bladder	1·1
mesentery	0·5
omentum	0·3

						Per cent.
Wounds of the abdomen .	.	.	.	.	.	8·4
Proportions : Non-penetrating	.	.	.	.		4·0
Penetrating	.	.	.	.		3·0
Indefinite	.	.	.	.		7·0
Mixed or various .	.	.	.	.	.	5·9

(*e.g.*, rupture of hepatic artery, bullet wound, and multiple injury.)

This gives some idea of the relative frequency and proportions of these injuries, the total number of cases being about 2,500.

Before the time already mentioned there are few reliable records of recoveries from these internal injuries ; it is true that in people who were examined *post-mortem* cicatrices of limited extent were very occasionally found in the liver and spleen, but the history of their formation was not always to be obtained. Most surgeons willingly admit that some of the less severe ruptures of the solid viscera can and do get well without operation ; this is within our own experience, but without operation very many are hopeless, whilst ruptures of the intestines are most deadly. Dr. Le Conte ("Annal of Surgery," Vol. I., 1903, p. 526) quotes Petry as giving a list of 160 cases of ruptured intestine where 93 per cent. died and 7 per cent recovered, but only after formation of abscess associated with a fæcal fistula. Other collections give an even higher mortality up to 97 and 98 per cent. Le Conte estimated the operative mortality from this cause as from 50 to 60 per cent. in 1903. Every year has added to our knowledge, and the results in life-saving are not only better now, but there is prospect of further improvement. Some of our critics forget that we are dealing with patients who are not only suffering from a ruptured bowel or other internal organ, but perhaps from two or more of these injuries, or from a severe crush affecting the lungs also, or fracture of the pelvis, ribs, or other bones—injuries which of themselves would be severe without the one which really offers the greatest danger to life.

To those who think our best results are but meagre I would recommend a perusal of this section of the reports of a hospital before the commencement of the period, or a paper in the *Lancet*, on the " Recollections of a Hospital Surgeon," written about 1889.

This paper was written by a man of eminence, and recounts

his experiences in this branch of surgery.   It is most instructive reading.   To the account of more than one out of his 19 cases of fatal rupture of the intestine he adds remarks to the effect that had he operated it seemed' possible that the injury to the gut might have been repaired.

Another table shows the various ways in which some patients were injured before they came under observation, and the particular part on which the stress of the injury fell.   It is compiled from records of cases to be found in hospital reports, the *Lancet*, the *British Medical Journal*, and the paper by Messrs. Berry and Guiseppi.[1]

Causes and Situations of some Internal Ruptures.

	Duodenum.	Jejunum.	Ileum.	Large Intestine.	Intestine Total.	Spleen.	Bladder.
Run over in street . .	12	27	11	7	57	5	3
Kicked by horse . .	1	13	8		24	2	4
Crushed	6	5	5		19	—	—
Struck by moving object .	4	13	7		26	3	2
Fall on hard object . .	1	5	7		14	5	4
Fall of weight on abdomen	—	6	5	—	11	1	3
Fall from height . .	1	4	—	1	6	6	2
Other causes, mostly unknown . . .	1	7	—	—	8	1	4
	26	80	43	16	165	23	22

If it is possible to ascertain the exact part of the body struck by the force which caused the injury, then one can make an approximate guess as to the organ ruptured, for it is generally lying beneath, between that point and the spine, and incision over this area gives most direct access to the damaged structure.

You must not expect to find local signs of injury to the skin, for there may be none.   This is of importance from a medico-legal aspect, for not long ago a jury, with the sapience

[1] Transactions of the Royal Society of Medicine for 1909, etc.

which appears to be almost the prerogative of coroners' juries, refused to believe that a kick from a man had produced a rupture of the gut because there was no mark of the kick.

In all abdominal injuries it is advisable to follow a certain routine in the examination of the patient. Ascertain when the last meal was taken, when the bladder was emptied, and if the patient was in good health before the accident. Inquire as to the position and extent of pain, and then examine the abdomen carefully for dulness, and see if this is fixed or shifting. Find out if there is rigidity of the muscular wall, whether it is general or local, and the amount of tenderness, its position and extent. You should note also the state of the pulse and the temperature.

Further, the patient should be re-examined nearly every hour, and no morphine given unless it has been decided to operate.

TRAUMATIC RUPTURE OF THE INTESTINE.

I have previously, when writing on the subject of traumatic rupture of the intestine without external wound, directed attention to the similarity existing between these injuries and perforations of the intestinal canal which constitute such a large part of the " acute abdomen." In the perforations from disease there is the initial " peritonism " at the moment of perforation, which corresponds to the injury and the symptoms immediately following the injury, in the case of rupture ; the effect of the escape of intestinal contents is much the same in the production of a spreading peritonitis in the two, but the peritonitis in the healthy person appears to be more rapidly fatal. Probably in him the fluid containing bacilli is in a con-centrated form, for little escapes, whilst his injured peritoneum is unprepared to cope with the vigour of the invasion. When it is recognised that in about 50 per cent. of these cases there is a " period of repose " before the development of the more characteristic symptoms, then our house surgeons will treat these patients with the same respect as they do now a man who gives a history of chronic indigestion and a recent acute pain in the stomach.

With regard to the symptoms which may result from rupture of the intestine, there has been much written on the subject by various authors, and it is comparatively easy to take a series of cases and analyse the recorded symptoms in each. The result obtained will be fairly accurate as regards the obvious manifestations of the injury, such as shock, vomiting, pain, and perhaps rigidity, which are common to nearly all injuries in which the viscera are damaged. There is, however, such a difference of opinion between those who examine the abdomen as to what are to some comparatively unusual signs, that little reliance can be placed on statements which vary so greatly. Yet these minor symptoms may be most valuable with a clear history, for in all, I repeat, it is important to diagnose the lesion as early as possible, before the onset of peritonitis, and every symptom that may be of use in bringing about an early diagnosis is of importance.

I do not propose to consider the value of all the individual symptoms in detail. Mr. Berry has recently done so, and his conclusions in the main confirm those expressed by Mr. John Croft and Mr. Makins, though founded on a recent and therefore more extended review of the subject. From the practical point of view, we need not consider those cases which are admitted with intense shock, from which they never rally. The others can be arranged in fairly typical groups, as they present themselves in actual practice :—

A. In the first of these there is shock, vomiting, acute abdominal pain, with great tenderness over the part struck, and board-like rigidity of the abdominal wall. All these symptoms are present, but they vary somewhat in their intensity ; at one time shock is the main symptom, at another it is the pain, and so on. With these there should be found a certain amount of localised dulness on percussion. This group forms about 50 per cent. of all cases.

Multiple Ruptures of the Small Intestine : Rupture of Mesentery : Resection : Anastomosis. (Death six days later.)— A stableman aged 24 admitted on August 10, 1892, suffering from the effects of a kick in the abdomen by a horse, about half an hour earlier. He was received in a very collapsed state, but had not vomited. The patient was a man of slight build, suffering much pain in the abdomen. His face was white and anxious-looking, and his pulse small and feeble. Below and to the left of the umbilicus was a bruise, not clearly defined, where the hoof of the horse had struck him. The abdomen was extremely hard to the touch, somewhat distended and motionless. There was dulness on percussion over the front of the abdomen. Clear urine was withdrawn by catheter. Soon after admission he commenced to vomit. At 3 p.m. he was still suffering from shock, very cold and shivering with anxious face, and was lying on his right side with limbs flexed. The abdomen was fixed like a board, very hard and very tender. The dulness over the front of the abdomen was more extensive, but did not invade the epigastrium or pass into the flanks.

Intraperitoneal rupture of the small intestine with rupture of the mesentery or omentum with extravasation of blood was diagnosed, and at 8 p.m., when operation was performed, on sufficient recovery from shock, this diagnosis was fully confirmed. The mesentery was bruised and lacerated, and hæmorrhage was still going on from it. There was rupture of the small intestine in two places within a distance of 8 inches, the gut having been divided as cleanly as with a knife. Only a small amount of intestinal contents had escaped, amongst which were one or two partly-digested beans. The intestine was contused, and in one or two places the peritoneal surface was torn. Thirteen inches of the bowel, including the damaged mesentery, were removed, the section being made beyond the ruptures where the bowel appeared healthy. Union was effected by lateral apposition, and the mesentery was sutured. Another rupture involving almost the entire circumference of the gut was then discovered, about 12 inches away ; the edges of this did not appear bruised, and end-to-end anastomosis with Senn's plates was done without resection. Saline infusion to the extent of 5 pints was given. Progress was satisfactory until 6.15 on the evening of the 15th, when vomiting returned, with severe abdominal pain and local signs of peritonitis. The wound was reopened, and, the end-to-end union having been found broken down, an artificial anus was made, his condition not permitting of more prolonged treatment. He died a few hours later. At the necropsy it was found that the first rupture had occurred 20 inches from the pylorus. Extensive hæmorrhage into the right lung was also discovered.

RUPTURE OF THE SMALL INTESTINE WITH RUPTURE OF THE MESEN-TERY : SUTURE. (Recovery).—A small boy, aged 5, was admitted on December 31, 1910, having been knocked down by a tram which was drawn by a horse. It is not certain if the horse trod on the boy or not. He was very sick afterwards and was taken to a doctor, who could find nothing definite. His father thought the boy looked very ill and brought him up to the hospital, where he arrived three hours afterwards. He was then looking very white, and his nostrils were working very rapidly. On examination of the abdomen there was seen an abrasion with faint bruises of the skin above and to the outer side of the left anterior superior spine. There was dulness on percussion in the left flank up to the edge of the rectus, and the muscles were rigid but not board-like. The pulse was rapid, 128, but not feeble. Temperature 97°.

He arrived whilst I was at the hospital, so that no time was lost, the boy being taken directly to the theatre. The incision was made to the left of the middle line and the rectus muscle pulled outwards. On opening the peritoneum free bright blood was found in the left flank. About 3 feet from the ileo-cæcal valve the mesentery was torn longitudinally, and some vessels were bleeding freely. A perforation the size of an ordinary hydrocele trochar was found in the antimesenteric border of the gut, at the same level. This was closed by a continuous Lembert suture of silk (No. 1). The tear in the mesentery was closed after ligature of vessels and the abdominal wall closed in layers. He developed some bronchial pneumonia, but it gradually subsided. On January 5 a large quantity of clear fluid came away from the lower part of the wound, evidently peritoneal, and continued to flow for a few days. The temperature became normal as the lung signs improved, and he left hospital on January 23, 1911, having quite recovered.

B. In the second group there is no evident shock, and perhaps the patient walks to the hospital, or goes home, congratulating himself that he has had a " narrow escape " ! He may have vomited soon after the accident, which made him feel faint, but there are no marks of injury on the abdominal wall, or they are but slight. He has considerable local pain, and there is rigidity of muscle, sometimes confined to the side of the abdomen which was struck. There is tenderness on pressure, and perhaps localised dulness, but the man feels that he will soon get over it, and probably remains under treatment with reluctance, or neglects to call in medical advice on his return home.

This group forms about 35 per cent. of the total number of cases.

In a case which I communicated to the Pathological Society in 1885, in which there had been extensive laceration of the small intestine, the patient, a man of 25, an ostler, had been kicked by a horse at 5 p.m. the day before admission to hospital. He seemed unable to move for half an hour, but then went on with his work until 6.30 p.m. He had food on reaching home, but vomited it almost immediately, and was restless during the night. However, he returned to work in the morning at 6 o'clock : was unable to resume his work after a slight breakfast, because of the onset of pain and vomiting. He passed into a state of extreme collapse, and died twenty-seven and a half hours after the kick. There was an extensive rupture of the small intestine, and intense peritonitis.

In the following case we were much hampered by the alcoholic condition of the patient. In the first place, the vomiting was mistaken for the results of drink ; in the second place, he was very intolerant of discipline ; and in the third, his general condition was very unsatisfactory from chronic alcoholism.

On the night of April 4, 1898, a man aged 27, who was crossing Whitehall when in an intoxicated condition, was run over by a two-wheeled van. He was taken to a hospital near, but was refused admission, so was brought to St. Thomas's about three-quarters of an hour later. He could give no coherent account of the accident, but complained of pain in the abdomen, where there were marks of wheels. Pulse fairly good ; temperature normal. A scalp wound had been already stitched up, and he was admitted because of his drowsy state. At midnight his temperature was 100·2°. He commenced to vomit a clear fluid smelling strongly of alcohol, and this continued all through the night till 9 o'clock on the morning of the 5th, when he complained of pain over the abdomen, which was very sensitive to the touch and very resistant. Pulse 160 ; very small. I was asked to see him at 2 p.m., when his condition was practically the same, but there was still no local change to be found on percussion. Immediate operation was performed, at which a large quantity of sero-purulent fluid was evacuated, and a rupture measuring ⅜ inch in length in the long axis of the bowel was found 12 inches from the ileo-cæcal valve. Eight Lembert sutures were sufficient to close it. There was a good deal of lymph on the surrounding coils. The abdomen was cleansed with sterilised water, and a drainage tube passed into the pelvis through a second opening ; the upper wound was closed. Ten days later the upper wound yielded, two days after removal of sutures, and there was protrusion of small intestine. This protrusion was washed and replaced, the wound being again sutured. The patient, who had been a heavy drinker and suffered from albuminuria, was difficult to manage, having on one occasion got out of bed soon after his operation and walked about the ward during the night. Following on the second application of sutures, the wound suppurated, and he ultimately died on April 30 with lung symptoms. At the *post-mortem* examination the abdomen was almost normal, with the exception of a small retro-hepatic abscess on the right side. The gut was firmly healed. The lower lobe of the right lung was collapsed.

C. In a third group the symptoms are rather indefinite ; there is a history of abdominal injury, probably of the kind which sometimes produces a rupture of the intestine, but the shock is trifling ; there is no vomiting, local pain is slight or absent, there is little tenderness, no rigidity of muscle, whilst percussion shows no change. After a variable time there may be a rising pulse, with that change in facial aspect which indicates to the experienced eye the presence of grave peritoneal inflammation. It may not be easy to say at what moment this commenced, but " a change has taken place." It may develop after an attack of vomiting, as in the case under the care of the late Mr. Walsham. This surgeon, who was patiently watching for symptoms, in a case of this kind, found a complete change after the patient had vomited, and, operating at once, gained a well-merited success. In yet another patient the onset of serious symptoms may be sudden and unexpected, caused by the giving way of a portion of the contused bowel.

In some instances, especially where there is a definite history of the kick of a horse or mule, it will be judicious to operate at once, as recommended by Mr. Bernard Pitts, without waiting for symptoms.

Should the escape of intestinal contents be very restricted, possibly in consequence of the smallness of the perforation, the symptoms may be limited to occasional sickness, with uneasiness in the abdomen, gradual distension and general tenderness, caused by a slowly extending inflammation of the peritoneum, which may become localised, and result in the formation of an abscess. It must be remembered that meteorism may follow an injury to the abdomen without any rupture of the intestine or internal organ.

A rigid condition of the abdominal muscles is a very important sign ; it practically always means serious underlying damage. Cases in which it is present may, in rare instances, recover, but it is a sign which should be regarded as of great value, and in most as an urgent indication for operation. Mr. Croft compared it to the protective contraction of muscles round an inflamed hip-joint. Hartmann has also shown its value.

No deduction regarding the value of localised dulness on percussion can be drawn from published cases. In the large majority the condition of the abdomen on percussion is not mentioned, and appreciation of the slighter degrees of abdominal dulness is not universal.

Mr. Bernard Pitts thinks that dulness at the site of contusion may be due to collapsed intestine, as a result of a temporary paralysis following the injury. It has been ascribed to escape of intestinal contents ; this may be so, but it is rare to find much feculent fluid present when the abdomen is opened soon after an injury, although blood may be found which has come from a rupture of the mesentery or a tear of the omentum. An extensive extravasation of blood under the peritoneum of the anterior abdominal wall will also cause dulness which does not move with alteration of position, but this is a very rare complication. If there is a history of localised contusion, such as that produced by a kick, and in addition to dulness under the part struck there is also fluid in one or both flanks, the mesentery is torn, and, whatever the opinion as to the state of the gut, the indications for operation are evident—first, to prevent further bleeding, and, secondly, to repair the injury, which may have placed the gut in danger of gangrene by deprivation of its blood supply. When the injury has been less localised, such as that resulting from a fall or from being run over, it is possible that there may be a complication in the shape of rupture of one of the solid viscera in addition to damage of the bowel and its mesentery.

It has been observed that local tenderness is usual, but there may also be a sharp superficial tenderness extending from the rupture towards a dependent part, indicating the direction taken by fluid of great irritative properties, in its course to the flank or the pelvis.[1] In one patient with rupture of the splenic flexure this sign was present, and was caused by the escape of offensive fæcal fluid from an opening behind the bowel through minute lacerations in the peritoneum, and its spread down to the pelvis along the inner side of the descending colon, and at the operation some of it was sponged out of the pelvis. A similar tenderness may be found in examples of the recent rupture of a jejunal, or of a stercoral ulcer ; it is found some-times at the margin of a spreading inflammation started by a diseased appendix, and more generally diffused, in acute hæmorrhagic pancreatitis. Even when other symptoms are slight, this alone should indicate caution in prognosis.

There is another symptom which may possess more importance than has hitherto been accorded it, and that is a marked rise of temperature within a short time of the injury. It was present in one patient before the bowel gave way (on the second day) ; here 103° was recorded within a few hours of the injury, whilst the usual local signs were still absent. There is probably some absorption through the lymphatics from the lacerated parts of the gut and mesentery, for it is not found in many of the cases in which the opening is of large size and the escape of feculent fluid presumably greater ; whilst in the case to which I have alluded the rupture was a secondary one.

On October 8th, 1904, a boy aged 14 was admitted at 7 p.m. with a history of injury to the abdomen. At 3 p.m. he was walking along a row of iron posts, and when stepping from one post to another his foot

---

[1] See p. 50.

slipped and he fell, striking his abdomen on the post in front. He fainted, was taken home, where he was sick several times, and complained of great tenderness in the abdomen. He could not pass his water. When brought to the hospital he was still suffering from shock, and complained of pain in the lower part of the abdomen. This on examination was found to move fairly well, was not markedly rigid, though some rigidity was present about the lower part of the left rectus. There was tenderness around and below the umbilicus, but this appeared to be rather superficial. There was no area of dulness in front and no shifting dulness in the flanks. The liver dulness extended from the sixth to the ninth rib. A considerable quantity of clear urine was drawn off. Pulse 100, of small volume ; temperature 99°.

It was stated that for two or three days before the accident the boy had had a cough and sweating at night, and had talked of going to the hospital for medicine.

October 9.—He was sick at 9.30 last evening, but since then has not vomited. During the night the temperature went up to 103°, and the pulse rose to 120. This morning the temperature was 101°, pulse 110, and the patient seemed very comfortable. Urine normal. There was no diminution of liver dulness, and no increase of rigidity of the abdomen. He said that he had no pain unless the abdomen was touched. At 3 p.m. he had quite recovered from the shock, and presented the aspect of one suffering from reaction. He was flushed, with red lips, bright eyes, and dilated pupils ; the pulse was 110, and he was dozing comfortably, lying on his back. The thighs were not flexed on the abdomen, but were placed straight. His temperature, which had been 103° during the night, had fallen to 100°. The pulse was not wiry, he was not restless, and the vomiting had ceased. On examination of the abdomen there was no abrasion or mark to be seen. It was normally distended without any visible peristalsis. He could draw a deep breath without pain. On palpation there was no rigidity of the muscles, but he complained of a general tenderness, not excessive. The percussion note was normal throughout, the liver dulness being satisfactory ; it was thought that the note was less clear in the flanks, but this was put down to the greater thickness of the muscle there, for it did not alter with position. The opinion given then was that we had no evidence of complete rupture of the gut, but that it was quite possible it was severely contused, and that it might give, when immediate operation would be required. This opinion was founded on the account of the case up to 3 p.m., not on the local condition. About 5 p.m. he again complained of sharp pain in the abdomen, and the pulse rate increased to 136. At 7 p.m. the abdomen was rather more rigid, and there was some diminution of liver dulness. At 9.30 p.m. he vomited a considerable quantity of greenish fluid, and the abdomen was slightly more rigid, especially about the upper part of the left rectus. The pulse was 120 ; the liver dulness was less evident, but there was no dulness in the flanks.

Median section was performed at 12 midnight by the resident assistant-surgeon, who found evidence of recent peritonitis, with some free fluid in the pelvis, which had run down the descending colon. In several places the small intestine was distended and showed signs of bruising, with small hæmorrhages into the mesentery. Near the upper end, where the flakes of lymph were most abundant, a small recent perforation was found. This was sutured with two rows of Lembert sutures. The abdominal cavity was freely washed out with warm saline solution, and the wound closed. He improved for a time, but on the 10th was restless and vomited considerably during the afternoon, whilst later the abdomen was rather distended.

He died at 5.30 on the 10th, the pulse having become very rapid and weak, after a restless night.

The perforation was situated 57 inches from the commencement of the intestine. The sutures had held perfectly, and the *post-mortem* examination only showed localised peritonitis, which had probably commenced before operation.

The absence of liver dulness as a sign of ruptured intestine is rarely seen, and if one may judge by published reports of cases, much invaluable time has been lost waiting for it to develop. It does not require a large amount of gas in the peritoneum to produce this symptom, but the contraction of the injured section of bowel prevents the escape of intestinal contents including gas, the condition of the gut not being quite the same as it is in perforation from disease.

Emphysema of the sub-peritoneal tissue is recognised mostly in cases of rupture of the duodenum, during the course of an operation for that lesion ; the gas may make its way through the inguinal canals, and distend the scrotal tissues when operation has been delayed. It is also found when the large bowel has been ruptured behind the peritoneum. The crackling which is felt by the fingers in these circumstances may assist in the localisation of the rupture after the peritoneum has been opened. The only cases of ruptured gut in which blood was found in the vomit were those in which the duodenum had been lacerated ; in no instance was there any blood passed by the bowel.

Something must be said about general treatment in cases of internal injury, but no hard-and-fast rule can be laid down. We must be guided by general principles, and are in a very much better position than formerly, because of the recognised value as an aid against shock of saline fluid, injected into the subcutaneous tissue, passed into a vein, or allowed to enter the rectum continuously. We must not forget, however, in injuries of the solid viscera that hæmorrhage is the chief danger to life, hence permit no more delay before the operation to arrest it is carried out than is absolutely required.

It has been recommended by some surgeons that when there is rigidity of the abdominal wall warm applications should be made to the part, so that if the rigidity is due to injury of the abdominal wall alone it may have a better chance of passing off and the patient be saved a possibly useless operation. It is hardly necessary to say that this treatment should not be continued for any great length of time, if there is any possibility of rupture of the intestine, because peritonitis is known to begin within six hours in many of these cases.

I may refer again to Messrs. Berry and Guiseppi, who show not only that the mortality is less when early operation is performed, but that the best results are obtained when it is done between seven and twelve hours after the accident. This is practically the same conclusion as that to which Siegel came, and is explained by the fact that the shock is passing off, and peritonitis is still localised, if it has commenced.

By operation in cases of ruptured intestine is here understood abdominal section, a search for the injured gut, and its repair by suturing. The incision should be a long one to give easy access to the intestine, and its central point should be placed at the level of the umbilicus. In some it may be necessary to excise the contused and lacerated part, and perform an anastomosis, but in the majority a double layer of sutures, applied as already advised, will suffice. The formation of an artificial anus in the small intestine is to be much deprecated. In about 10 per cent. there is more than one lesion ; forgetfulness of this fact may lead to serious trouble. The surgeon had better satisfy himself on this point before he begins to apply sutures.[1]

It appears to me that some of the more recently published cases of recovery in this branch of surgery have shown an advance in the after-treatment, founded on the principles which guide us in perforative peritonitis. The patient has been placed in the " Fowler position," drainage employed, and saline fluid administered continuously by the rectum. Messrs. G. H. Edington, W. Sheen, and W. G. Nash recorded successes in 1908, whilst Dr. Radcliffe introduced saline into the cæcum

[1] See p. 40.

after appendicostomy at the rate of two gallons in twenty-four hours. The effect of this is instructive, as the patient recovered, " perspired, passed urine freely, and at the end of the time had some incontinence, passing fæces with a moderate quantity of saline fluid. Moreover, there was fluid continuously welling up through Keith's tube, so that the pad over the tube had to be changed every half-hour."

A table on p. 52 shows the result as regards actual recoveries, but does not show how many were relieved by operation. In Mr. Croft's first case the patient died a month later after resection of the artificial anus which had been formed in the first instance. Another patient, also in the series from St. Thomas's, lived for a month, and still another some six days, dying ultimately from peritonitis due to the giving way of a stitch.

Rupture of Duodenum.

Rupture of the duodenum is one of the more rare results of injury to the abdomen. The history is nearly always that of " run over in the street," caught between a moving and a stationary object as in a buffer accident, or struck by an opponent's knee during a football match, and it is evident that the damage was inflicted above the umbilicus. Occasionally the peritoneum is torn and intestinal contents escape into the peritoneal cavity ; more frequently the tear is in the posterior retro-peritoneal part of the bowel, and extravasation takes place in and around the rupture to a rapidly increasing extent. As this extravasation contains a certain amount of pancreatic secretion, there is a swift change in the state of the cellular tissue of the part. It may be sufficient to produce a fixed dulness continuous with that of the liver if the patient survives for a day or two.

The signs of "peritonism" are severe, the shock being especially great, so much so that occasionally it has been necessary to abandon an operation for the relief of this injury, because the state of the patient has made it evident that any continuation of the exploration would prove fatal before he could leave the operating theatre. In addition, there may be board-like rigidity of the upper abdomen with great tenderness on pressure, emphysema of the abdominal wall, blood in the vomit, and on opening the abdomen localised ecchymosis of the peritoneum, and sometimes fat necrosis of the kind seen in acute hæmorrhagic pancreatitis.

Some of these patients die from the shock, others, and the more numerous, as a result of inflammation of the retro-peritoneal cellular tissue ; therefore it is well to arrange for drainage of this region.   The recorded cases of recovery after operation are very few indeed.   Those of Messrs. Godwin and Moynihan were at or near the duodeno-jejunal junction.   If it is possible to find the opening in the peritoneum, the bowel underneath must be examined and treated by suture if this opening is small and accessible.   Mr. Lawford Knaggs, who opened a discussion on this subject at the Royal Society of Medicine,[1] describes a case in which he sutured the opening, which was 1 inch from the pylorus, with a continuous suture through the mucous and muscular coats, and applied inter-rupted Lembert sutures outside that.   At the necropsy twenty-four hours later these had held.   The drainage was provided for in this case by three tubes, one in the right flank to the kidney pouch, one into the pelvis, whilst the retroperitoneal space was drained through the abdominal incision.   In this, the second of two cases related by Mr. Knaggs, the patient was a man of 20, and operation was performed more than twenty-four hours after the injury had been inflicted.

If there is complete rupture above the entrance of the bileduct into the second part of the duodenum, the best method of treatment is to close both ends and perform a gastroentero-stomy after the method of Mayo, or by the ordinary anterior method which takes less time for its performance.   Cholecyst-enterostomy must also be performed when the complete lesion is below the bile papilla.

When a complete rupture has taken place below the duodeno-jejunal junction, a modification of the operation of gastro-jejunostomy " en Y." of Roux may be possible, but the proximal limb may be very short and require some skill to adapt it to the efferent loop.

These are suggestions of possibilities, but in actual practice there is rarely a chance of doing more than pack and drain, on account of the excessive collapse.

[1] See Vol. V., No. 9, p. 243, Transactions.

Rupture of the Large Bowel.

Rupture of the large bowel by force, from within, has been occasionally seen. Dr. Andrews[1] has drawn attention to the effect of compressed air in causing this accident, and published a most instructive case in which he had to excise a portion of the sigmoid and do a lateral anastomosis. He collected fifteen other cases from American sources. The air hose which leads to the compressed air supply need not be applied directly to the anus, but produces its effect through the clothing. Rupture is usually in the sigmoid and may be multiple. All the cases not submitted to operation died ; as in other cases, operation must be early. In the days when intussusception was treated by means of air injections into the bowel, rupture of the gut was not unknown. It may be torn also by an attempt to introduce the sigmoidoscope or to pass a large bougie through a high non-malignant stricture, when the patient is under anæsthesia, not from perforation by the bougie, but from pushing the inelastic stricture upwards. In cases where enemata have been forced into the peritoneal cavity it is usually difficult to say whether the damage has been caused by the nozzle or from too forcible delivery of the fluid into an obstructed rectum.

Rupture of the Descending Colon, with Lacerations of the Overlying Peritoneum.—A woman aged 33 was brought at 12.15 a.m. on July 14, 1907, having been run over by a horsed omnibus, the wheel of which passed over the abdomen about the level of the lower ribs. When admitted she was pale and collapsed with a feeble pulse, 120, and a temperature of 97°.

During the night she was sick once, suffered much pain, and was evidently worse in the morning. I saw her at 10 a.m. Much of the shock had passed off, and she was lying somewhat propped up in bed with quickened respiration and pulse. She was complaining of pain in the left side of the abdomen over the lower ribs, and the abdomen was not moving well with respiration. There was rigidity especially marked on the left side, with excessive tenderness extending in a line from the site of the injury towards the pelvis. She had passed urine of normal appearance, but the bowels had not acted. There was no evident bruising of the skin.

Ten hours after the injury operation was carried out through the left rectus sheath with displacement of the muscle inwards. At the first inspection there was little visible beyond a scratched appearance of

[1] " Surgery, Gynæcology, and Obstetrics," January, 1911, N. Y., *Lancet*, Vol. I., 1911, p. 524.

the peritoneum over the situation of the splenic flexure. A bruised state of the descending colon was seen, it was not extensive, but there was no abrasion or tear of its peritoneum or alteration in the normal consistency of the part. Some free gas could be felt in the mesocolon, and a mounted sponge passed into the splenic region showed a dark fluid with fæcal odour. Compression of the descending colon between finger and thumb whilst they were moved towards the flexure caused some bubbling of gas and escape of a small quantity of fæcal fluid through the small tears of the peritoneum about the splenic flexure. Incision backwards at the angle just below the ribs carried through the peritoneum behind the splenic flexure opened up a cavity outside the bowel in which there was some solid fæcal matter which had escaped from a hole the size of a penny, at or below the splenic flexure. This cavity extended upwards into the retroperitoneal tissue behind the spleen and could hardly be cleansed, for the fæces were ground into the cellular tissue. The edges of the rupture were brought together with interrupted silk sutures, the margins being inverted. The peritoneum was cleansed, and some ounces of offensive blood-stained fluid removed from the pelvis. The wound was closed, the peritoneum being sutured so as to shut off the septic area behind the bowel which was drained.

The sutured bowel partly gave, and a fæcal discharge appeared from the lumbar opening on the fifth day—there was also some rise of temperature, and as this did not subside, 25 c.c. of anti-coli serum was injected into the axilla on the ninth day. Improvement was satisfactory, but the temperature kept above normal, so on the fourteenth day 25 c.c. of the poly-valent serum was injected. Some fæcal matter with pus continued to come away for nearly five weeks, the amount was becoming smaller from day to day, and the wound had quite closed before September 7, when she left the hospital.

The mortality attending rupture of the intestine when the patients are placed under the best conditions is shown in the table on p. 52. These are all hospital cases—ninety-seven operations with twenty-one recoveries. In this table are included all the cases submitted to operation, whether successful or not, but a truer estimate is obtained if only the cases for the last ten years are taken.

I have not made a separate heading of *Rupture of the Mesentery*, because it is usually a complication of the more severe lesion, rupture of the intestine. The symptoms are also similar, and although a surgeon may be certain there is a laceration of the mesentery, he cannot be certain there is no accompanying lesion of the intestine. They are serious because of the danger of interference with the blood supply of the intestine. They may also be the cause of extensive hæmorrhage into the peritoneum. Should the separation from the bowel be extensive or there is accompanying rupture of the intestine, the part must be excised and the ends united with sutures.

Table Showing Results of Operation for Traumatic Rupture of the Intestine.

	St. Thomas's Hospital, 1886—1910.		Berry and Guiseppi (London and other Hospitals, 1893—1907 inclusive).	
	Cured.	Died.	Cured.	Died.
Small intestine—				
No operation . .	—	6	—	37
Operation . . .	5	20	8	49
Large intestine—				
No operation . .	—	1	—	5
Operation . . .	5	1	3	6
	10	28	11	97

St. Thomas's Hospital   .   . 31 operations, 10 recoveries.
Other hospitals 66   ,,   11   ,,

RUPTURE OF THE PANCREAS.

The pancreas is another organ which occupies a protected position in the upper abdomen, so it is very rarely injured by anything short of a stab or gunshot wound ; still there are a few cases on record where such has occurred, and the possibility of it must be recognised in cases of contusion in the epigastric region.

A laceration of this organ gives rise to no special symptoms beyond those of shock and effusion of blood into the peritoneal cavity. When peritonitis supervenes it is apt to be ascribed to other causes.

Should exploration be decided upon in consequence of the urgency of the symptoms, which are referred to the region of the stomach, a median incision should be used, and after examination of the stomach. liver, and spleen, the gastro-hepatic omentum should be torn through and the lesser sac of the peritoneum examined.   Blood may be seen coming through a tear of this omentum, or it may be seen below the greater curvature of the stomach.   If there is extravasated blood in this sac, the wound should be packed off and the space cleansed with sterilised saline.   Hæmorrhage from a laceration should then be arrested by the application of ligatures of catgut to the bleeding points.   Should this method fail to arrest the bleeding, deep sutures to bring the parts together should be tried, care being taken to avoid the ducts if they have been cut.   If the laceration is in the tail of the pancreas, it will be well to cut this off beyond a ligature, at the surgeon's discretion.

Should it be possible to close the rent, additional sutures of catgut should be also employed to draw together the peritoneum covering the gland so that the damaged organ may be quite shut off from the peritoneum.

The peritoneum must be thoroughly cleansed.

In every case provision should be made for drainage; the best plan is to close the opening in the gastro-hepatic omentum and make one in the gastro-colic omentum, through which a strip of gauze the required size can be passed.   In more than one recorded case a plugging of the wound combined with drainage has sufficed.

A complete rupture of the pancreas was successfully treated by Professor Grave.[1]

The patient, a man of 24, had been crushed between the buffers of a train.

There was some little pain after the accident, no vomiting or nausea, no shock, whilst the temperature and pulse were normal.   The abdomen was tense, and there was some tenderness in the epigastrium.   Three hours later vomiting of coffee-grounds material, later of some blood, set in, with severe pain.

A complete tear of the pancreas was found, the edges of which were about an inch apart, and sharply cut as if with a knife.

The torn edges of the organ were brought together with exact apposition, and with three posterior and three anterior fine silk sutures through capsule and parenchyma the defect was repaired and the hæmorrhage stopped.   Gauze packing was put in and became saturated with secretion in two days.   This packing was removed after eight days and a new loose one inserted.   In two weeks a drain was inserted.   The fistula closed in six weeks.

Of twenty-four subcutaneous injuries, thirteen died without

[1] "Beitrage sur Klin. Chir.," 1905.

operation ; eleven were operated on and seven recovered ; this operation merely consisted in exposure of the wound and drainage, any blood which had been effused being cleared away.

Dr. Randall has obtained success after suture of a laceration of some 2 inches in length. He employed drainage.

Rupture of the Liver.

Rupture of the liver is an extremely fatal accident, and the symptoms which ensue are usually marked and serious. Shock is present, frequently passing into collapse and death. Short of this there are vomiting, rapid pulse and respiration, pallor, etc. In this accident rigidity of the abdominal wall is very evident, so that it may appear board-like. Tenderness becomes localised to the hepatic region, and there is shifting dulness in the flanks with the ordinary symptoms of loss of blood, according to the amount of it which is effused—the man becoming restless with a rapid weak pulse, sighing respiration, and what is called " air hunger." Jaundice may be a late symptom, and is therefore of no use in the *early* diagnosis, which is so very important.

There is, as might be expected, much variation in the size of the rupture, which is usually on the convex surface of the right lobe ; the combined statistics of Mayer and Ogston give three right lobe to one left lobe as the proportions.

Shock in this injury may not be evident when the patient first comes under observation.

Fatal Case in which Shock was Delayed.—When leaving the Royal Free Hospital some years ago, I saw a woman of 59 brought in, who had been run over in the street a few minutes earlier.

She was excited, and resented examination. There was no mark on the abdomen, no dulness in the flanks, or rigidity of the muscles. It was difficult for us to induce her to remain in the hospital, yet three hours later the abdomen was full of blood, and she did not survive for many hours the operation to arrest the bleeding. The liver was extensively torn posteriorly and the kidney showed a recent laceration ; there were other injuries also present.

I must repeat that all cases of abdominal injury should be carefully examined during their stay in the hospital, for secondary symptoms give very few signs which enable them to be detected.

FATAL CASE IN WHICH THE SYMPTOMS WERE SLIGHT.—In 1911 a man who had been injured in a motor car accident was in the hospital for about ten days and then went to a convalescent home, apparently well.   Soon after his arrival there he was transferred to a hospital, where it was noted that in addition to jaundice there was a considerable effusion in the peritoneum.   A large quantity of this was withdrawn by aspiration, but the patient died from peritonitis.   It was found that there had been a rupture of the liver.

RECOVERY AFTER GAUZE PACKING.—In July, 1912, a boy was admitted who had been run over and received fractures of the right ribs over the hepatic region.   For two days there were no symptoms of importance.   He vomited on the third day, the abdomen became somewhat distended and tender, whilst the temperature rose and the pulse increased in frequency.   No definite dulness could be found on percussion, but incision on the right side gave exit to about a pint of fluid blood which was becoming septic, and a rupture of the back of the right lobe was found from which blood was flowing.   He recovered after this place had been plugged for thirty-six hours.

The records of cases which are published give no reason for thinking that there is any special disease of the liver that predisposes to rupture, although it is stated by a Russian veterinary surgeon, Dr. Grymer, that rupture of a lardaceous liver is a comparatively frequent cause of death in horses. Hæmorrhage is the most common cause of a fatal ending, yet Dr. Homer Gage considered that 14 per cent. proved fatal from peritonitis, caused by the continued presence of blood in the peritoneum.   Dr. Hogarth Pringle, who contributed a paper to the " Annals of Surgery " (a paper which is full of interest to the surgeon) on traumatic hepatic hæmorrhage, considers that, if the severe cases are to be got through at all, the operation must be an immediate one for the majority.   That some of these cases can be saved is shown by the statistics of Ferrier and Auvray, and by the cases which are published in the literature of this country, though these are few in number. He suggests that when the peritoneum is opened, the hepatic and portal vessels should be immediately grasped with finger and thumb, and held by an assistant whilst the effused blood is cleared from the peritoneal cavity and the necessary manipulations are carried out on the liver.   He has practised this in two cases, and says that perfect control of the bleeding areas of the liver was obtained and a clear field for operating.

There can be no doubt that at the operation the first thing is to arrest the hæmorrhage, which appears to increase directly the peritoneum is opened. In these cases the incision should be a large one, the operator quick and decided in his movements, and the immediate arrest of hæmorrhage the first care. There is a difference of opinion as to whether the laceration should be closed by means of suture, or whether the surgeon should be satisfied with gauze-plugging of the area from which the hæmorrhage comes. Dr. Hubbard recommends that in some instances the packing of the wound shall be done through the pleura, after a flap has been made from the chest wall.

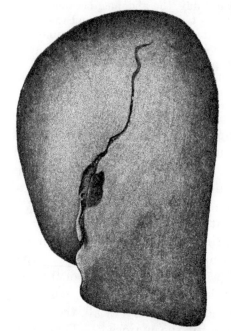

If hæmorrhage from the area affected cannot be arrested, then in the majority of cases a long strip of aseptic gauze should be employed to plug the wound. This should be placed in position gently, but firmly, and its amount proportioned to the size of the cavity from which the bleeding comes Masses of gauze should not be employed, otherwise adhesions form between intestinal coils, which may cause obstruction later. I have had to operate for such a late complication of a treatment which was successful in saving life in the first place.

Fig. 5.—Extensive Laceration of Liver, Hæmorrhage: 432, St. Thomas's Hospital Museum.

There are some wounds in which it is best to insert stout catgut sutures by means of a round-bodied needle which is a size or two smaller than the suture. This method of treatment should be attempted only when there is ready access to the laceration, and the condition of the patient permits of the time required. A ready and simple method is to place strands of catgut on both sides of the laceration on the surface of the liver, otherwise the sutures are apt to cut their way through the liver substance. Intermediate sutures may also be inserted in the ordinary manner, on which there is no tension.

Since writing the above the following case under the care of Mr. Rutherford Morison [1] has been published which bears out what has already been said, and emphasises the possibilities of success in the most extensive of these injuries :—

A miner aged 17, crushed between two objects five hours before admission to the Royal Victoria Infirmary, March 17, 1913. He felt very faint, and on being released fell down in great pain and very ill. The abdominal pain, so severe at first, gradually passed off, and he had none when he arrived. His complaint then was of pain over the lower ribs on the right side, and he was tender there. The only sign discoverable was some rigidity over the right side of the abdomen. He looked well, his pulse was 80, and his temperature was normal. He was examined by several different authorities, and all agreed that there was nothing to indicate a serious lesion or the need for an operation. Next morning he had not slept and was in great pain. His colour was good, he was sweating freely, his tongue was moist, and his pulse of good quality and only 80 to the minute. His abdomen moved very little with respiration, it was markedly *rigid and tender* all over, and there was *shifting dulness in both flanks and the hypogastrium.* Mr. Morison continues his account :—

"It was now evident that some serious intra-abdominal lesion was present, and the problem whether this condition was due to ruptured intestine with general peritonitis or to intra-peritoneal hæmorrhage was fully discussed. My view was in favour of peritonitis, as, though I knew a large intra-abdominal hæmorrhage might exist with very little disturbance, I could not believe that a hæmorrhage large enough to cause dulness so marked could fail to produce evident anæmia."

Operation (seventeen hours after the accident).—On opening the abdomen blood poured out. This was traced to the liver. Remembering Hogarth Pringle's valuable hint, I passed my left forefinger into the foramen of Winslow, and with my thumb in front compressed the hepatic artery, portal vein, and bileduct, arresting all hæmorrhage at once. The wound was found to be in the right lobe of the liver extending from the coronary ligament through the free margin and involving so much of the whole thickness of the organ that the portion on the right seemed to be attached to the left part by only a narrow band.

The tear was sutured in four tiers with thick catgut. The first line of mattress sutures commenced about 1½ inches from each side of the tear, and caught the bottom of it, the next were introduced about 1 inch from the edge, the third ½ inch, and a final continuous suture brought the fibrous capsule together. Before the sutures were tied any relaxation of the hold upon the gastro-hepatic omentum was followed by active hæmorrhage, but as soon as the sutures were tied the wound

[1] *British Medical Journal*, Vol. I., p. 8, 1914.

was quite dry. The peritoneum was washed clean. Intravenous infusion on table.

A drainage tube was left in the hepatic pouch for the first ten days, but nothing escaped from it, and the wound healed by first intention. Except for a curious rise in temperature every evening (up to 102°) the patient made a good recovery, and went home well fourteen days after the operation.

Mortality after Rupture of the Liver.

Mayer . . . Out of 207 cases, 86·6 per cent. fatal.
Edler (1887) . . ,, 547 ,, 85·0 ,,
Fraenkel . . ,, 31 ,, 45·0 ,,
Tilton (1905) . . ,, 25 ,, 62·5 ,,

Thole-Dantzig gives the mortality after operation—

If performed during the first twelve hours, 55 per cent.
If performed during the second twelve hours, 67 per cent.
Beyond, 78 per cent.

RUPTURES OF THE GALL-BLADDER AND BILIARY PASSAGES.

Traumatic rupture of the gall-bladder is a very rare accident, but is occasionally seen. If the bile is diffused throughout the peritoneum there will be evidence of free fluid slowly increasing without symptoms of hæmorrhage. There may be an injury of the liver also, when the symptoms of liver laceration will mask those of injury to the gall-bladder. Of the few cases which have been published the following is a good example in which the effusions became localised.[1]

The patient was admitted into Cashel Union Hospital under the care of Dr. T. Laffan. She was a married woman, aged 50 years, who had been trodden on by a cow while in the act of milking it. She felt something give way inside, and after suffering for some time from all the symptoms of acute inflammation was sent to hospital on September 15, 1898.

On admission the patient was in an alarming state, being almost moribund. She was deeply jaundiced and all the symptoms of peritonitis were present. The effusion was, however, circumscribed, presenting the appearance of a considerable tumour in the epigastric and adjacent regions. The patient was put under chloroform, and with the assistance of Dr. T. O'Connell, Dr. G. Cook, and others laparotomy was performed. A large quantity of bile, pus, and some liquid fæcal matter were evacuated. The cavity was washed out with antiseptic

[1] *Lancet*, 1900, Vol. II., p. 1497.

solution, a drainage tube was inserted, and the wound was sutured, with the exception of the opening for the tube. The patient was so weak and the parts being so matted as to require a regular dissection to unravel the point of rupture, it was deemed more prudent to make it an operation *de deux temps* if necessary. The necessity for a second operation, however, did not arise, as after an uneventful period the wound entirely closed, all discharge ceased, and the patient made a perfect recovery.

At first there is usually shock with faintness, perhaps local pain and vomiting, and a slow accumulation of bile takes place in the peritoneal cavity, with production of limiting peritonitis and the deposit of much plastic lymph. Jaundice may appear early or late, and bile is absent from the fæces. There appears to be no indication for immediate operation, and when operation is performed, it is usually for the evacuation of fluid which has accumulated on the right side of the abdomen. The abdomen is asymmetrical, for the bile is never generally diffused in the peritoneum.

If the rupture is quite recent the gall-bladder may be sutured as in some cases of cholecystotomy. It is usually safer to drain it, or, failing this, place a tube down to the rupture, packing off the peritoneum after it has been cleansed.

Ruptures of the bileducts are very rare, and openings in the common duct can very seldom be found. Those which have recovered have been treated by aspiration of the collection of bile which has formed in the peritoneum, and this operation has been repeated on more than one occasion ; but, if it is considered best to explore, it may be possible to suture the duct, at least partially, if it can be found.

Henlin is said to have recommended abdominal section in these cases in 1767.

If the opening cannot be sutured it would be best to place a drainage tube down to the duct, pack off with gauze, and perform a cholecystenterostomy. If the patient is very bad a temporary cholecystostomy should be done and later the junction made with the small bowel ; it would also be well to make a lateral communication between the afferent and efferent portions of the loop selected.

Only one example of this injury has come under my immediate care, and in this the impression given by the slowly increasing collection of fluid was that it was very heavy.

Traumatic Rupture of the Common Bileduct : Laparotomy.[1]

A boy aged 6 was admitted to the Royal Free Hospital on August 15, 1893, having shortly before been run over by a hansom cab.

He was a well-developed lad, suffering slightly from shock and complaining of spasmodic pains in the abdomen. The only mark of injury was slight grazing of the skin on the left side of the chest, running downwards and to the right. He vomited soon after admission, but did not bring up any blood. Temperature 97·6°. The abdomen was not rigid and no special tenderness could be elicited.

On the 16th he seemed fairly well, but still had spasms of pain in the chest, chiefly on the right side. During the night he had been restless and fretful and vomited twice. His bowels had not acted and the temperature was 98·4°.

On the 17th, in the afternoon, he was lying on his back with his thighs flexed on the abdomen ; there was no rigidity, tenderness, distension, or alteration in the percussion note. He vomited twice and his temperature rose to 101·2°. Urine, sp. gr. 1,020, very red in colour, but no blood or albumin present.

18th.—Still restless, with frequent vomiting : bowels have acted normally. Respiration mainly thoracic. Was drowsy in the afternoon. Vomited three times and bowels acted three times. Temperature, 2 a.m., 101° ; 6 p.m., 102·3°.

On the 19th slight jaundice noticed ; continued restless and looked very ill : vomited four times. Less complaint of pain. Highest temperature 100·2°. There was more vomiting on the 20th, and only 3 oz. of urine were passed. Slight dulness noticed on right side of abdomen. The temperature did not exceed 98·4°.

On the 21st there was evident change. He looked very ill, with sunken eyes, was deeply jaundiced, vomited frequently in the effortless manner of a patient with peritonitis. His pulse was rapid and weak, and emaciation was marked. The abdomen, however, was not what might have been expected—the impression given was that of " flaccid distension," it was larger than normal, moved with respiration, but chiefly in the upper part, was but slightly tender and without any rigidity. On percussion there was an area of dulness extending from the hepatic region into the right iliac fossa ; there appeared also to be dulness on the left side in the flank. On the right side the dulness extended forwards to the right linea semilunaris, and changed but slightly on movement. He vomited in the manner already described during the examination, was restless, and gave an occasional deep sighing inspiration. The temperature was 97·2°.

The fluid in the peritoneum was supposed to be extravasated bile, with some inflammatory effusion, and it was supposed that there had been a rupture of one of the biliary ducts, not a rupture of the liver or of the gall-bladder. We could not obtain permission to evacuate this until 6 p.m. of the 26th. On incision through the peritoneum, which

---

[1] Transactions of Clinical Society, 1894, p. 144.

was stained a deep yellowish red, a large quantity of pure, odourless bile ran away. The intestines were congested, but there was no lymph on them. A drain was placed into the space from which the bile had come, but no attempt at fuller exploration was permitted by his bad general condition.

He died on the 28th, apparently from exhaustion. Bile was absent from the motions only on the last two days of the illness. At the *post-mortem* examination the whole of the small intestines were found injected, and to have on them layers of lymph ; this was especially marked on the right side. The liver and gall-bladder were intact, but about half an inch beyond the junction of the cystic and hepatic ducts the common bileduct was found torn completely across, but the aperture was difficult to find. No other traces of injury were discovered.

Erhardt's experiments are of interest as showing the effect of the bacillus coli (which is present in the common bileduct) on the peritoneum, when mixed with the bile after its escape from the biliary passages, both in the production of a plastic peritonitis and the prevention of cholæmia.

RUPTURE OF THE SPLEEN.

Rupture of the spleen is mostly met with in malarious districts, where it is so commonly diseased ; it may also occur during the course of an attack of typhoid fever. In this country it is nearly always the result of a severe injury, and none of our recorded cases of operation have been for rupture of a diseased spleen, so far as could be ascertained without microscopical examination. In one instance which Dr. C. Wheen has found in our medical publications there was evidence of disease of the blood on examination.

It is unnecessary to enter to any extent into a consideration of rupture of the diseased spleen, for although it would be interesting, it would be chiefly so from a medico-legal point of view. Much of interest on this subject can be found in papers by Dr. D. G. Crawford, in the *Indian Medical Gazette* (1902 and 1906). Some of the accounts given by medical men in charge of hospitals in tropical countries, or by those attending hospitals where patients are admitted from malarial districts, are quite startling. A patient with a large spleen " turns in bed," is playfully " dug in the ribs " by a jocular friend, someone throws a grain of mustard seed at him or flicks him with a cane, and death ensues in a period of time measured by minutes. Playfair gives seven to eight minutes as the average duration of life after rupture of a malarial spleen, and the late Surgeon-General Coull-Mackenzie said that 68·9 per cent. of his cases died under half an hour. If the abdomen is examined after death it is found to have been flooded with blood, as if the sac of an aneurysm of the aorta had burst into the peritoneum. There is rarely time for more than a guess as to the cause of the symptoms—none for treatment. Rarely is the rupture of a malarial spleen survived even for a few days.

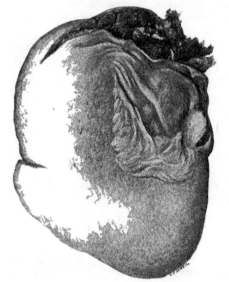

Fig. 6.—Traumatic Laceration and Contusion of the Spleen. Removed during life on account of hæmorrhage: 444, St. Thomas's Hospital Museum.

Dr. White Hopkins, who spent some years in Sarawak, has brought to my notice a weapon which I have called the "lethal cross," but in Malay the real name of which is "larang" (meaning forbidden). He says it is used only in southern China, and generally in the Malayan countries and islands, Malay States, Java, Sumatra, Celebes, etc. The weapon is unknown in northern China, for the reason that an enlarged spleen is not so common as in the southern or tropical portion. It is heavy and made of an iron bar 16 inches long, with a cross-piece, the ends of which turn towards the point. The blunt end terminates in a nut which gives it a knobbed appearance. It is carried with the shaft up the arm of a long sleeve, clutched between the second and third fingers at the cross, leaving the knob extending. It cannot be seen in consequence of the size and shape of the sleeve. The Chinaman waits for his victim at night, and, accosting him, deals him a sudden and unexpected blow in the abdomen, not being particular as to the exact part which he strikes. The victim without a groan falls dead on the spot.   His pockets are rifled, and nothing more is known of his assailant.

Dr. White Hopkins adds, " from my experience in Sarawak, an enlarged spleen amongst the Chinese is found in about 90 per cent.   I would go further, and say that every China-man has an enlarged spleen.   But the ratio of enlargement would be as follows :—The whole of the abdomen involved with a hard nodulous enlargement would be 60 per cent., perhaps more ; a partial enlargement, occupying three-quarters of the abdomen, would be about 25 per cent., and the remainder, from a half to a quarter enlarge-ment."   If a Chinaman is found with a larang upon him he is at once tried and imprisoned, because it is known what

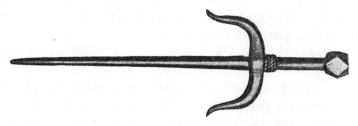

FIG. 7.—The Larang.

intention he has.   It is rarely found, except in the case of intoxication, or the finding of a Chinaman in close proximity to a dead man.

I do not know of any other instance in the history of the peoples of the world in which similar advantage has been taken by the criminal of the pathological opportunities of the district in which he lives.

Rupture of a normal spleen is found as the result of consider-able violence, and is met with clinically under two conditions. From its position under the shelter of the ribs, where it is well guarded, especially in the adult, it is a comparatively rare injury.   It is not surprising to find that amongst the published cases there is an unduly large proportion of young people, whose ribs are more elastic and yielding, no less than fifteen out of twenty-three being under 20 years of age, nearly all of whom were " run over " in the streets.   It was formerly held that there must be adhesions between the spleen and diaphragm before rupture can take place, but this theory has been disproved in recent years. Rupture of this organ is not always fatal ; healed cicatrices have been found during necropsies by Ayres, Neville Jackson, D'Arcy Power, and others. There are some cases in which life is said to have been much prolonged after this injury, but, unfortunately, the condition of the abdomen, as given in the report, does not always carry conviction that the diagnosis was correct. Statistics are, therefore, of little value, but Edler computed the mortality at 82·3 per cent. in the uncomplicated cases.

The symptoms produced may be immediate and alarming, or they may be delayed in their development. Barrallier summed them up in these words : " *péritonisme*," " *l'hémorrhagie*," " *syncopie*," but probably referred to the rupture of a malarial spleen. Rupture of the malarial spleen may be compared to the rupture of an aneurysm, and that of a normal spleen to the wound of a large artery.

The amount of shock varies very considerably when a healthy spleen has been ruptured, and does not help in the diagnosis, but I am inclined to think it greater as a rule when the spleen rather than when the liver has been ruptured, unless the laceration of the latter is deep or extensive. There may be no local evidence of contusion, but if the injury was to the splenic region, more especially if the overlying ribs are broken, then the great probability is that the spleen has been torn, and the symptoms will be shock, " air hunger," and the signs of free fluid in the peritoneum.

Pain may be severe, but on the other hand it may be absent, and there may even be no tenderness. The chief reliance must be placed on the presence of blood in the peritoneal cavity soon after an injury, and the general effect of the escape of this blood on the patient. It is strange that in many recorded examples of rupture of the spleen there is no statement as to the presence or absence of dulness in the abdomen during the progress of the case, or, in fact, any note to show that those in charge were aware of the very large accumulations of blood which were revealed at the *post-mortem* examinations. In one or two cases, in which operation was performed abroad, it is stated there was no dulness, and, a paragraph or so later on, that a great deal of blood escaped when the peritoneum was incised. In ruptured spleen there is the shifting dulness of the effused blood, whilst the immediate vicinity is occupied by a fixed clot which gives the impression of an increase in size of that organ. All cases should be closely observed and operation performed if there is rapid increase of the effusion or of the symptoms of loss of blood.

Some of the cases which were successfully treated presented a less urgent group of symptoms, there being apparently a small amount of intraperitoneal hæmorrhage at the commencement, but recurrences during the following days rendered the state of the patient precarious.

The clotting of the escaped blood in and around the laceration appears to close the vessels for a time, but secondary hæmorrhage has been known to prove fatal three weeks after the accident.

If the patient survives, and no relief is afforded during the first day or two, to the other abdominal signs and those depending on loss of blood are not infrequently added increasing distension, vomiting, pain, restlessness, and other symptoms of peritonitis, which has for many years been known to follow large effusions of blood into the peritoneum.

It is advisable to remove the spleen, and empty the peritoneum of the blood which has invaded it. The use of a plug of gauze is useful in rupture of limited extent, but with such a soft vascular organ great pressure may produce sloughing. In one case (the notes of which were read before the Clinical Society), that of a big, heavy man, where the spleen was very adherent to the diaphragm, I passed a ligature round the splenic vessels and so arrested the hæmorrhage. Saline infusion was most useful and bleeding did not recur, but he only survived operation four days. Dr. C. Wheen has tabulated the successful cases of excision for this injury, done by British surgeons, and it is interesting to find that Mr. C. A. Ballance not only obtained the first operative success, but has the credit of two out of the twenty-three recoveries which have been published in this country, and Mr. B. Pitts obtained a third success. In all three cases there was marked enlargement of the lymphatic glands afterwards, on the surface of the body, when the patients had recovered from the immediate effects of the loss of the organ.

A.A.   F

The abdominal incision should, if a diagnosis has been made, be placed in the splenic region below the left ribs. An incision in the middle line does not give satisfactory access to the spleen, although it is very useful if general exploration is indicated, because the surgeon is uncertain of the nature of the lesion which is present. When it is recognised that the spleen is the source of hæmorrhage the operator should immediately secure the pedicle by temporary means. Either a clamp should be placed on it or it should be held by the fingers whilst the required extension of the incision is made. As a rule the laceration is of the hilum and vessels entering by that part, and it is easy to increase the size of the lacerations by violent dragging on the spleen.

It is worthy of note that, in the examples of ruptured spleen during the course of typhoid fever, operation has mostly been performed for supposed perforation of the small intestine. A laparotomy of the lower abdomen has been first performed, and then a second incision made over the spleen, when it was found to be the source of the symptoms.

In many of the ordinary traumatic ruptures this is done and the spleen removed through the second incision. Dr. Auvray has advised a long incision in the left side, the upper extremity of which slopes backwards over the lower ribs, the cartilages of which are excised to give more space. The increased shock which such a resection would cause is against its employment as a routine practice.

The pedicle of the spleen should be clamped, the organ removed beyond the clamps, and interlocking ligatures applied carefully before the clamps are removed. If plenty of tissue is left beyond there will be no fear of secondary hæmorrhage, but if the tissue beyond is possibly inadequate, larger vessels in the face of the stump should be secured separately.

RUPTURE OF THE KIDNEY.

Contusions of the kidney leading to laceration of that organ are amongst the most common of abdominal injuries, but on account of its protected position the extent of the damage does not often require surgical interference. It is not uncommon to find hæmaturia develop in a patient who has been run over in the street and complains of lumbar pain and tenderness.   There may be some swelling in the region of the kidney and slight rise of temperature, but a few days' rest in bed enables the patient to resume his work again without any disability.   A watch must, however, be kept on such cases, for serious suppuration may ensue with few symptoms or a hydro-nephrosis or urinary cyst develop later.

The more severe injuries are, however, of considerable gravity although retroperitoneal, even when the lesion is not accompanied by serious damage to surrounding parts. In these the shock may be severe and the pain great, a more or less rapid extravasation of blood forms a swelling in the peri-renal tissue, and the escape of urine when the laceration extends into the pelvis of the kidney renders the occurrence of suppuration probable.   Suppuration is not an unusual complication from the proximity of the large bowel, which is itself often bruised.   The amount of hæmaturia varies, but is not often an indication for operative interference, unless at the same time there is a rapid development of swelling in the region of the kidney.

Tuffier[1] found that these contusions of the kidney were complicated by other lesions in 20 per cent. of cases which he had collected.   He also found that the deaths in uncomplicated cases were 43 per cent., whilst in the complicated cases death followed in 87 per cent.   During the ten years 1903—12 inclusive there were forty cases of uncomplicated contusions of the kidney admitted to St. Thomas's Hospital which recovered without operation.

In five others it was thought advisable to operate and the kidney was removed in four ; of these one died ; in one a lumbar incision was made and the patient recovered.

Of the more complicated cases, twelve in number, the liver was also ruptured in six (of these two had also a rupture of the lung).   The spleen was also ruptured in four, one of which recovered after excision of both spleen and kidney.   In another there was also fracture of the skull, whilst in one there was rupture of the peritoneum over the kidney and an extensive hæmorrhage into the abdominal. cavity ; the kidney was removed and recovery followed.

It requires considerable force to produce a rupture of the

[1] "Arch. Gen. de Med.," 1888—9.

overlying peritoneum, especially in the adult, and when this complication is present the symptoms are much the same as those produced by a ruptured spleen, there being signs of extensive hæmorrhage into the peritoneal cavity with evidences of injury in the kidney region. There will probably be a hæmaturia of varying severity, with the general symptoms of loss of blood.

In the case of a man who had been run over, and which proved rapidly fatal, under my care in the Royal Free Hospital the peritoneum was full of blood and blood-clots. A completely lacerated left kidney was found partly displaced through a tear in the peritoneum and was removed. The patient died from the rapid and excessive loss of blood, the amount being greater than that seen after injury to the other abdominal viscera.

INTRAPERITONEAL RUPTURE OF THE KIDNEY.—A girl aged 8 was admitted on March 24, 1911, having been run over about midnight by a motor car. It was stated that one of the wheels passed over the abdomen.

On admission she was conscious and looked well, but had a pulse of 120. The abdomen was tender generally, but there was no definite area of tenderness. Pain was referred to the umbilicus. On percussion there was slight dulness in the flanks, and the muscles on the right side of the abdomen were slightly rigid.

She vomited soon after admission, at which time the urine was normal ; three hours later it contained a trace of blood.

At 4 p.m. she was pale, restless, appeared to be suffering from shock, and had a rapid pulse. There was tenderness in the abdomen, chiefly referred to the outer margin of the right rectus. The abdominal wall was but slightly rigid. This diminished during the next two hours, but the dulness in the flanks had increased, and there was considerable tenderness over the kidney region.

At 6 p.m. an incision was made over the right rectus and the muscle displaced inwards. There was a considerable quantity of fresh blood in the peritoneal cavity, which came through a rent in the peritoneum over the right kidney. This opening was plugged with gauze, the patient turned over, and the kidney removed through a lumbar incision. In it there was a large rent extending from the hilum three-fourths of the distance to the outer side. The peritoneum was cleansed, the opening sutured, and the anterior wound closed. The lumbar incision was filled with gauze. Intravenous saline was given during the operation, and afterwards saline (with brandy) was given *per rectum*. Two days later the lumbar incision was closed with sutures. Five days after operation a quantity of sterile fluid was drained from the peritoneum, there being a considerable amount of distension. The tube was left in for four days. She left hospital having quite recovered on April 20.

Operation when undertaken for the treatment of a ruptured

kidney should be by the lumbar route, a pillow being placed under the opposite loin ; the incision should be free, so that no time is lost in securing the pedicle after the collection about the kidney is opened ; there must be plenty of room to carry out the manipulations.   For this reason some recommend an opening which does not follow the usual direction of a nephrectomy incision, but extends from the middle of the twelfth rib to the iliac crest a little in front of the middle ; it is then prolonged to the anterior superior spine.   Extra-vasated blood is often met with in the muscles, and sometimes the effused blood is found making its way to the outer side of the spinal muscles.   If it is possible avoid opening the lumbar fascia until the muscles are clearly divided over it, the fascia can be then quickly cut and the kidney pedicle compressed with the left hand, whilst with the right accumu-lated clot is cleared away.   Let the wound be well opened up with retractors, and ascertain the origin of the bleed-ing, and the exact position of the kidney.   It is not well to apply a clamp too hurriedly to the pedicle, as the vena cava may be injured.   If it is possible to apply forceps to the bleeding points, do so, and replace them by ligatures if you can.   Usually it will be best to separate the kidney from its capsule and bring it up to the surface as before incision in nephrolithotomy ; it is not difficult to pass the finger through the lacerated capsule.   In some cases it will be found possible to pass thick catgut sutures into the substance of the kidney and so close the wound and arrest bleeding, but when there is a complete transverse rupture, as when there are many frag-ments, removal of the organ will be much the safest.   Try to separate the main part of the kidney quickly with the fore-finger, bring it to the surface, and ligature the pedicle with catgut in two portions.   It will be advisable to use a pedicle or aneurysm needle for these ligatures, and pass them so as to secure the ureter and vessels separately.   The kidney is cut away about $\frac{3}{4}$ inch beyond them.   It is sometimes easier to pass them after the clamps have been removed, and if the kidney is properly under control there is no danger from hæmorrhage while this is being done.

If silk is used for the pedicle, then the ligatures must be left long.   Efficient drainage must be provided.

When there is reason for thinking that the peritoneum overlying the kidney has been ruptured, no time must be wasted ; the danger to the patient is the rapid effusion of blood into the peritoneum. The abdomen must be opened as in the case described and the kidney excised as soon as possible. It will be necessary to give much saline during the operation and take every precaution to diminish the amount of shock ; as hæmorrhage is going on internally there is no time to prepare the patient ; every minute permits increased loss of blood, and the sooner this is arrested the better the patient's chance of recovery will be.

On completion of the operation in these cases the peritoneum should be sutured over the stump of the kidney and the abdominal wound closed. If drainage is required, it should be carried out through an incision in the lumbar region. It is a good plan to leave some saline solution in the peritoneal cavity.

Intraperitoneal Rupture of the Urinary Bladder.

Intraperitoneal rupture of the bladder is still a very fatal injury, in spite of the fact that surgeons do not fail to operate whenever the lesion is diagnosed, or there is reason to fear that it has occurred. In 1886 Mr. Rivington wrote : " No indubitable case of recovery after intraperitoneal rupture of the bladder is on record." In the same year Ullman collected 143 cases, and of these only two had recovered, whilst Sir W. MacCormac operated successfully in two instances, abdominal section being performed and the rent sutured in each case. This was nearly one hundred years after Benjamin Bell proposed that the abdomen should be opened and the bladder sutured for this injury.

The patient probably presents himself at the hospital with a statement that he has had an injury to the lower part of his stomach ; that since that time he has been unable to pass urine, or has done so in small quantities, and that it is blood-stained. I shall always remember the first patient on whom Sir W. MacCormac operated so successfully, the " pioneer case," when he first came to St. Thomas's Hospital :—

Going into the casualty department about noon in the pursuance of my duties as resident assistant-surgeon, I found a big, strong, healthy-looking labourer, standing up near a couch readjusting his clothing, whilst the dresser of the week was turning away with a porringer (con-taining urine of normal appearance) and a No. 8 catheter. Noticing that the amount of urine which had been drawn off (about 1¼ oz.) was small in quantity for a man applying for relief of retention, whilst the size of the catheter suggested the absence of stricture of the urethra, a few inquiries were made, 'and we learned that the patient had not been able to pass urine since the previous evening, when, running after his boy, he had hurt himself against a post in the alley. Throughout the night the abdominal pain had been severe ; he had wandered about his room, whilst his frequent efforts to pass urine had failed absolutely. He partly undressed again and laid down upon the couch for re-examina-tion. Percussion showed the presence of such a large quantity of free fluid in the peritoneum that in the absence of symptoms of hæmorrhage it could only be urine which had escaped through a rent in the intra-peritoneal part of the bladder. The abdomen was rather distended without hypogastric dulness. A catheter was again passed in the ward, and 95 oz. of urine came away ; it was obvious that this quantity could not have been retained in the bladder, and renewed examination of the abdomen now showed great diminution in the amount of free fluid. The rent in the bladder measured 4 inches in length.

I have dwelt on this change in the dull area found in the abdomen after an instrument has been passed, and fluid with-drawn by it, because it has not received attention adequate to its value às an aid in diagnosis. Another useful sign would be a contracted state of the bladder, rendering movements of the catheter difficult, whilst perhaps only an ounce or two of blood-stained fluid is withdrawn.

Of intraperitoneal rupture of the bladder it must also be remarked that shock is most unreliable as a symptom : in Sir W. MacCormac's second case, which was also under my observation, the patient, a heavy man, who had fallen from a height of 20 feet in a sitting position, presented no appearance of shock and so few signs of injury that the house surgeon, a most able and careful man, did not find justification for his admission until he applied again on the following day. Yet the rent in the bladder was 2 inches long. This is all the more interesting, as this house surgeon had been on duty with the first case and recognised the possibility of this lesion.

The result of injection of sterilised saline in measured amount into the bladder, which is allowed to flow out again, may be tried, but the forcing of air into the peritoneum may give a serious addition to any shock already present, and nothing is gained by it. In the majority there will soon be rigidity of the lower abdominal muscles, followed by the symptoms of peritonitis. At times these symptoms are delayed. Dr. Quick's case, which was successfully operated on by Dr. Thompson on the eleventh day, is an extreme proof of this. Dr. Quick's patient performed his work as a labourer an entire day after the injury, which was incurred during intoxication, and was not compelled to take to his bed until the second day was well advanced. Here the laceration admitted the end of a thumb.

The symptoms of peritonitis may be very insidious in their onset, and in this class of case, more than in any other, the pulse will prove an invaluable guide. Failing strength, rapid pulse, and, later, vomiting, may be the only symptoms of extensive mischief. Ashurst states that amongst the patients who were intoxicated at the time of the accident the mortality was over 43 per cent., whilst amongst the sober it was less than 28 per cent.

The shock may pass away during the unconsciousness of intoxication and the patient know nothing of any injury received when in such a state. There is a record of a series of soldiers who died from peritonitis after this injury. The men had taken a wrong turning when drunk and fallen from a window to the ground outside the barracks when attempting to enter a lavatory after return from leave. The cause of the accident was discovered by placing a guard over the lavatory.

Some cases may give less definite symptoms. In both patients under the care of Sir W. MacCormac there was a normal temperature, no vomiting, and the patients walked to the hospital. The second man had little pain, but there was no distension of bladder, as there should have been when he applied on the second occasion, considering the duration of the retention. Tympanites and the presence of urine in the peritoneum do not prove the existence of peritonitis.

A patient with this injury may live for five days, apparently improving, and then die quite suddenly.

Mortality after Operation for Intraperitoneal Rupture of the Urinary Bladder.

1886.   Ullman, 143 cases with two recoveries.
1901.   Alexander and Jones, 54. (Before 1893, a mortality
            of 63·5 per cent. after 32 operations ; between

1893 and 1903, a mortality of 27·5 per cent. after 22 operations.)

1906. Ashurst, 110, between 1893 and 1903, a mortality of 42·72 per cent.

1907. Quick, 29, between 1893 and 1903, a mortality of 24·1 per cent.

Occasionally a bladder has been ruptured by the injection of fluid preparatory to the operation of suprapubic cystotomy. Here there is the sensation of something giving way as the fluid passes into the cellular tissue around the bladder ; if the injection is continued an abnormal swelling may appear above the pubes, which gradually diminishes in size.

An extraperitoneal rupture of the bladder is often associated with a fractured pelvis, but is not restricted to such cases. There is the history of a likely injury and a complaint of inability to pass urine. A catheter if passed goes into a contracted bladder and a little urine is found which may contain blood. No dulness is found in the flanks, nor does a distended bladder show above the pubes as time passes. Signs of inflammation of the cellular tissue around develop and are most marked on the side of the rupture. There is a rapid pulse and respiration, with symptoms of inflammation and suppuration as the extravasated urine decomposes. An irregular swelling appears above the pubes, which is sometimes tympanitic, and is not diminished when the bladder is emptied.

Operation is the only treatment permissible ; this must consist of cœliotomy, with cleansing of the peritoneum, and of the application of sutures to the rent in the bladder, which must not penetrate the mucous membrane. It has recently been suggested that a plug should be placed over the laceration in the bladder without suturing of the rupture, and the pelvis drained through a suprapubic opening. There may be instances when this would be the only available procedure on account of the desperate state of the patient, and it has been successfully employed.

It is necessary to describe more fully the operation in the intraperitoneal ruptures. A median cœliotomy is quickly performed and the peritoneum opened freely. Extravasated urine with peritoneal exudation is removed as much as possible, and the intestine pushed out of the way with sterilised gauze. The

Trendelenberg position may be of assistance at this stage. After the rent has been localised it may be difficult to reach ; the incision must be carried well over the pubes, and should there be insufficient room the recti muscles may be detached on each side. Silk sutures (No. 1) should be passed by means of a small round-bodied needle in a holder after Lembert's method, about ¼ inch apart, taking up the peritoneum and muscular coats only. The end ones should be placed beyond the rent in the bladder, which is usually vertical and about 2 inches in length ; all should be passed before any are tied. Their introduction is facilitated if the one nearest the abdominal incision is passed first. After they have been tied an injection into the bladder will show if the line is watertight. Some surgeons recommend a double row, one to bring the torn edges together, the other to bury the first one in a broad fold. The sutures are cut short, and the bladder resumes its normal position. The peritoneum is cleansed, especially in the flanks, where fluid may have escaped notice ; and the wound closed, without drainage. If the patient suffers from retention during the after-treatment a sterilised catheter should be passed, and it is well to have a supply, prepared by Herring's most efficient method of sterilisation, ready for use.

In cases of extraperitoneal rupture the space of Retzius should be freely incised and drained, for sloughing of the cellular tissue will follow wherever the urine has gone. This cellulitis requires free incisions. It is sometimes possible to pass a drainage tube directly to the opening in the bladder and so prevent any further diffusion of urine. This opening must be left to close by granulation ; it is seldom possible to employ sutures.

Peritonitis is the most common cause of death, and early operation is the best preventative ; but even in early cases it may occur from extravasation of infected urine ; infection at the time of operation ; infection from a dirty catheter ; or from an imperfect suturing of the rent.

THE AFTER-EFFECTS OF ABDOMINAL INJURIES.

It usually happens that when a patient has survived the immediate effects of an abdominal injury his condition rapidly returns to the normal, since he is in excellent health at the time of the accident, and his vitality has not been sapped by previous disease or prolonged ill-health—hence convalescence is rapid and recovery complete.   Nevertheless, injuries to the abdomen are in certain cases liable to leave behind them traces which, scarcely noticeable at first, or perhaps not apparent at all, later on acquire alarming proportions.   The number of patients who suffer from such sequelæ is no doubt small considering the great frequency of abdominal injuries of all sorts, particularly in industrial communities, but the lesions themselves are often of a serious order.   Since abdominal injuries are nearly always due to the localised impact of violence, and not to general contusion, so the lesions produced are local lesions, and the nervous system as a rule is spared—hence one great feature characteristic of those who suffer from the sequelæ is their immunity from traumatic neurasthenia.

In the following sections, the effects of injuries to the abdominal wall are considered first, individual viscera being dealt with subsequently.

The Abdominal Walls.—The anterior suffers more frequently than the posterior abdominal wall, ventral herniæ resulting from stab wounds or following exploratory incisions, while direct rupture of one of the abdominal muscles is very rarely responsible.   The muscle which is most liable to rupture is the rectus abdominis below the umbilicus, and the fact of its rupture may be taken as indicating that the blow was not altogether unexpected, the muscle in fact by its violent contraction having broken the force of the impact and thereby shielded subjacent viscera from injury.   In operations upon ventral herniæ which arise in this manner, it is often found that only the deeper layers of the abdominal wall have given way, while the more superficial layers are still intact.   McGavin has reported a case in which rupture of the rectus took place on the left side, a ventral hernia followed, and at operation intestine was found lying between the ruptured muscle and its anterior sheath.

Retroperitoneal cysts, apart from those in connection with the liver and spleen, have been observed, in which trauma was held to be responsible ; most of these have been blood-cysts. They probably arise by progressive enlargement of hæmatomata.

Cases of diaphragmatic hernia due to injury are not common ; they are generally due to buffer accidents, severe blows on the upper abdomen or lower part of the chest, or to stab wounds through the lower intercostal spaces. The signs and symptoms are those due to interference with the functions of the stomach, the viscus most commonly involved (see pp. 236— 238). When the diagnosis is made operation should be undertaken for the closure of the defect, as strangulation may at any time bring the case to a fatal termination.

In those cases which follow stab wounds of the chest the hernial protrusion may find its way through the diaphragm, across the phrenico-costal sinus, and thence through one of the lower intercostal spaces. Gerster reports thirteen cases of this nature, in only one of which had strangulation taken place ; in another a man had been struck three years previously on the left side of the chest by a plank, and the hernia had appeared shortly afterwards. It had never given rise to any inconvenience. The swelling was easily reducible when the patient lay on his right side, but reappeared on coughing.

The Stomach and Intestines.—The commonest sequelæ of injuries to the gastro-intestinal tract are cicatricial stenosis, external fistula, and intra-peritoneal abscess formation ; and of the last two, perforating wounds more frequently lead to the former and contusions to the latter. Alexis St. Martin, the famous hunter, suffered from gastric fistula following a gunshot wound of the abdomen, an accident which earned him the right to immortality, since it enabled him to become the first subject for direct gastroscopy. Fistulæ are formed in a similar manner in other parts of the intestinal tract, but occasionally they arise somewhat differently. It may happen that a viscus has undergone partial rupture, one or more of its coats remaining intact, and in such a case an abscess forms in the neighbourhood of the lesion owing to emigration through the weakened spot of bacteria from its interior. Such an abscess may extend till it reaches the surface, when it is either opened or else bursts externally, sometimes leaving a fistulous track through which intestinal contents leak to a greater or less extent. In examining such a fistula it is important to observe the condition of the skin round about its orifice, since this point affords valuable information as to the portion of intestine involved.   Thus a fistula arising high in the intestinal tract has a more serious digestive action on the surrounding skin than one arising lower down, while the character and odour of the discharge should supply confirmatory evidence. Occasionally an abscess ruptures into a neighbouring viscus and forms an internal fistula ; such fistulæ have been observed between the stomach and the colon, and may lead to serious consequences by short-circuiting long stretches of the intestinal tract.   External fistulæ have a tendency to close spontaneously, but they may require operative interference, and then form a menace to life by subjecting the patient to the risks of general peritonitis.

In the St. Thomas's Hospital Reports for the year 1904, there is a case of fæcal fistula following abdominal contusion.   The patient, a carman aged 52, was run over by a wagon two months before admission, the wheel passing over his abdomen.   An abscess formed and was incised, when a quantity of stercoraceous pus was evacuated ;   the wound had discharged fæcal matter ever since.   As the surrounding skin was much excoriated, careful treatment was carried out and operation postponed for four weeks.   At the end of this period the local condition had so far improved that operation was no longer feared. The abdomen was accordingly opened in the middle line above the umbilicus and the ileum anastomosed laterally to the transverse colon : the wound healed by first intention.   Eighteen days after operation two stools were passed by the rectum, and on the twenty-second day the edges of the fistula were freshened and sutured together.   Seven days later the bowels were acting normally, but there was still some discharge from the fistula, and the patient went home relieved, but not cured.

In the light of more recent experience, it seems probable that a better result might have been achieved in this case if the ileum had been divided and the distal end closed, with implantation of the proximal end into the colon.

Injuries to the stomach are rarely followed by cicatricial deformities excepting at the pyloric end, where stenosis may occur as the result of previous laceration, the inflammation to which it gave rise, or the operation performed for its treatment. Such stenosis is liable to cause gastric dilatation with its attendant evils, but the prognosis is good if the patient is willing to undergo operation ; as in this class of case, gastro-enterostomy affords certain relief.   It is an open question how far injury may be responsible for the aggravation of previously existing gastric ulcers or for the formation of new ones, but it seems more than probable that if injury plays any part at all it can be only an exceedingly small one.

Intraperitoneal adhesions are not likely to be formed merely as the result of hæmorrhage, since extravasated blood is absorbed, and appears to have no other effect than the production of temporary agglutination of peritoneal surfaces ; but adhesions are undoubtedly formed whenever denudation of peritoneum occurs as the result of injury, and their action is protective in that they strengthen an otherwise weak spot in the visceral wall. But, their object once attained, they cease to be of value and henceforth become a source of danger, since they may under suitable conditions be directly causative of acute intestinal obstruction. Cases of intestinal obstruction are common in which peritoneal adhesions have been responsible, such adhesions having formed after abdominal injuries or their operative treatment ; but it must be confessed that in most of these cases the adhesions were due to operation and not to the injury itself.

Simple stricture of the small intestine has been known to follow injury, but here again operation plays the greater part, since the stricture most frequently occurs at the site of suture of a perforation or at the line of an axial anastomosis, but it is possible that cicatrisation of a contused wound of the bowel may itself be responsible for stenosis.

Traumatic appendicitis is recognised by some, and if cases of recurrent attacks of pain in the right iliac fossa attributed to injury may be regarded as due to that injury, then chronic appendicitis must be included among the sequelæ of abdominal trauma.

The duodenum, owing to its fixed position, is particularly liable to contusion, though its depth from the surface renders it less likely to suffer in stab wounds. One result of its rupture is the escape of bile and pancreatic juice into the retroperitoneal tissues with consequent abscess formation, and here again fistulæ may ensue, or duodenal stenosis and gastric dilatation follow. If the peritoneal surface of the duodenum be damaged and the case does not immediately prove fatal, the formation of a subphrenic abscess is exceedingly likely.

The Mesentery.—The sequelæ of mesenteric injuries are

few and rare.   Laceration of the mesentery may be followed by cicatrisation and consequently by kinking of the bowel; destruction of its peritoneum may court the formation of adhesions, and extravasation of blood between its layers may ultimately form one variety of the mesenteric cyst.   But the most important of all the lesions, by virtue of its attendant risks to life, is mesenteric perforation.   Perforations of the mesentery due to injury are a perpetual menace, inasmuch as

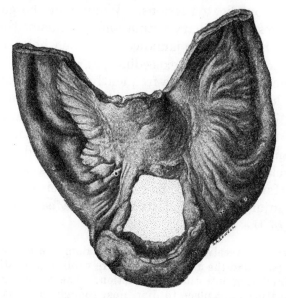

FIG. 8.—Opening in the Mesentery of the Small Intestine, which caused Intestinal Obstruction: 341, St. Thomas's Hospital Museum.

at any moment they may snare and incarcerate a wandering coil of bowel and initiate acute intestinal obstruction.

The Liver, Pancreas, and Spleen. — Perhaps the most characteristic sequela of an abdominal injury affecting the solid viscera is the formation of cysts; if infection occurs abscesses result, but, except in the case of the liver, sterile cysts are far more common.   As in the case of the hollow viscera, adhesions are more often due to the operation than to the lesion which prompted it, particularly as operations for the rupture of solid viscera so often entail the introduction of gauze packing into the abdomen.

A boy was admitted to hospital with signs of hæmorrhage and a history of abdominal trauma ; at operation a rupture of the liver was found and packed with gauze. He made a good recovery, but was readmitted a month later with obstructive symptoms. The abdomen was opened and an omental band found obstructing the small intestine. The case was too far advanced to admit of any hope and the patient died. At the necropsy nothing further was discovered beyond the healed scar in the liver.

Perforating wounds of the liver may lead to hepatic abscess, while subphrenic abscess occasionally follows ruptures, though rarely in uncomplicated lesions. Wounds of the gall-bladder sometimes result in biliary fistula and wounds of the ducts in stricture with obstructive jaundice. On the whole, the sequelæ of injuries to the liver are exceedingly rare.

The pancreas suffers more frequently and presents a greater variety of lesions ; among the sequelæ may be found lesions in the gland itself as well as lesions in the neighbouring tissues. Although it may seem incredible, prolapse of the pancreas through an abdominal wound has been observed. Inflamma-tory sequelæ have been recorded by various writers ; thus Fitz and Hansemann describe cases of necrosis of the pancreas following injury, while Rolleston reports a case of abscess of the head of the organ :—

A woman of 50 received a blow on the abdomen which was followed at once by pain, and the next day by severe vomiting, constipation, and collapse simulating intestinal obstruction. The vomiting continued, and constipation gave place to diarrhœa, though this was not severe. Two months after the injury an abscess developed in the right hypo-chondrium, and a fortnight later the patient died. At the necropsy there was found an abscess in the head of the pancreas with fat necrosis in the subperitoneal tissues.

Cysts of the pancreas due to injury have been classified as " true " and " false," the latter arising by closure of the foramen of Winslow and cystic dilatation of the lesser sac, and the former by dilatation of the lesser ducts behind an obstruc-tion of the main duct or of one of its large branches and brought about either by direct injury to the duct or its stenosis by involvement in scar tissue. Pancreatic fistula is caused by the incision of a true cyst or of a pancreatic abscess, and rarely by retroperitoneal rupture of the duodenum. False cysts or pseudo-cysts of the pancreas are due to the effusion of blood and pancreatic juice into the lesser sac after a partial rupture. A case of this nature was admitted in 1906, the account of which is as follows :—

On June 13, 1904, I saw a master butcher, aged 50, with Dr. Shelswell, of Mitcham, for an epigastric tumour. The history given was that twenty years before he had had several ribs broken and been severely crushed by a cart against a wall, so much so that he was nearly killed. For some time he had suffered from pain in the epigastrium and attacks of faintness, and three days before, when returning from market, had a severe attack of abdominal pain and became so ill that he was taken to the house of the medical man from the station. There was also a history of strain during lifting a heavy weight four years before. He then had pain in the epigastric region, was jaundiced for two or three days, and shortly after the strain noticed blood in the motions. There had been some swelling in the epigastrium for two years, but beyond gradual increase in size it had caused no pain.

He was a big, heavy man, complaining of pain in the epigastrium where there was a considerable prominence dull on percussion, which appeared to be due to a swelling as large as his head. It pulsated freely, but pulsation ceased when it was lifted off the aorta. There was well-marked fluctuation, and the outline was very definite. The cyst was punctured where most prominent and 6 oz. of brown fluid drawn off. The puncture suppurated and the cyst refilled; he complained of a good deal of pain and lost weight. The fluid was examined, and the report stated : " The fluid is red-brown in colour, slightly alkaline and coagulates on boiling. Sp. gr. 1,022 : No sugar or ferments : slight deposit, with blood cells and granular matter.

On admission later the sinus was healed and a swelling could be seen presenting characters similar to those present when the patient was first seen. Distinct movement was observed when he changed his position. The cyst was now opened and 7 oz. of offensive fluid escaped ; after thorough irrigation it was drained. After operation the temperature rose twice, while the discharge became more offensive, and it had not settled completely when the patient left the hospital with the wound unhealed. The Cammidge reactions A and B were negative. The wound continued to discharge for ten months after operation and then healed, though the man was too weak to work. In 1906 he was readmitted after several attacks of severe epigastric pain with rigors. Beneath the scar of the previous operation could be felt a firm mass extending transversely across the abdomen, while below, in the umbilical region, was a large cystic swelling dull on percussion and pulsating. The temperature and pulse were normal, no abnormal constituents were found in the urine, and the bowels acted regularly. The old wound was reopened and a cyst encountered at a depth of ½ inch from the surface, 24 oz. of the same red-brown fluid being liberated. Again the cyst was drained and irrigated daily ; the discharge was abundant but inoffensive. Convalescence was uninterrupted, and when the patient left the hospital the sinus had almost closed.

A.A.   G

When first seen in consultation the resemblance of the cyst to an aneurysm of the abdominal aorta was very close. The stomach appeared to be displaced downwards and the cyst came forward to the abdominal wall, to which it appeared closely applied.

Injuries to the spleen are more common in those countries where malaria is prevalent. Small lacerations heal, and give rise to no symptoms other than such as may be accounted for by the presence of adhesions, but if infection occurs, as is more likely to happen in stab wounds, then an abscess may result. Trauma has long been held responsible for certain cysts of the spleen, and not without cause, since there is abundant evidence to support the contention.

In Fowler's series [1] there were no less than five cases of splenic cyst in which a definite injury had been received less than one year previously. Léjars mentions a case in which a woman was seized with severe pain in the epigastrium, with diarrhœa and vomiting, three years after an accident in which she was injured ; a cyst was found in the splenic region containing 1½ litres of fluid ; the wall of the cyst was rough and fibrinous and suggested a hæmatoma of long standing. Heurtaux also records the case of a woman, aged 27, who developed a splenic cyst eight years after an injury, and here again the cyst had evidently arisen by progressive enlargement of a hæmatoma.

While the majority of these cysts thus belong to the category of blood-cysts, the view is held by some that certain of the serous cysts may also be of traumatic origin by inclusion of peritoneum during the healing of splenic lacerations.

The Kidneys, Ureters, and Bladder.—Though the onset of symptoms of nephroptosis is sometimes attributed to injury, this factor cannot be held responsible for the condition. It is more than probable that in all such cases the condition has been latent, and has only been brought into prominence by the general functional disturbance and the possible medical examination following the injury. Injury is also said to play some part in the production of chronic nephritis, but here again sufficient evidence is lacking to prove the assertion. Stab wounds of the loin, if penetrating the kidney, often lead to urinary fistulæ, partly owing to the introduction of septic organisms from without and partly to the decomposition of extravasated urine. Urinary fistulæ may also result from stab

[1] "Annals of Surgery," 1913.

wounds of the ureters or bladder or from extraperitoneal rupture of the bladder with urinary extravasation ; or, again, they may follow operations for the exposure of ruptured kidneys. In all cases in which renal fistulæ fail to heal under treatment, nephrectomy is the only available course to pursue. Stab wounds of the ureters are rare, but contusions are less rare ; hence numberless examples of their sequelæ are on record, and in these, in nearly all cases, the ureter has undergone cicatrisation at the point of injury and hydronephrosis has resulted. While true hydronephrosis may be formed in this manner, the so-called " traumatic hydronephrosis " is formed quite differently ; this variety of cyst indeed is not a hydronephrosis at all, but a cyst of extravasation, an encapsulated collection of extravasated urine arising months, or even years, after an injury in which the kidney underwent partial rupture. In these cysts the kidney may sometimes be felt, of normal size and not apparently diseased. Examples may be quoted from the St. Thomas's Hospital Reports :—

A man was admitted having been run over on July 28, 1896. He sustained fractured ribs and abdominal injuries, the exact nature of which was not evident, but no signs of renal injury were observed. He was readmitted on September 3 with an enormous fluid swelling occupying the left side of the abdomen and extending beyond the middle line. The overlying skin was red, smooth, shining and tense. At operation $8\frac{1}{2}$ pints of urinous fluid were withdrawn ; the kidney and ureter appeared normal. The patient made a good recovery.

Another interesting case was that of a man, aged 24, who was admitted as an urgent case under the care of Dr. H. P. Hawkins on November 21, 1899. He stated that he first felt ill on the 18th, had pain in the left side, and was unable to go on duty. Next morning he was worse, had an attack of vomiting, and the pain was more severe. The abdomen was much enlarged, especially across the umbilical region ; there was no movement on respiration in the lower and very little in the upper part. On percussion an area of dulness was found all over, excepting for a small space in the upper part under the right costal margin. Over the whole of this area there was a fluid thrill, but the dulness did not change with alteration in the position of the patient. There was much tenderness on the right side. The general effect was that of a large flattened encysted collection of fluid, and it was not possible with this history to give an opinion as to its nature. After the operation, when he had recovered from the fever (103·6°) and upset of the acute condition, he remembered that he had been kicked in the abdomen some twelve years before ; the injury was severe, but he could not say anything about the condition of the urine at that time. On opening the peritoneum in this case, the same evening, a shining surface having the appearance of intestine presented itself. On exploration with the hand it was found that the collection of fluid was retroperitoneal, passed down into the pelvis, nearly into the right lumbar region, close to the kidney, whilst the spleen could not be felt. The small intestine was pushed to the right, and the descending colon crossed the swelling from above downwards near the middle line of the body under the median incision. A large quantity of brownish urinous fluid, slightly turbid, flowed away under considerable tension on insertion of trochar and canula. This opening was sutured and the median incision closed. Through a lumbar incision the full evacuation of cyst was completed, some solid fleshy material coming away with the last pint or two of the fluid. Over 8 pints were removed. The wall of the cavity was thin and everywhere adherent, so that no attempt was made to remove it. A large drainage tube was inserted. The fluid contained urea and a little pus, but no crystals. The kidney was not felt. The sinus did not close for some weeks after he left the hospital, but he quite recovered and resumed duty as a policeman.

In another case the course of events was much more rapid. A clerk, aged 24, was admitted on March 8 and left on April 9, 1901.

Five weeks before admission he slipped and fell on the pavement, striking his right side. This injury was followed by severe and continuous pain in the side struck and on the right side of the abdomen, which lasted for a fortnight. During this time he had vomited several times daily, usually soon after food. At the end of the fortnight he felt well and resumed work again. On the third day after going out the pains recurred and were much more severe for two days, and then disappeared. There had been no hæmaturia and he thought he was quite well, but a swelling had appeared in the side.

Nearly the whole of the right side of the abdomen (except the lower part) was dull on percussion, the dulness being continuous with that of the liver, and extending as far as the umbilicus towards the middle line. It did not change with alteration of the position of the patient.' There was well-marked fluctuation in this area. The left side was normal, but over the lower part, near the groin, there was a little superficial swelling, and the upper and inner part of the left thigh was also swollen and very painful on pressure. The urine was strongly alkaline, but in other respects there was nothing abnormal found on examination. On March 9 a lumbar incision was made and the cyst emptied of about 4 pints of urinous fluid. On the posterior surface of the kidney a depression or pit just admitting the tip of the finger could be felt. This was regarded as the site of a recent rupture. Drainage was employed and the man recovered.

If the history of a renal injury is suppressed by the patient, as it was in another case, the collection of fluid may be mistaken for an ovarian cyst.

An unmarried woman, aged 34, was admitted on October 19, 1900. She had been treated in another hospital for the results of a cycling accident in April, during which she had been run over by a van.   In September she had been under my care for malposition of fragments at the site of a fracture of the leg.   She was under care then for three weeks and noticed a swelling in the abdomen, but, not wishing to be detained, did not say anything about it.   She could not say if her kidney had been injured in April, but she remembered that about a week afterwards she had a (vague) sort of pain on the right side, and a little later noticed a swelling there, which did not change for a long time.   This cyst was opened and drained through the loin.   It contained almost 3 pints of dark-brown fluid.   The kidney occupied a place on the anterior wall of the cyst, which was partly lined with fibrous material.   She was under treatment for about three months before the sinus closed.

These cases show the necessity for occasional examinations after contusions of the kidney region, although no sign of actual rupture of the kidney has been found.   I remember a man in whom, after a ruptured kidney indicated by the usual signs, no tumour could be found three weeks afterwards, at the time of discharge, but a fortnight later he was admitted to another hospital for a cyst which required operation.

PART II

PERITONITIS, PERFORATIONS, AND OTHER LESS COMMON CAUSES OF THE ACUTE ABDOMEN

PERITONITIS.

THE acute inflammation of the peritoneum which so frequently forms a part of the acute abdomen varies greatly according to the cause on which it depends, the rapidity of its spread, and the part where it has its origin. It also varies according to the number and virulence of the particular organisms which have found their way into it, the power of absorption of the peritoneum, and the resistance of the individual.

In this section it is not necessary to dwell very much upon the symptoms of an inflammation which has to be considered in almost every part of our subject, whether it follows an injury, intestinal perforation, appendix perforation (Fig. 9), intestinal obstruction, or invasion from some ascertained external source such as that by the Fallopian tubes. Here I only wish to mention the general symptoms which are met with in peritonitis and refer to those varieties in which no gross cause can be found, but in which there is an acute bacterial invasion by some organism which has probably obtained entrance through the blood-stream.

The patient complains of pain in the abdomen, mostly in the umbilical region, becomes feverish, complains of chilliness, and probably vomits. The temperature rises and the pulse increases in frequency. The position soon assumed by the patient who has gone to bed, feeling very ill, is a very characteristic one, for he lies on his back with arms thrown above the head and the thighs flexed on the abdomen. When examined a few hours afterwards there is much tenderness sometimes amounting to hyperæsthesia, especially when there is an inflammation which is extending. The complaint of pain may be less insistent, whilst its past severity is often indicated by the amount of redness, and even vesication of the skin which has resulted from the applications which have been made. The respiratory movements of the abdomen are limited or almost arrested, and there is still occasional vomiting. There is also rigidity of the abdominal muscles ; this may be localised at first, but may become general. The face is flushed, there is a furred tongue, and usually constipation. Percussion may yield here little information until there is some exudation of fluid or of lymph. In the former instance it may be free in the peritoneal cavity and vary with the patient's position, or it may be patchy or localised to one spot, as in the latter. The patient will often be restless, and call out or groan when the paroxysms of pain become severe.

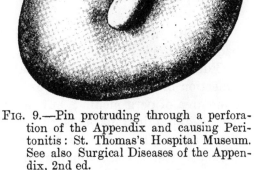

Fig. 9.—Pin protruding through a perforation of the Appendix and causing Peritonitis : St. Thomas's Hospital Museum. See also Surgical Diseases of the Appendix, 2nd ed.

Later the expression of his face changes, he is listless, dark lines appear below the eyes, which appear to have sunken, whilst the cheeks are hollow. The lips become dry, and the tongue dry, brown and coated. The breath is offensive. Effortless vomiting continues and is now copious, whilst the ejected fluid becomes brown-coloured, bad smelling, and even feculent. Examination of the abdomen shows an amount of distension which is apparently increasing, and the wall of the abdomen is moving less than ever. There is, however, no peristalsis to be seen, and the surface looks smooth ; palpation is painful and much resented by the patient. It is still rigid, mostly resonant, but in the flanks there may be dulness which can sometimes be traced across the middle line above the pubes ; if this is so, a fluid thrill may be elicited. The temperature is raised, not necessarily very high, but it may be normal, or subnormal, even when the inflammation is of the most severe type, with a general diffusion of pus. Such a low temperature with a rapid pulse is of very serious import. The constipation is probably relieved by an enema, and the patient passes flatus without any difficulty until the distension of the intestine is due to paralysis of the bowel wall caused by the general poisoning which has supervened.

It is always of bad import in a case of peritonitis to find that the patient has lost all pain, and has commenced to hiccough. With these symptoms there may be a clearness of intellect which disguises the real state of the man from his friends, whilst the frequent pulse becoming almost or quite imperceptible warns the medical attendant that the clammy, moist hand which he took on entering the room was indeed a true witness of the patient's state as already indicated by the nurse in charge.

A return of the restlessness and sighing respiration are also bad symptoms.

Œdema of the abdominal wall may indicate a localised collection of pus or an extravasation of fæces into the underlying area of peritoneum ; but there is another form of œdema of the abdominal parietes to which I drew attention some years ago. This may be seen when the general peritonitis is very acute. It accompanies an inflammation of the cellular tissue, and is caused by an exudation which has passed into the subperitoneal cellular tissue and come out along the inguinal canals ; it may spread into the scrotum, and laterally towards the anterior superior spines, but not into the thighs beyond the attachment of the deeper layer of the superficial fascia.

It may be stated at once that a localised inflammation of the peritoneum is not always a dangerous thing, and few abdominal operations which are carried out under the most perfect aseptic conditions are without a limited peritoneal reaction which amounts to an inflammation. In the same

manner all cases of inflammation of the appendix are accompanied by some peritonitis which is a result of the relation
which that organ bears to the general peritoneum.

Most attacks of peritonitis can be traced to some form of
organism or to some definite lesion, but it is not always so ;
there are some cases in which no organism is discovered on
examination by the bacteriologist and no gross lesion found
when the abdomen has been carefully searched. Here the
symptoms may be so severe and threatening that operation
is performed, and rightly so ; it is unlikely that a fluid inflammatory exudate would remain sterile for many hours. Operation
may save the life of the patient, and should not be delayed.

N. R., a married woman aged 24, was admitted ✕ March 22 and
left April 11, 1912.

She stated that she had not been feeling well for a month ; there had
been vomiting at intervals, with a slight aching pain in the abdomen.
For a fortnight there had been intermitting pains and diarrhœa and
occasional vomiting. Two days before she had suffered from pain in
the lower part of the back, which in the afternoon had extended all over
the abdomen, and was chiefly in the middle and right side. It was also
tender. Vomiting had been fairly constant for twelve hours.

On admission she had a somewhat distended, rigid abdomen, with
tenderness mostly to the right of the umbilicus—generally resonant on
percussion. Pulse, 104 ; temperature, 101·4°. An incision was made
over the right rectus and the muscle displaced inwards. There was a
quantity of brown-stained fluid in the pelvis and below the incision,
which was not offensive. The peritoneal surfaces of some of the coils
of the small intestine had a good deal of lymph on them. There was
nothing abnormal found to account for the fluid. A drainage tube was
inserted into the pelvis and removed on the fifth day as there was no
discharge. The temperature was normal then and no further rise took
place. She recovered completely. Dr. Dudgeon reported the fluid to
be sterile.

In another case there was no exudation of fluid in the
peritoneum, but the abdomen was opened and the operation
gave great relief.

J. G., a coachman aged 55, was admitted ✕ on July 12 and left on
August 2, 1911.

There was no history of any previous abdominal attack. Twenty
four hours before admission he was seized with violent pain in the
abdomen, which became generalised, not particularly acute in any one
region. There had been occasional retching but no vomiting. The
bowels had not acted for two days.

The face was flushed, features pinched, with an anxious expression.

Pulse, 100; respiration, 18; temperature, 99°. The abdomen was slightly and symmetrically distended, rigid, and acutely tender all over. The percussion note was tympanitic and examination gave no evidence of free fluid.

Incision in lower right half of abdomen showed a normal appendix; a second incision over the stomach revealed nothing abnormal. There was no free fluid. During his residence many examinations were made of the patient, but no cause for the attack was found. There was no continuation of the pain after operation.

The advantage of early operation was evidenced by the unsuccessful result of a similar line of treatment carried out for a patient, M., aged 55, on December 31, 1904. ✳ The abdomen was distended, with tenderness over the sigmoid. Temperature 98·8° (pulse 96). There was no fluid or cause found. The illness had commenced on December 27, the day after taking three pints of cider. Abdominal pain, constipation, and vomiting. The man, who was very ill, died next day. At the necropsy, beyond the peritonitis, which was purulent in the pelvis, nothing abnormal was found. Judging from the other cases an earlier operation might have saved him.

Of the varieties of peritonitis which result from an acute bacterial invasion through the blood-stream the following must be mentioned.

A. *Pneumococcal.*—This form of peritonitis is not frequent when compared with the peritonitis which follows gross lesions of the alimentary canal. As a rule it is not difficult to differentiate the two unless by any chance the signs of the infection are most marked in the right iliac fossa when the patient comes under observation for the first time. The patient is most frequently a child (Barling gives 73 per cent. girls), whose parents tell a history of some recent chest trouble. The child was apparently well when a complaint of pain in the stomach was made; vomiting followed, with fever and diarrhœa. There are found some of the usual signs of peritonitis already mentioned, and the child looks flushed and ill. Distension of the abdomen is often present with general stiffness and resistance of the muscles, and this may be associated with dulness in the flanks.

Operative interference is indicated, and the appendix examined in the first place. A perforation should also be sought for in the adult, in the stomach or duodenum. The best incision will be one through the right rectus sheath with outward displacement of the lower part of the muscle. The exudation, which is abundant, should be removed with gauze strips and soft sponges, and a good-sized drainage tube placed in the lower part of the wound to the bottom of Douglas's pouch. The child must be placed in the Fowler position and saline fluid given *per rectum.*

In this, as in all forms of peritonitis, it is well to obtain a culture from the fluid (odourless in pneumococcic cases) which is present, so that a vaccine may be prepared for future use.

There may be signs of pneumonia present, and herpes of the lips. Barling divides this type of inflammation of the peritoneum into three clinical types :—(1) Acute cases presenting marked abdominal features from the first, but with no other pneumococcal lesions elsewhere. (2) Cases in which, simultaneously, or almost so, with the onset of peritonitis, a pneumonia develops. (3) Chronic septicæmic cases.

It is only right to add that Dr. Hector Cameron is against operation excepting in cases of residual abscess. I can but think, however, that in the majority it would be wisest to drain and so get rid of one source of the toxæmia which is the great danger to life. A case which was under the care of my colleague Mr. Betham Robinson[1] gives an excellent clinical picture of primary pneumococcic peritonitis and shows the value of vaccine treatment, combined with operation.

D. W., aged 8, was admitted on April 22, 1908, under the care of Dr. Sharkey.

She had always been a nervous child, subject to bilious attacks. Three years before she had measles, and two years before influenza with symptoms very similar to those of the present illness, abdominal pain, and vomiting.

On the day before admission she seemingly had been in perfect health. At 8.30 a.m. on the 22nd she was suddenly taken ill with free vomiting, faintness, and slight abdominal pain centred round the umbilicus ; she was very thirsty and feverish. Fifteen hours after the onset, she was admitted looking ill and complaining of severe abdominal pain and vomiting. The face was very flushed, the eyes bright but not sunken, and the tongue furred generally but rather dry at the tip. The pulse was 130, regular and of small volume ; temperature, 103·8° ; and respirations 36. The chest moved well and equally, and there were no abnormal physical signs detected in heart or lungs. Abdominal movement was restricted below the umbilicus ; there was definite distension, but it was everywhere resonant. Palpation proved an almost universal tenderness, more marked round the umbilicus and in the right lower quadrant ; here there was some increased resistance, but no distinct lump could be felt.   *Per rectum* there was a boggy feeling, especially on the right side, as if there was something in Douglas's pouch.

Mr. Robinson saw the child at 11 next morning, her pulse then being 150 and temperature 103·4°.   The abdomen moved fairly well on respiration except on the right side below ; here and across the bladder region she was tender.   There was a little rigidity over the right rectus both below and above the umbilicus.   An immediate operation was decided on, as her condition suggested a perforative peritonitis dependent probably on a gangrenous appendix.

Operation.—The right rectus was displaced inwards.   On opening the peritoneum a greenish-yellow fluid escaped, of gummy consistency, with a few flakes of dirty-white lymph in it.   Although this was generally diffused through the cavity, and the intestines and omentum were smeared over with it, yet they did not otherwise appear to be in any way altered from the normal ; the appendix was absolutely healthy.   A good deal of fluid had collected in the pelvis and in the right kidney pouch.   There was no sign anywhere of glueing together of the intestinal coils by early adhesions.   The right Fallopian tube was very definitely injected.   (Subsequent inquiry elicited no evidence, past or present, of any vulval or vaginal discharge.)   The glands along the iliac vessels and at the bifurcation of the aorta appeared to be a little enlarged.   The peritoneal fluid was quite odourless.   Drains with wicks were placed in the pelvis and in the kidney pouch, and the main part of the wound was closed in layers.   She stood the operation very well, and was put back to bed in the Fowler position and given $\frac{1}{10}$ grain of morphine.   Saline was ordered *per rectum.*

After the operation there was a gentle drop in the temperature to 99° at 8 o'clock the next morning, with a corresponding marked reduction in the pulse-rate.   She was feeling much more comfortable, and there had been very little pain and no vomiting.   She was given milk and water frequently in small quantities.   On April 25 her condition was very satisfactory, but both pulse and temperature had again risen a little.   As her bowels had not acted, she was put on magnesium sulphate in the evening.   The next morning there was a very slight result after an enema.   The wicks were removed from the tubes, and a considerable discharge of turbid fluid came away.   Calomel, 2 grains, given at night, followed by magnesium sulphate in the morning ; this resulted in four actions during the day.   On this day (April 27) the temperature again began to go up, and, as the clinical report showed that the peritoneal effusion was a pure culture of the pneumococcus, it was decided to use pneumococcic vaccine.   On May 5 both drainage tubes were removed and gauze drains substituted.   The discharge did not cease altogether.   On May 27 a counter-opening was made in the loin and a piece of gauze pulled through from front to back.   This soon had a marked effect both on the discharge and the temperature.   On June 6 the front wounds were healed, and on the 10th the drain was left out behind.   By this date her temperature had been normal for a week.   She was able to leave the hospital on June 15.

B. *Streptococcic.*—This is a very fatal variety of peritoneal inflammation, and is most commonly seen in cases of puerperal infection. There is little to be found in our literature which enables me to give an authoritative account of it ; most of the references are to cases which were treated with vaccine but in which the exact bacillus at work had not been proved by the usual tests. In a case of streptococcic peritonitis published by Dr. Horldidge, of Pinner, the entrance of the germ was by way of the appendix, and vaccine was most useful when complications arose during the progress of the case after operation. This bears out the experience of others in appendix cases, but the *Streptococcus pyogenes aureus* in the fluid surrounding an acute appendicitis always makes the prognosis grave. Whether a delay of a few hours in the examination of peritoneal fluid may give this germ a chance of killing off the active bacteria, and so appearing of greater importance than it really is entitled to, I cannot say.

The following is an example of recovery, treated on the lines advocated, and I do not think that there can be any doubt as to the exact nature of the germ which caused the peritonitis.

A married woman, aged 60, was admitted ✶ on April 21 and left on June 30, 1911.

On the morning of April 15 she woke up at 4 o'clock feeling very ill. She had great pain and felt that a cord was being drawn in around her body. She had diarrhœa all day, but was not sick. The two following days she was better and was able to do a little work in the house, but on the 19th she was not so well and went to see a doctor. She was in great pain, but did not suffer from diarrhœa. She was advised to come to the hospital.

On examination the patient was lying on her back with her knees drawn up, in very great distress. Face pale and anxious, features pinched. Tongue furred and dry. Pulse, 108, poor volume and tension ; respiration, 28 ; temperature, 102·8°.

The abdomen moved very badly all over and was noticeably distended, with general rigidity of muscles. Tenderness was present all over, especially at a spot under the right rectus, just above the level of the umbilicus. The note was tympanitic in the umbilical region, but there was shifting dulness in the flanks. Liver dulness normal. Pelvic organs appeared quite normal.

↳ The same afternoon operation was performed, an incision being made through the right rectus, the upper part reaching the area of greatest tenderness. On opening the peritoneum a quantity of clear fluid escaped, and a great deal more was found in the pelvis extending also into the left flank. Scattered about on the surface of the peritoneum were flakes of yellow lymph. The appendix was removed, although examination showed it to be apparently normal. Nothing abnormal was found in any part of the abdomen beyond this fluid, etc. Two good-sized drainage tubes were placed in the abdomen, one being passed upwards under the liver, the other into the pelvis. The wound was closed in layers as far as the tubes. A bacteriological report on the fluid removed and examined in the clinical laboratory was " Streptococcus."

Some discharge continued from the drainage tubes, and later from the wound until about May 11, there being gradual general improvement. About this date an abscess was found in the right buttock which was aspirated, the aspiration being repeated more than once ; ultimately it was incised. For a long time this discharged, the active germ being reported as the *Streptococcus pyogenes*. A vaccine was made and used :

May 16 : 11,575,000 cocci.		June 2 : 23,000,000 cocci.	
19 : 10,000,000 ,,	$\frac{1}{3}$ c.c.	6 : 23,000,000 ,,	1 c.c.
23 : 15,400,000 ,,	$\frac{2}{3}$ c.c.	12 : 23,000,000 ,,	,,

There was nothing special to report on the case beyond continuation of fever about 101—102° at night until the middle of June and the fact that the abdominal wound was very slow in healing, so much so that it was again sutured in the lower part on June 12.

A more general infection of the blood of which the peritonitis formed only a part, but was very severe, was the case of a lady, aged 50, seen with Dr. A. E. Godfrey on May 7, 1913.

She visited Dr. Godfrey on May 3, complaining of pain about the right shoulder and general feeling of illness. She thought she had caught cold. He sent her to bed, and on his visit next day found the temperature raised, and a complaint of some pain in the left side of the abdomen. In the afternoon she had a rigor. Temperature, 105°. There was no vomiting, and examination *per rectum* showed nothing abnormal. On May 6 she had increased and general abdominal pain and another rigor. On the 7th, at 11 a.m., she was looking very ill. Pulse, 130 ; respiration quick. Tongue dry and furred. She complained of some pain in the left side. The abdomen was somewhat distended ; generally resonant ; very tender, and the muscles hard set. The liver dulness normal.

At 2 p.m. there was some friction in the left chest. Dr. Z. Mennell gave anæsthetic and Dr. Godfrey assisted ; the right rectus was displaced outwards. A quantity of odourless pus, generally diffused, looking like mucopus, escaped. Nothing was found to account for it, the internal organs being generally normal. Dr. Dudgeon reported that the bacillus present was the *Streptococcus pyogenes*, and anti-streptococcic serum was given next day, but produced no influence on the progress of the disease. At 6 p.m. of the 8th she was worse generally, with evidence of spreading inflammation in the left lung. The face was pinched, pulse very rapid ; temperature still high, but no abdominal pain and no return of shivering. She died four hours later.

In a third case which had been sent to a fever hospital as a case of typhoid a child of 12 years of age was very ill on transfer. Here the appendix appears to have been first affected.

She came ten days after the commencement of symptoms, during which time she had been under treatment, with fever and some abdominal pain, etc. On admission, April 20, 1905, she was very ill with general peritonitis. Pulse, 140 ; temperature, 103°. Operation was performed and appendix removed, although it appeared normal ; there was pus and lymph all over the peritoneum. *Streptococcus pyogenes* was found, in pure culture, on the appendix and peritoneum near it. The wall of the appendix was acutely inflamed, and no mucous coat remained. She died from exhaustion next day. There were sheets of very recent lymph on the pleura—like those in the abdomen; lungs congested. Evidence of a general infection.

It is well therefore to remove the appendix in these cases, as the source of infection may be in it, but give no proof except on microscopical examination.

C. *Tuberculous Peritonitis.*—The ordinary forms of tuberculous peritonitis do not demand a consideration from us in discussing the acute abdomen in the same manner as do the forms of peritonitis which are due to other organisms. The manifestations for which the surgeon is called in are, with the exception of local suppuration, included under other headings.

(A) There may be obstruction of the bowels, following adhesion of a coil of the bowel to another coil, to the omentum or to the abdominal wall.

(B) Perforation of a tuberculous ulcer (see p. 186).

(C) The formation of strictures of the bowel. In a case under care in 1913, in which the cæcum was excised for hyperplastic tuberculosis, there were no fewer than eight strictures found in various parts of the small intestine which produced no symptoms.

The peritoneum when tubercle is present may, in cases associated with abdominal pain and irregularity of the bowels, give rise to a suspicion of chronic intussusception from the presence of one or more tender swellings. In the neighbourhood of the transverse colon the rolled-up peritoneum may be somewhat sausage-shaped.

Tuberculous glands in the mesentery may not only cause trouble by producing adhesion of a neighbouring coil of bowel, but when suppuration extends beyond the capsule of the gland a localised peritoneal abscess forms, and a fatal peritonitis may ensue if the pus is not satisfactorily limited by adhesions. These glands in the iliac fossa may be mistaken for an enlarged and inflamed appendix, and the possibility of an attack of acute appendicitis must be remembered where tuberculosis of the peritoneum is present already.

An example of the complicated abscess of tuberculous peritonitis is furnished by the case of A. U., aged 16, who was under care from February 12 to March 2, 1910.

There was a tuberculous family history and she had been under treatment for "something wrong with the left lung," during which time she had had a feverish cold. Three days before she came in there had been a sudden pain in the lower abdomen, and she was very ill on admission with a pulse of 132 and temperature 102°. There was suppuration in the lower abdomen not distinctly defined, and a fulness on the right side of the rectum. At the operation the intestines were found irregularly matted together, and there were intermittent spurts of gas and offensive purulent fluid from the deeper parts of the wound, showing undoubted perforation of the bowel wall. Whether this resulted from ulceration or giving way of the bowel during examination it is not possible to say. More searching exploration was not considered advisable. A tube was inserted, and for some days there was a feculent discharge, but it gradually diminished and the wound closed satisfactorily. When she was discharged we could find no evidence of tubercle anywhere.

THE INFLUENCE OF DISEASES OF THE APPENDIX VERMIFORMIS ON THE PRODUCTION OF THE ACUTE ABDOMEN.

It is difficult to exaggerate the importance of this part of our subject, the cases which come under this heading presenting the largest of all the groups which are met with in practice. It is of the greatest importance, therefore, that you should have a good working knowledge of it from a clinical standpoint (Fig. 10).

In the year 1881 we find few records in the St. Thomas's Hospital Reports of diseases of the appendix ; five cases of peri-typhlitis were under care and one case of general peritonitis. What are the recent records, not of all diseases of the appendix, but of the acute inflammations of that small part of the alimentary tract ? Mr. Rouquette, the Surgical Registrar, has given me a summary of the cases under treatment in our wards from 1903–12 inclusive.

These are as follows :—

	No. of Cases.	Recovered.		Died.	
		M.	F.	M.	F.
1903—1907 . . .	472	208	128	102	34 .
1908—1912 . . .	1052	546	353	98	55
Total (1903—1912) .	1524	754	481	200	89

This shows that of these cases 62·6 per cent. were males and 37·3 per cent. females, whilst the mortality rate was less during the second half of the term—1903–7, 28·8 per cent. ; 1908–12, 14·5 per cent. The percentage of deaths was always higher in the males, but in the second half of the period taken it was less than half that during the first five years, having fallen from 32·9 per cent. to 15·2 per cent. This may be rightly ascribed to the fact that the importance of early operation has become more generally recognised both within and without the hospital. These few figures from one hospital out of many will convince you of the need for special study of this branch of the subject, and no excuse is necessary for treating it somewhat fully. You cannot give t$_{oo}$ much attention to the investigation of the manifestations of acute appendicitis, for it will meet you at every turn of your professional career

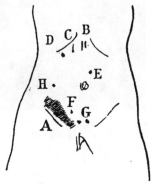

Fig. 10.—Diagram to illustrate by Shading the relative Proportions of various Perforations of the Hollow Viscera : A. Appendix. B. Gastric. C. Duodenal. D. Biliary. E. Jejunal. F. Typhoid. G. Tubal. H. Stercóral.

unless some discovery is made which will make it less prevalent.

As students you cannot spend too much time in the wards ; more than that, you cannot examine too many of these acute cases. Do not be satisfied that what you are told by the physician or surgeon in charge is all that can be learnt of the case. Examine for yourselves, and try to draw a conclusion, before the abdomen is opened, as to the nature of the lesion present.

You must endeavour to decide, firstly, whether the case is one of acute appendicitis ; and secondly, if it is, what is the condition of the peritoneum. You must also endeavour to estimate its effect on the individual, for these cases do not die simply as a result of the inflammation—they die from the toxæmia. Some of the apparently mild ones are very insidious in their progress, and the toxins developed produce their fatal effects rather suddenly and unexpectedly, in spite of operation, if deferred too long. You should all be able to recognise a case of acute inflammation of the appendix, although you cannot always say what is the exact lesion of the appendix on which the symptoms depend.

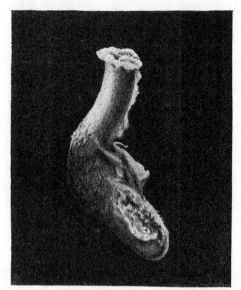

FIG. 11.—Appendix (half size) showing localised Gangrene with Perforation secondary to a Fæcal Concretion from a Child of 3½ years, with General Peritonitis, first attack (from " Surgical Diseases of the Appendix Vermiformis," 2nd ed.).

In the early stages of a serious injury, acute invasion, or marked lesion involving the peritoneum, there will be a combination of symptoms to which the term " peritonism " has been applied. The patient will suffer from local pain, vomiting and shock. There is then most usually an interval of varying duration, when the resources of the individual are being drawn upon to enable him to rally from the shock, repair the lesion, and fight the invading bacterial horde. Probably a peritonitis will immediately commence, and other symptoms be superadded as the inflammation extends and the toxins produced by the invading bacteria become to a certain extent absorbed.

To the state which accompanies such symptoms the designation " Acute Abdomen " has been applied, and the intensity of the symptoms will vary very much in different circumstances when disease of the appendix is the primary cause of them (Fig. 11). It may be added that the nature of the lesion will also make a difference and the patient will react in a different manner according to whether he is old, middle-aged, or a child. Then again there will be a difference according to the position which the appendix occupies, whether it is pelvic, iliac, retro-cæcal, or lying to the outer side of the cæcum.

The amount of pain will vary ; it may be severe though transient, referred to the iliac fossa, unaccompanied by appreciable fever, or more than a temporary increase in the pulse-rate. There may be little tenderness, and that of short duration, yet at removal of the appendix the surface may be coated with recent lymph.

At other times the patient may call out with pain, having been awakened from sleep, and become quite collapsed, so that the administration of stimulants is necessary to bring him round ; this pain may continue for hours and then pass off quite suddenly.

The pain is described differently by patients : all agree that it is bad ; usually it is referred to the region of the umbilicus, and passes from that region to the right iliac fossa, where it becomes localised to the spot in which the individual appendix is lying. When it is in the pelvis the pain will be less clearly defined, but is said to be low down, and is often increased by pressure on the right lower rectus. Vomiting is usually present, coming on soon after the onset of the pain ; if it continues, the attack is probably of severe character. In many attacks of appendicitis there is no vomiting in the early stage, but there is almost always a feeling of sickness ; yet even in these cases operation is best.

To these symptoms there are added those of fever, a quickened pulse and respiration, with a raised temperature ; this is mostly about 101°—103°, but may be higher. The patient looks ill, has a furred tongue and foul breath, whilst the bowels are usually constipated ; in severe cases diarrhœa is

common. If the abdomen is examined, you find diminished
respiratory movements, chiefly in the lower part. It feels
stiff, even rigid, especially about the lower part of the right
rectus, which is doing its duty, that of guarding the inflamed
part from all injurious movements or pressure.

Tenderness may be widely spread, but is most easily elicited
on pressure over the iliac fossa, or, if the appendix is in the
pelvis, on rectal or vaginal examination. Frequency of
micturition and dysuria are present with the pelvic appendix.

It is very seldom that one can find any tumour in the iliac
fossa within twenty-four hours of the onset of the acute
attack ; the rectus muscle prevents even a distended appendix
of considerable size from being felt ; there is often a sensation
of fulness beyond the muscle, and from the rectum a tender
lump may often be demonstrated. When under an anæsthetic
an enlarged appendix may be felt in the iliac fossa at an early
stage. Some inflammations due to the appendix quickly
subside although they begin very alarmingly, whilst others
continue, and if untreated cause a spreading inflammation with
suppuration, which may extend throughout the whole peritoneum. Often the suppuration becomes localised. The
larger number, luckily, undergo resolution, the pain subsides,
the temperature falls, and convalescence begins at the end of
two or three days. As the rigidity of the muscles is diminished
a swelling is felt about the appendix, which indicates a localisation of the whole process, and the illness is for the time practically over. In a few days this swelling has quite disappeared.

Unless the medical man draws attention to this swelling it
is very probably not noticed by the patient, and when asked
in a later attack if there had ever previously been any swelling
the answer is given in the negative. Although the temperature
and pulse may be normal, the patient is not well until this
swelling has quite gone.

When the symptoms and local signs do not subside but
increase because the inflammation is spreading, the patient
often shows signs of increased suffering. He becomes anxious
looking, the pulse increases in rapidity, the respirations are
slightly more frequent than normal and more shallow, the
respiratory movements being chiefly costal. The tendency
in young people is to throw the arms above the head and keep

them there. The abdomen is more or less motionless, tender on palpation over a larger area, though mostly so in the appendix region ; slight percussion is also resented. Exudation around often gives a dull note in the appendix region and also in the right lumbar region. There is possibly evidence of free fluid, shifting dulness in the flanks, which later extends across above the pubes. Vomiting is almost invariably present, and after that of the onset has passed off a little becomes distressing. The tongue is usually furred, and the breath often foul ; the bowels are difficult to move, but sometimes an offensive diarrhœa is present. When it is a late symptom it is called " septic diarrhœa." There is always some disturbance of the alimentary canal. The urine is usually scanty and high coloured, at first normal ; later it may contain albumin, but rarely blood.

There are, however, hardly any two cases that are alike in the exact cause of the illness and in the power of resistance of the individual. So that in one patient the general symptoms are of the greatest importance, and must be relied upon as an indication for treatment, whereas in another the local signs indicate the dangerous nature of the illness.

You will naturally ask, " What are the signs and symptoms to be specially noted, after the onset of " peritonism," to which importance should be attached ? Make all your examinations in one routine manner ; in the first place look with attention at the patient's face, for you may learn much from it. The colour, in a case of acute abdominal disease, will vary very much, from that of a healthy person to the dusky flush of one whose respiration is embarrassed ; the expression, from a placid indifference to that of a man in mortal agony. Sunken eyes, with dark circles round them, a pinched face, and anxious expression, are very ominous. If the nostrils are working rapidly you may be sure that the heart is also going too fast, and there is very serious and advanced disease present.

The pulse-rate is a very important indication as to whether the case may be safely left, it is imperative to operate, or there is no hope. If some hours have elapsed since the commencement of the attack, and the pulse-rate is much too high, there is nothing to be gained by postponing an operation, it must be done. Every hour lost renders the success of it less probable. Any acute abdominal case with a pulse-rate of over 100 should be carefully watched ; if it continues to rise beyond this the patient requires surgical aid, although other symptoms may be improving. The temperament must be considered in estimating the significance of a quick pulse, for occasionally a patient may be unduly excited by the medical visit or be suffering from a neurosis.

The temperature is often most misleading ; there may be the most widely diffused septic peritonitis, with a normal or subnormal temperature. Usually, as I have said, there is a rise at first, but it should begin to fall within forty-eight hours. A low or subnormal temperature with a rapid pulse is a very bad combination.

Restlessness is an unfavourable symptom ; so, indeed, is a state of manifest indifference and apathy.

Look for the marks produced by recent applications for relief of pain. These will give you some idea of its severity. Examine the skin for signs of inflammation or œdema. Find out the character of the pain, its most marked seat, and if it has moved since the first onset. Gently palpate so as to learn the condition of the muscles as regards rigidity, general or local ; also the presence of any local swelling or undue resistance behind the muscles. Percuss the abdomen throughout, but with a light hand, paying special attention to the flanks and to the parts above the pubes. If there is any dull area, try if it is affected by moving the patient, as the presence of free fluid is a sign of importance. Define the liver dulness. Observe also the extent of distension of the intestines, the presence or otherwise of peristalsis, and whether this is local or general. If there appears to be some distension of the bowel, find out if this is recent or increasing in amount. A distended fixed abdomen without any sound on auscultation and obstinate constipation must cause great anxiety. It is a late and unfavourable sign in a bad case. It is hardly necessary to remind you of the importance of the previous history, especially as regards attacks of abdominal pain. You must learn from the friends the condition of the bowels, if there is constipation or diarrhœa, and endeavour to avoid worrying the patient with those questions which the friends or nurse are quite capable of answering. In most cases your duty is not completed until you have learnt the state of the pelvic contents, as proved by rectal or vaginal examination. In some instances you will find inflammatory swelling on the right side, and in others an abnormal amount of tenderness. The extent of these will vary much with the nature of the case and the duration of the illness.

The number of acute abdominal conditions which are secondary to 'disease of the appendix naturally makes us, in the first instance, consider " the acute abdomen " from the point of view of that part of the alimentary canal. The relative proportion of the various factors in the causation of acute abdominal diseases is shown in the. statistics of the cases under care in St. Thomas's Hospital during the three years 1900–2 inclusive. In all there were 456 cases, of which 168, or 37 per cent., caused by inflammation of the appendix, formed the largest class.

If to these we add the following table compiled for the years 1903–12 inclusive, we find this statement much emphasised :—

Appendicitis and its complications	1,787
Intestinal obstructions (other than intussusception)	296
Intussusception	165
Perforations of the stomach	116
,, ,, duodenum	64
Other perforations of alimentary canal	7
Acute peritonitis (other causes)	50
Acute cholecystitis	53
,, pancreatitis	14

The acute inflammations of the appendix are therefore nearly twice as many as all the others put together.

The great importance of the *rôle* which the appendix plays is clearly shown by this table. The first four of the groups in this list are the most important of the acute illnesses and require special attention. They are worth consideration, in the first place, from the question of age, for, given certain difficulties in diagnosis, the probabilities will be in favour of intussusception during the first ten years of life, acute disease of the appendix between the ages of 15 and 30, perforations of the alimentary tract from 15 to 40, and intestinal obstruction from the age of 30 upwards, with increasing frequency to a maximum between 50 and 60.

It may be conceded that some cases of acute appendix disease are rather difficult to appreciate in their early stages, whilst others are so severe that they can be called fulminating. The latter cry for operation ; the others do so also, but unless you are listening carefully the cry will be unheard. An indefinite pain with a history of indiscretion in diet may make the relatives regard the illness as an ordinary stomach ache, for which the treatment is in their opinion quite within their own competence.

I remember the case of a girl, aged 7½ years, who after repeated " bilious attacks " which had come on at long intervals complained of another attack, which was apparently similar in character, so far as the parents could tell. But she did not improve as they expected, and when her medical attendant was asked to see her he found a generalised peritonitis. An operation was performed as soon as possible, but the appendix was gangrenous, suppuration diffused through the pelvis and lower abdomen, and she died in less than a week from toxæmia with heart failure.

Instances of the danger of the domestic treatment of these " stomach aches " could be multiplied considerably, if necessary ; the following case is a good example :—

A boy, aged 6½ years, was admitted March 30 and left May 20, 1905. He first began to be unwell on March 27, about midday, and was sick on the 28th and 29th. He had some abdominal pain and constipation, but not very much pain. He was thought to have some stomach derangement and was given castor oil. Mr. E. T. Whitehead, who saw him on the morning of admission, thought seriously of his state, and when we saw the boy together about 12 o'clock he had diffuse peritonitis secondary to disease of the appendix. The state was as follows :—He was a pale lad, with light hair, lying in his bed partly turned to the right, and apparently quite comfortable. He did not look very ill, smiled when spoken to, and answered questions about his age, etc., quite readily. He drew a deep breath when requested to do so, and said that his chest did not hurt him ; he admitted that he had had some pain in the stomach. When requested to turn round on his face he did so easily and with a smile. The abdomen was somewhat distended, not rigid, but with greater resistance in the right iliac fossa than in other parts. In the right flank, running obliquely into the pelvis across the iliac fossa, was a well-marked area of dulness, evidently, from its shifting character, due to fluid. His tongue was moist and clean ; he had vomited the night before, but not that morning. The bowels were confined. He had slept naturally. The temperature was 99°, but his pulse was 140. At operation at 3 p.m. we found very offensive pus in the right flank and pelvis, quite unlimited by adhesions, and lymph on some of the coils of intestine, in the iliac fossa, and pelvis. The appendix was large, its walls were œdematous, there was a circular band of gangrene running round it about ¾ inch from its distal end, and in the mesenteric border of this part there was a perforation. On opening the appendix there was a concretion above and another below the gangrenous part.   The subsequent history was briefly as follows :—The bowels acted on the 31st after a turpentine enema, and improvement followed in the condition of the abdomen, but he suffered from vomiting. Until April 2 he was very ill, losing flesh and strength, with occasional vomiting of coffee-ground material.   His pulse had come down to 100 and his temperature was 98°, but he seemed to have "no rally."   On the 3rd this brown, offensive vomiting ceased at 3 a.m.   Later in the day five grains of calomel were given with good result, and he began to improve.   Making steady progress from this time, his condition no longer continued to be a source of anxiety to us.

It is the cases in which there is little pain that often give the greatest anxiety, a slow absorption of the poison goes on, and the patient appears to be now better, now not quite so well, and so the pendulum swings, until perhaps the return of vomiting with a rapid pulse shows that the illness is a very grave one.

Some years ago I saw a patient in one of our large public schools who was in this condition. A "stomach ache" had been treated for some days by the house-keeper with various domestic remedies which she considered appropriate. It was only towards the end of the week that the medical officer was told of the boy's illness, when he was transferred at once to the sanatorium. He had a diffused peritonitis with much fluid in the peritoneum. Permission to operate could not be obtained, and the patient died next day. This occurred in a school where the regulations are very strict and every boy is seen at once on complaint of illness being made.

A more common type of spreading inflammation of the peritoneum secondary to appendix disease is shown in the following account.   It also shows the effect of the toxins on the cardiac muscle :—

A schoolboy, aged 11 years, was admitted. ✗   His illness began four days before (January 21) during the night, with acute pain in the right side of the abdomen ; on the following day he was much worse.   He also felt sick, and vomited everything he took.   His bowels were constipated, and remained so until admission.   The vomiting and pain in the abdomen continued.   On admission he had a pinched, anxious-looking face, and complained of pain in the abdomen, chiefly in the lower part on the right side.   He was lying on his back, with his legs drawn up.   The abdomen did not move at all in the lower part, and there was only a slight movement in the epigastrium and upper part. On palpation, great tenderness was found all over the lower part, especially in the right iliac fossa.   The abdominal muscles were rigid, and a swelling was detected in the right iliac fossa, extending upwards from Poupart's ligament. This swelling could not be defined accurately owing to the muscular rigidity. On percussion, dulness was present over this swelling, and also in the left flank. The rest of the abdomen was resonant. The pulse was 100, the respirations were 20, and the temperature was 100·6°. This patient was restless, and protested vigorously against operation. When the abdomen was opened pus in considerable quantities was found free in the peritoneum. There was much deposit of lymph on the peritoneum covering the small gut, which was generally reddened ; in some places hæmorrhagic patches could be seen under this lymph. The purulent fluid filled the pelvis and extended into the right flank. The appendix was 3 inches long, thick and fleshy, with gangrenous mucosa. There was a concretion in the central part, and just below it a minute perforation, plastered externally with fibrinous lymph. The peritoneal cavity was washed out with warm saline solution ; a drainage tube was inserted, and also a gauze strip. After the operation the patient's sickness ceased ; his pulse gradually fell to normal, but was still 108 on February 8, fourteen days after operation. At first he was peevish and difficult to please, but left the hospital quite well on March 17.

You will perhaps be called upon to give your opinion in a case in which, for a time, there has been a very evident improvement and the friends of the patient naturally think the dangerous stage is passed and recovery assured. "He is so much better!" Here you must be guided by various considerations.

We may take as an example the case of a stout strong man, aged 35, who had suddenly improved about twelve hours after the commencement of symptoms. Dr. Yeld asked me to see him because he was not satisfied with the general condition. We found him (twenty-four hours) without pain, but with a pulse of 120. He protested very strongly against operation, and struck his abdomen violently with his closed fist to show how well he was and how free from pain. After much persuasion we convinced him of the need for operation, and found a perforated appendix with commencing suppurative peritonitis (spreading).

Another way in which acute symptoms arise is by the sudden rupture of an empyema of the appendix into the general cavity of the peritoneum.

F. B., a boy aged 11, was admitted under the care of Dr. Acland on September 29, 1909. It was stated that the patient awoke at 1 o'clock on the day of admission, complaining of severe general abdominal pain, worse in the right iliac fossa. There was no vomiting ; the bowels had been constipated for thirty-six hours previously. It was reported that the boy, who was said to have been always delicate, had been quite well on the previous day, and had eaten several apples. Although delicate he had had no previous illnesses, with the exception of an attack of abdominal pain four weeks prior to admission, which was unattended by sickness and localised itself in the right lower abdomen. On admission he was a thin, anæmic boy, with a six hours' history of abdominal pain. His pulse was 120, regular, of good volume and tension, Respiration, 20 ; temperature, 101°. The abdomen was poorly covered, and did not move well on respiration. On percussion the liver dulness was normal ; dulness was present in the right flank, which disappeared with change of position. Tenderness was general, but most marked in the right iliac fossa. At 10.30 a.m. when I saw him the pulse-rate was 132 ; temperature, 102° ; abdominal pain more acute. There was more dulness on the right side of the abdomen with some over the pubes, the amount of free fluid having increased. At this time the boy was pale, looked anxious and pinched. Operation was performed ten hours after the commencement of symptoms. An incision was made in the right side of the abdomen through the rectus muscle, the fibres of the muscle being separated with the handle of a scalpel. When the peritoneal cavity was opened much pus was found in the right iliac fossa and also in the pelvis. It was thick, yellow, and without offensive odour. A gauze strip was placed in the pelvis and another in the left flank through the abdominal wound, so as to absorb pus whilst the appendix was removed. Three rows of sutures were applied over the cæcal opening. The peritoneum in the region affected was dried by means of gauze strips, and the wound closed, with a rubber drainage tube passed through the lower angle into the pelvis. The greater quantity of pus was found in the right flank above the position of the appendix. Anti-bacillus coli serum (25 c.c.) was injected subcutaneously into the chest wall before the patient left the theatre. He was placed in a sitting position, and continuous instillation of warm saline fluid into the rectum commenced. The tube was taken out on the third morning and shortened, but its use was continued for ten days.

The appendix was unusually large, and presented a perforation towards the tip. When opened a stricture was found about the junction of the proximal two-thirds with the distal third, which completely closed the lumen of the tube at that point, forming in this way a cavity of the distal third, with which the perforation communicated, and from which pus was exuding when the appendix was found. The patient had had an empyema of the appendix, which had ruptured without warning into the general peritoneal cavity.

The diagnosis of the exact condition depended upon the extreme suddenness of the onset, the severity of the symptoms, and the large amount of fluid which was noted before the operation, although such a short time had elapsed since the commencement of the trouble. The history of a former attack of pain, as pointing to pre-existing disease of the appendix, was regarded as important.

You must not, however, be misled by a case in which a few hours after the onset of "peritonism" the patient appears to be better. Always suspect the acute attack which appears to have got well quickly ; a rapid improvement in general condition with entire loss of pain often means the giving way of an over-distended appendix. A lull is taking place before the septic fluid which has escaped from the appendix produces its effect on the peritoneum, but all the time absorption of poison is taking place, and the next stage is but a short prelude to a fatal ending.

I have seen a man of 32 in consultation who had a pulse of 80 ; respiration, 20 ; temperature, 98·6° ; the local signs but ill marked ; a rather rigid abdomen ; some tenderness on pressure over the right iliac fossa, but no distension. He had, however, a marked rigidity of the lower part of the right rectus. This was about eighteen hours after an attack of pain of a mild character, followed by a sudden severe abdominal pain six hours before, then the quiet period during which I saw him. A large appendix had perforated beyond a stricture, and there were four concretions in it. He had suffered from a previous attack, which had been diagnosed as appendicitis two years previously.

Almost all surgeons who have seen anything of the treatment of appendicitis recognise that to save life in the largest number of instances you must remove the appendix as soon as possible after the onset of symptoms. The public has not yet been educated to the need for this, but members of the profession recognise its great importance as a routine method of treatment.

Now that the acute " belly " cases are sent in at once to the surgical side, there will be less delay than there was when they had to pass through so many hands before they reached the operation theatre. I would endeavour to emphasise this question of time in the treatment—an hour saved may mean the removal of a distended appendix before the poisonous contents have escaped and fouled the peritoneum, not only in the cæcal region, but also in the pelvis, where there is such a large surface for absorption. There are undoubted records of recoveries from a general septic peritonitis, but they are not so numerous as published cases would have us believe. There is a difference between " diffused " and " general," which is, I am afraid, not always appreciated by those who write and talk about the disease. In many it is inadvisable to remove the patient to a surgical home ; an operation done on the spot may save weeks of illness and pain, especially if the journey involved would be a long and possibly shaky one. You can quite understand why the extra movement would be bad for a distended but still unruptured appendix, the wall of which is sometimes like moist tissue paper.

As a rule you can differentiate an acute appendix attack from other urgent affections of the abdominal contents. I will return to this subject later ; but this is the essential—to make up your mind whether the patient is suffering from a state which necessitates interference or not. If you are not certain and there is a reasonable probability that you are dealing with an appendix trouble, the wisest plan is to operate. Surgeons who see much of this disease can often tell you the exact state of the appendix on which the attack depends. This may be of great temporary importance, for the surroundings of the case may not lend themselves to the probability of a successful operation of any kind, especially one involving the peritoneum. Or again, there may be urgent private affairs to be settled before the risk of an operation is undergone.

Indefinite or subacute appendix symptoms coming on in patients of advanced years should excite the apprehension of any one under whose charge the patients may be. The signs of disease may be few, whilst the age and weakness of the patient make it inadvisable to do any operation excepting one of absolute necessity. Yet the most serious disease of the appendix may be present, and a fatal result inevitable, unless it is removed. Vague abdominal pains, with some rise of temperature and perhaps a little sickness, may be the only complaint ; perhaps even the medical man is not sent for until there is superadded a flatulent distension of the abdomen and a running pulse. The following account will show the type to which I am alluding :—

On September 10, 1909, I saw a man, aged 73. During the night of the 7th he was awakened by pain in the abdomen, but did not vomit. The pain was not severe, but he took some castor oil. Next day, the 8th, he sent for his medical man, who found him with a temperature of 100° and symptoms of a mild attack of appendicitis. On the 9th he was much the same, but his temperature was slightly raised ; he had vomited on the previous evening, and his tongue was becoming dry. Nothing abnormal could be felt *per rectum*. His condition at 2.30 on the 10th, when we saw him together, was as follows :—He was a healthy-looking man, with a normal temperature, good appetite, and a pulse of 88 ; his chief complaint was want of food, and he did not like being kept in bed. The only symptoms of anything wrong were a very dry tongue and some sharp, indefinite, superficial tenderness about the abdomen on the left side. The walls of the abdomen moved well, there was no rigidity, no tumour, and no abnormal dulness. He had no sickness, and his bowels had acted well the day before. Operation was not advised, but later vomiting came on, he became much worse, and died after an operation on the 12th, at which I was not present. The appendix was gangrenous, and two concretions were found outside in the pus which had accumulated in the peritoneal cavity.

It will be noted that there was no swelling in the iliac fossa, whilst a sharp general superficial tenderness could be elicited, although he had no pain.

THE DIAGNOSIS OF APPENDICITIS.

The diseases which may be mistaken, especially in their onset, for acute appendicitis may be grouped as follows :—

A. *Thoracic*, having their origin above the diaphragm. Acute inflammations of the lower part of the pleura and of the lungs.

B. *Abdominal.*—These may be divided into groups :

1. Pelvic, the most prolific group of all, has its origin in the female generative organs : of these we may mention salpingitis ; pyo-salpinx ; extra-uterine gestation ; torsion of the pedicle of an ovarian cyst ; rupture of an ovarian cyst ; torsion of the pedicle of a subperitoneal fibroid, or acute necrosis of a uterine fibroid.

2. Upper abdominal.—Perforation of duodenal ulcer ; perforation of gastric ulcer ; acute pancreatitis ; acute cholecystitis and perforations of gall-bladder ; biliary cohc.

3. Mid, abdominal.—Calculous affections of the kidney and ureter ; movable kidney, producing Dietl's *crises*.

4. Intestinal obstructions.

5. Acute inflammations of the peritoneum from infection through the blood-stream.

6. Gastro-intestinal affections. — Enteritis and gastroenteritis ; mucous colitis ; intestinal perforations.

7. General diseases. — Typhoid fever ; "abdominal influenza" ; hysteria ; lead colic ; malaria ; the *crises* of tabes dorsalis ; angeio-neurotic œdema ; Henoch's purpura.

Malignant disease of the cæcum and ascending colon.

Some of these are extremely rare conditions, and it is only necessary to remember their occasional occurrence. Others only simulate appendicitis when the inflammation has produced a localised swelling which can be felt.   Moreover, in discussing the diagnosis of acute appendicitis, it must be recollected that the appendix may be placed as high as the liver, in the iliac fossa, or in the pelvis, whilst the pain is often referred to the umbilicus in the early stage, only passing to the iliac fossa later.

It would not be advisable to enter into a long discussion of this large group of diseases which simulate acute appendicitis, but we must say something about the most important from a practical point of view, although they are again considered when we reach the special sections devoted to them.

Acute Pneumonia.—There are few surgeons who have not been requested to perform laparotomy for abdominal symptoms in this disease, which have simulated the acute abdomen. The difficulty has mostly arisen on account of sudden pain in the upper abdomen with rigidity of the muscles, some vomiting, and fever, symptoms found when a perforation of a gastric or duodenal ulcer has occurred.   In young people before the age when gastric and intestinal perforations mostly occur, the resemblance to acute appendicitis may be very close indeed.

An instance mentioned by Adams and Cassidy [1] may be referred to in which there was not only a rigid abdominal wall, but the site of the greatest tenderness was over McBurney's point.

A careful examination of the chest should therefore be made in all cases when there is any likelihood of such condition being present, as indicated by the rapidity of the respiration in comparison with that of the pulse-rate, which is seldom more than 100.   The late Mr. Barnard [2] in his communication on this subject pointed out that direct thoracic signs are often almost entirely lacking for twenty-four hours or more.

He mentions one case in which there were such definite abdominal signs that the abdomen was opened, when the pleurisy was associated with fracture of the ribs due to a known injury.

The medical diseases which must be considered here as they will not be referred to later are as follows :—

[1] "Acute Abdominal Diseases," p. 555.
[2] "The Simulations of Acute Peritonitis by Pleuro-Pneumonic Diseases," *Lancet*, Vol. II., 1902.

1. *Typhoid Fever.*—The statistics collected by Kelly and Hurdon show, from various sources, that amongst 330 cases of perforation occurring in typhoid fever, this perforation was situated in the appendix in 30. They point out that (1) appendicitis may be purely accidental, that is to say, appendicitis and typhoid fever, both of which are common maladies, may by accident be found concurrently in the same individual, or a latent and chronic inflammation of the appendix may be roused into activity by typhoid fever. (2) An appendicitis of a mild or of a severe type may arise from a typhoid affection ot the lymph glands or from an ulcer situated in the appendix, and may even go on to perforation. (3) Appendicitis may follow typhoid fever, appearing within such a brief time after the subsidence of the fever as to suggest a causal relationship.

It is a well-established fact that a true typhoid affection of the glands of the appendix occurs which may proceed to ulceration—and symptoms in the right iliac fossa may induce the surgeon to perform an operation for the removal of the appendix in the early stage of typhoid before there are any definite symptoms of that disease, or indeed any possibility of diagnosing it correctly.

If there are, in addition to fever, the usual signs of appendicitis, iliac pain, tenderness and rigidity of muscles, it would be best to operate, for it is far better to remove the appendix by an operation, which should not in any way distress the patient at this stage, than it is to let him run unnecessary risk. Curschmann has described a condition occurring during typhoid which he has called " peri-, or para-typhlitis typhosa," in which a minute perforation is found in the cæcum, or between the cæcum and colon. In these perforations swellings are found which closely resemble those produced by appendix inflammation going on to the formation of abscess.

Occasionally a patient with a concealed abscess or a suppurative peritonitis due to a diseased appendix comes under observation with the diagnosis of typhoid. These are usually those cases in which the fever has been slight and the local symptoms somewhat indefinite ; probably the appendix has occupied the pelvic position, whilst the iliac fossa has been free from evident change. The result of absorption of septic products may produce a " typhoid state." Widal's test must be tried and a careful daily examination made in doubtful cases. Examination of the abdomen will usually disclose the presence of free fluid in the peritoneum, and a definite general-ised rigidity of muscle in the lower part, with tenderness, and a rapid, feeble pulse.

2. *Abdominal Influenza.*—In more than one instance in which I have been requested to see a patient there has been a history given of attacks of abdominal influenza. Of the manifestations of this disease Professor Osler writes :—

" The gastro-intestinal symptoms may be marked ; thus, with the initial fever, there may be nausea and vomiting. Diarrhœa is not uncommon ; indeed, the brunt of the entire process may fall upon the gastro-intestinal mucosa."

He does not mention influenza when speaking of the diagnosis of appendicitis.

During the prevalence of influenza a patient with a slight cold may complain of a severe pain in the abdomen, and vomit. There will not, however, be the muscular rigidity or localised tenderness of appendicitis. Others in the house may have similar attacks. They are sometimes alarming, but not usually prolonged, and are accompanied with a rise of temperature.

3. *Hysteria.*—This disease may simulate appendicitis, as most of us know, but it should not be possible to make a mistake.

A nurse once came to have her appendix removed ; she had not had an attack of appendicitis but had been nursing a boy who died from acute suppurative peritonitis, and she was determined to avoid any illness of that kind. After the operation she left London and went to the seaside for a change. When there she was seized with an acute " agonising " pain in the right lower abdomen. Operation was per-formed on the spot, and the right ovary and tube removed ; these had been normal at the first operation, and she could not tell me of any disease of the parts removed. Some months later I was summoned to the country to see her for severe abdominal pain, and found every preparation made for operation. The symptoms were not quite of the recognised type of hysteria, and some surprise was expressed when I refused to operate. She lived, however, and developed manifestations which convinced all of the nature of the acute attack. Had the appen-dix not been removed I think it would have been excised during one of the attacks of pain which she had later.

A.A.

Professor Osler [1] says :

" There is a well-known ' appendicular hypochrondriasis.' The worst cases of this class which I have seen have been in members of our profession, and I know of at least one instance in which a perfectly normal appendix was removed."

4. In *Lead Colic* the pain is general, paroxysmal and relieved by pressure. There may be vomiting without any rise of temperature. The occupation of the patient, the presence of a blue line on the gums, with other symptoms of lead poisoning, should prevent any mistake.

5. In the gastric crises of *Tabes Dorsalis* there may be severe pain in the epigastrium and vomiting, and the attack may last for some days. The attacks are variable and may be extremely severe. The loss of eye and knee reflexes with the history and presence of other symptoms should make the diagnosis clear. These attacks more frequently give rise to a mistake in the diagnosis of stomach perforations than in those of the appendix.

6. A malarial attack is very uncommon in this country, being rarely met with excepting in those who have lived in a foreign country or one of the colonies. Severe abdominal symptoms in the subjects of malaria may simulate appendicitis, and without operation and examination of the appendix it will perhaps be difficult to say with certainty at the first visit. If the symptoms mentioned above (local pain, tenderness, rigidity of muscle and fever) are kept in mind, there should not be very much difficulty.

THE RESEMBLANCE OF DISEASES ARISING IN OTHER ORGANS.

1. Of the pelvic causes of the acute abdomen which produce a resemblance to acute appendicitis, the majority are easily demonstrated on vaginal or rectal examination, the presence of a tumour being readily found. Sometimes a tumour rises out of the pelvis. Should a cyst of small size rupture, then the exact condition may be difficult to name, but vaginal examination should show a tender swelling on the right side if the appendix is pelvic and inflamed.

2. Of all the conditions which arise in the upper abdomen

[1] " Principles and Practice of Medicine," p. 440.

the one which causes most difficulty is the perforated duodenal ulcer, a large number of cases having had an incision made in the first place over the appendix. In this group the possible history of attacks of pain which have been in the upper part of the abdomen, perhaps with vomiting of blood and melæna, should be investigated. The subject will be more fully dealt with later (see p. 163).

. 3. A few words may be said here about the affections of the kidney which may produce difficulty in diagnosis from acute appendicitis :—(1) Renal colic, pain on the right side which shoots down to the iliac fossa, pubes, and even testis, producing vomiting and more or less collapse. The pain is very severe, can be traced to the right kidney, and there is increased frequency of micturition with hæmaturia. A calculus may be seen with the X-rays. (2) When a stone has been arrested at the entrance of the ureter it may cause a condition of pyonephrosis, which may simulate the retrocæcal abscess. (3) Sudden impaction in the right ureter lower down may give great alarm, but rarely reproduces the clinical picture of acute appendicitis which we have already given.

A case of calculus of the left kidney is worthy of reproduction, for it shows how very closely a cross transference of symptoms may resemble an attack of acute inflammation of the appendix (Fig. 12).

MULTIPLE CALCULI IN THE LEFT KIDNEY PRODUCING SYMPTOMS RESEMBLING THOSE OF ACUTE APPENDICITIS. NEPHRECTOMY.—A female patient, aged 30, was seen with Dr. A. E. Godfrey on June 12, 1912. She was suffering from an acute abdominal illness and gave the following history. About four years previously she had a similar attack with pain in the abdomen, and was ill for fifteen weeks. Two years ago she had a repetition of the symptoms, and suffered off and on for a year. She was under the care of a medical man, who advised her to have the appendix removed. On the 7th of June she became ill again with pain in the right lower abdomen and vomiting. The pain continued, and two days later she vomited again. Dr. Godfrey saw her on June 10. On the 12th she was complaining of pain in the same part of the abdomen, with resistance to pressure and tenderness. The temperature was 102°, and the pulse rapid. On this date there was still a temperature varying from 100° to 102°. She looked ill, had a furred tongue, with offensive breath, and pulse 100. The abdomen did not move well, and she complained of pain which was limited to the right lower part, where there was tenderness and rigidity of muscle. Nothing abnormal was found on examination, beyond this, and rectal examination was negative. The bowels were constipated. In a day or two the symptoms subsided, but returned with severity, so she was sent into hospital on the 19th.

The abdomen was then very tender all over, but not rigid. Nothing abnormal could be found. Temperature, 100·6°. Pulse 120. Tongue still furred and breath foul. Sp. gr. of urine, 1012. Acid, heavy deposit of urates, no albumin. The appendix was removed, it was normal. Examination of right kidney, ovaries and tubes showed them to be healthy, the uterus was retroverted. After the operation she vomited a good deal, almost continuously for two days, but the temperature came down to normal. The Widal test for typhoid was negative. On the 26th she was examined very carefully by the resident assistant physician, who found no evidence of disease of the chest. The vomiting which continued appeared to be functional, whilst the temperature, which was still irregularly high, might have been due to a sore throat of which she was complaining. She was removed to a small ward in charge of special nurses. July 5, the patient had ceased to vomit. General condition improving. Had been complaining of pain in her right loin for a few days, and there was a trace of albumin in the urine, with some pus cells. She continued to complain of pain in the right loin, so on July 17 she was sent to the X-ray department to have the right kidney examined. The report was returned : " There are six shadows in the left kidney region. The right kidney is normal."

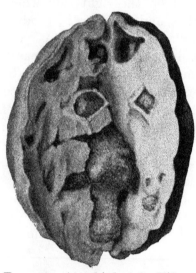

FIG. 12.—Atrophied left Kidney containing Calculi, which produced symptoms resembling those of Acute Appendicitis.

This examination was confirmed six days later. She was still complaining of pain in the right side of the abdomen. The sp. gr. of urine, 1015, pus being present with blood corpuscles in large quantities, and also epithelial casts. On July 24 the left kidney was excised. It was full of stones, and there was very little secreting tissue left. Its appearance when cut open is well shown in the illustration (Fig. 12). It only measured about 2½ inches in length, the surface was somewhat irregular, but smooth, and the capsule non-adherent. The largest stone was lying in the renal pelvis and practically filled it. The smaller stones were scattered throughout the substance of the organ. At the upper end there was a small cystic space containing a rounded stone. After the operation she improved quickly, but even on August 3 she still complained of occasional pain in the right side. She left on August 15.

In October she complained of pain along the course of the left ureter, and had some fever and sickness. There was tenderness over the ureter. Nothing abnormal was shown on examination by the X-rays, and the symptoms subsided.

In his interesting address (on reflex pains in diseases of the abdominal viscera), Mr. A. E. Maylard refers to the occasional transference of pain in renal calculus to the opposite kidney, an occurrence well recognised for years (Fig. 13). In this case there was not only a transference of pain, but a state of pyrexia, probably due to a temporary blocking of the renal pelvis, which for a time prevented the escape of pus into the urine. The diseased kidney was too small to be felt. When seen at our first consultation, had the case been one of appendicitis, there should have been evidence of swelling either in the iliac fossa or in the pelvis. In the absence of this we did not feel justified in recommending operation.

Quite recently a female patient was sent into the

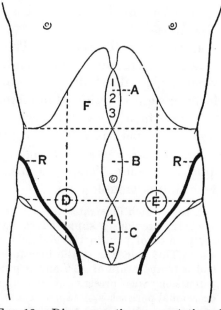

Fig. 13.—Diagrammatic representation of Seats of Maximum Reflex Pain in Disease of Abdominal Viscera. A. Stomach and pancreas. B. Small intestine and vermiform appendix. C. Large intestine, rectum, uterus. D. Vermiform appendix, right ovary and tube. E. Vermiform appendix, both ovaries and tubes. F. Gall bladder, cystic and common ducts, and duodenum. R. Kidneys and ureters. 1. Gastric ulcer towards cardiac end. 2. Gastric ulcer midway between cardiac and pyloric ends. 3. Gastric ulcer at pyloric end. 4. Large intestine down to splenic flexure. 5. Large intestine from splenic flexure to anus. (After Maylard.)

hospital for acute appendicitis, in whom we found a very movable and painful right kidney. She had complained of severe pain in the right lower abdomen a short time before admission. There had also been a rise of temperature with sickness. The presence of the swelling, which was very tender, had appeared to confirm the diagnosis, which was not rendered easier by the nervous apprehension of the patient. Here the extremely movable character, position, and shape of the swelling should have given the clue as to its nature, as well as its presence so soon after the beginning of symptoms. It is of common occurrence.

4. *Intestinal Obstruction.*—The sudden onset of pain in cases of acute obstruction due to bands, twists, internal herniæ, with vomiting, localised distension and visible peristalsis, without fever or signs of localised inflammation, usually make a clinical picture which does not very closely resemble appendicitis. Again, the pain is relieved by pressure, the muscles are not constantly in a state of rigidity, and distension somewhat quickly ensues. There is also complete constipation and vomiting is troublesome.

A case which illustrates this occasional difficulty was that of a boy, aged 12, previously supposed to have been quite healthy, who had complained of pain in the abdomen for two days, and had been very sick. This pain was in the iliac fossa, was increased by pressure ; he had a temperature of 99°, and a pulse of 130. A shifting dulness on percussion was present in the right flank. There was, however, occasional peristalsis, complete constipation, and an absence of rigidity of muscles. We found a loop of small intestine compressed by a well-developed band which passed from the inner side of the ascending colon to the mesentery of the small intestine near. It was attached to an old tuberculous gland which was one of a group. Strangulation had not been complete, and there was an abundance of clear fluid in the peritoneal cavity which had exuded from the obstructed loop. He' has grown into a healthy man and has had no further abdominal trouble.

When a patient is advanced in years, the temperature is little, if at all, elevated ; there is early distension and much sickness without anything that is definite on examination of the abdomen ; a state is present which requires surgical interference, unless it is evident that the patient is in a condition of collapse and cannot from the nature of the pulse bear the necessary manipulation. In these cases in the early stages the great iliac tenderness with some rigidity, and the rapid pulse, should supply the necessary warning. An extension of the area of tenderness (sharp superficial tenderness) is always a serious symptom, especially if there is no great complaint of pain.

In a paper recently published[1] I have described cases which prove that it is possible for a surgeon to give an accurate opinion as to the nature of the pathological process on which the symptoms of an acute attack depend.   It is not possible in every case.   Furthermore, I hold very strongly that the operator should endeavour to estimate the stage to which the disease has already advanced and its relationship to surrounding parts.   This knowledge can become of practical value only after a considerable experience of operative work in this branch, with a careful examination of the appendices removed.   It is not enough to say that the appendix was gangrenous, we must try to come to a conclusion in every case as to why it became gangrenous, and whether the gangrene was a general or local process.

The Treatment of Acute Inflammation of the Appendix.

The advantages of cutting short an illness presenting such dangers as pertain to an acute attack of appendicitis make the importance of immediate removal obvious.   The attack is arrested, divested of its greatest dangers, a possibly fatal result averted, and no weakness of the abdominal wall should follow.   Moreover, no further attack need be feared.   If we could stop an attack of typhoid fever by excision of part of the ileum I have no doubt the operation would be eagerly welcomed, yet a neglected attack of appendicitis is more dangerous and distressing than one of typhoid.

The operation which yields the most satisfactory result is that in which a temporary displacement of the rectus is done. The wound can be safely extended to any required distance, permits of thorough isolation of the parts affected, examination of the parts around which should be felt, and is not followed by any weakness of the abdominal wall.   This wound may be closed in the usual way without drainage, unless there is pus in the pelvis, the operation being a belated one.

It is performed as follows in the adult.[2]   An incision is made on the right side of the abdomen, midway between the

---

[1] *Lancet*, Vol. I., 1914, p. 1379.
[2] See Battle and Corner, "Surgical Diseases of the Appendix Vermiformis, etc."

umbilicus and anterior superior iliac spine, about 4 inches in length (Fig. 14). The inner lip of this incision is drawn towards the middle line, and the anterior sheath of the rectus muscle incised for the full length of the wound. The outer edge of the sheath is drawn towards the anterior superior iliac spine, by means of two pairs of artery forceps which are left on for the operation. With the knife the fascial attach-ments of the muscle to the sheath are divided, and the muscle drawn in-wards. If there is one of the lineæ transversæ in the part of the muscle to be displaced, it must be cut where it joins the sheath, and a small artery will usually require to be caught at this point. The deep epigastric artery is not usually seen, being drawn inwards with the muscle. Some branches of the twelfth intercostal may be seen, but division of them will do no harm. The posterior layer of the sheath, fascia trans-versalis, and subperi-toneal tissue, and peri-toneum are lifted up as

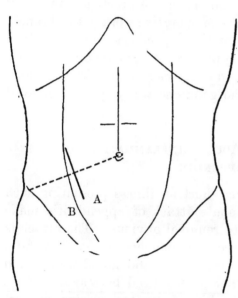

FIG. 14.—Incision for Appendicectomy by the method advised by Author. To illustrate the position of the skin incision with regard to the rectus muscle: A. Line of incision. B. Linea semilunaris.

one layer and divided vertically for the whole length of the wound. Nothing is much worse than an attempt to excise a sloughing appendix through a wound which is of inadequate size. Forceps should be placed on the edges of the peritoneum so that manipulation shall not displace it unnecessarily. Four-inch plugs should now be introduced, and if there is any free fluid the first should be passed into the pelvis and the second towards the kidney pouch. As this method opens the area to be dealt with to the inner side, you can fully protect the rest of the peritoneum by gauze packing before any search is made for the appendix, unless the mischief is already diffused. This is of importance, for frequently pus is found under the caput cæci when lifted, or escapes from an appendix as its separation is being effected, although every precaution may be taken by wrapping it in gauze as soon as possible. In every case care must be taken to secure the arteries in the meso-appendix, although in some instances of gangrene the vessels may be thrombosed. It is seldom possible in the acute cases to put a ligature on the meso-appendix to include the whole of it ; the thickening which has taken place as a result of the inflammation does not permit of this ; you must place forceps on the meso-appendix, beginning at its distal part and apply ligatures after the appendix has been cut away beyond. The separation of the appendix from the cæcum can be done with the clamp in the usual way, but not in every instance ; the coat-sleeve method is then employed, a ligature put on close to the cæcal origin, and the appendix divided between it and the thumb and fore-finger of the operator, which prevent the escape of any septic material as the division is made.

This ligature is then buried in the wall of the cæcum, and in cases where suppuration is present it is advisable to use three tiers of continuous Lembert sutures ; a single line of enclosing suture may give, and a fæcal fistula form. Where there has been no escape of pus from the appendix, the area from which the appendix has been removed should be cleansed with saline and any excess of fluid removed by the introduction of a plug into the bottom of the pelvis. Where there has evidently been a localised suppuration about the appendix, and it is thought possible to close the wound without drainage I have thought the application of peroxide of hydrogen (15 vols.) useful as a means of destroying septic material which may still remain. The wound is sutured in layers from behind forwards, in the usual manner. If a drainage tube is placed in the wound it should be brought out at the lower end and be of adequate size.

If the disease has been progressing for more than forty-eight hours and there are no signs of localisation of the septic inflammation, an incision through the rectus muscle is preferred by many. In this the muscle is divided about the middle of its lower segment and the two halves separated. I think my-self that it is better to cut cleanly through the muscle parallel to its fibres rather than roll them away from the selected line, so often it is found that they refuse to unite when they come together again afterwards. In this method the operator must tie several vessels in the muscle substance and secure the deep epigastric vessels in the lower part of the wound, dividing them between ligatures where they cross the line of the incision. In these late cases it is well to pass a large plug into the pelvis so that it may soak up the fluid which has gravitated there ; you will thus get rid of excess of fluid without wasting any time. This plug should be changed during the course of the operation ; but it is a mistake to wash out the pelvis with fluid of any kind, as the manipulation performed will probably tend to diffuse the septic material, breaking down defensive barriers which are already doing good work. The operation should be performed quickly on definite lines and with a light touch. In these cases of more extended mischief drainage should be provided, but it is not often that a tube is required elsewhere than in the pelvis. If the renal pouch is involved, then a tube passed into it may make for greater security, and this may be passed in some instances through a separate incision in the loin ; but the insertion of multiple tubes is not advised.

It is good that you should have a standard of what is the best to be done in cases of this kind where the septic inflamma-tion is becoming generalised. Remember that the danger to the patient is due to absorption of toxins by the lymphatics of the affected part of the peritoneum, and if you can diminish the amount of poison which is there or only check its increase you will give the forces on which you must ultimately rely to save the patient a chance of coping with the situation. Many patients have died as a result of too much surgery— the operation has been prolonged beyond endurance because it has been felt necessary to take away the appendix, and that appendix has possibly been very adherent, awkwardly placed, and the bleeding difficult to arrest, or the patient stout and intolerant of the anæsthetic, and perhaps the operator short-handed. The bruising and disturbance of parts has caused an increased local absorption which has been more than the already exhausted individual could withstand, and the heart has failed.   There are many of the late cases which will respond to surgical treatment if the intra-abdominal tension is relaxed by the introduction of a drainage tube through an incision of moderate size and no attempt is made to remove the appendix, or give a general anæsthetic.   The use of rectal infusion of sterilised saline and the Fowler position (Fig. 15) should be combined with this treatment.

In later cases the peritoneum may be converted into an abscess cavity containing many pints of pus, and sometimes recovery is effected when the aid of the surgeon has been refused, for the pus is discharged by the bowel.

I have known most unfortunate results to follow interference when the case is settling down, but has not become quiet ; therefore I am strongly against operation under such circumstances.   If the case is first seen after four or five days have elapsed, the inflammation is localised, and the general condition satisfactory, do not interfere unless obliged.   It is the spreading suppuration that causes anxiety.

Occasionally the collapse resulting from the attack is so extreme that operation is only possible after intravenous infusion of sterilised saline.

Mr. C. P. Childe has written an interesting paper[1] on the question of the position of the incision in operations for acute conditions of the abdomen, and it is well worth perusal by all surgeons.   In this he points out that nearly all the diseases for which the surgeon is required to operate, which cause the acute abdomen, have their origin between two imaginary lines, the one on the left drawn from the seventh cartilage, an inch to the left of the sternum, to Poupart's ligament ; the one on the right drawn from the anterior superior spine perpendicularly upwards to the lower border of the thorax.   The incision which he recommends in cases where the abdominal condition is obscure is one which is placed midway between these lines. This would, however, come directly over the rectus muscle, the outer margin of which (the linea semilunaris) is found at the junction of the inner three-fifths with the outer two-fifths of a line from the anterior superior spine to the umbilicus. The incision through the rectus is not a bad one in acute

[1]. The Area of "Acute Abdominal Conflux" and the "Incision of Incidence," *Lancet*, 1907, Vol. I., p. 936.

abdominal cases, and I have often used it ; but there must be
a clear understanding of the line which corresponds to the
edge of the muscle, if the operator wishes to take that. The
conditions which most frequently produce the acute abdomen
vary somewhat at different ages ; but taking an average of
a large number of patients, a diagram may be drawn which
expresses fairly well these positions and the frequency of their
occurrence by means of shading (see Fig. 10).

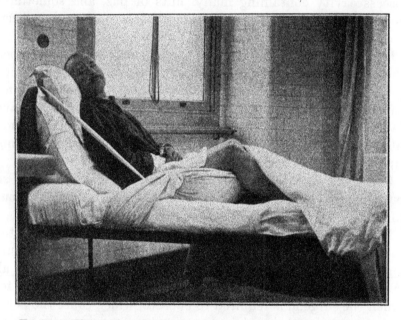

Fig. 15.—The semi-recumbent position advised in Acute Abdominal
conditions, known as "The Fowler Position."

In Fitz's table of acute intestinal obstructions no less than
67 per cent. had their origin in the right iliac fossa.

It is now customary to place the patient in bed in a sitting
attitude—" the Fowler-position " (Fig. 15). The object of this
is to encourage the gravitation of fluids towards the pelvis, thus
limiting the infection to a part where the local resistance
is high and drainage feasible. The pressure on any barriers
of defence is also lessened. The maintenance of the position
may be facilitated by the fixation of a bolster, padded block,
or stretcher across the bed, just below the level of the buttocks.
It is kept in place by straps or bandages passing to the

head of the bed on each side.   In any case in which the patient's condition is not good at the completion of the operation, a pint of warm saline, containing an ounce of brandy, should be administered by the rectum before he leaves the table.   As a routine, after the patient is arranged in bed, the continuous instillation of saline is commenced.   A perforated pewter tube or Jacques' catheter is introduced into the rectum ; the end of this is attached by means of rubber tubing to

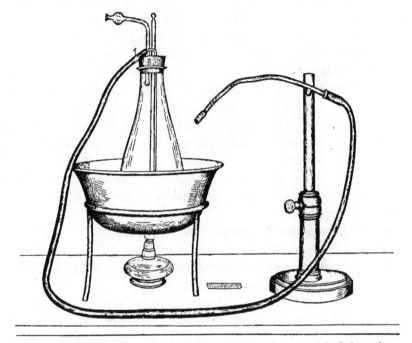

FIG. 16.—Simple Apparatus used for the Continuous Administration of Fluids *per rectum*.

a reservoir containing the fluid, kept at a temperature of 105°.   The flow is controlled by a screw-clamp on the tube. The vessel should be about 1 foot above the level of the rectum (Fig. 16).   Other more elaborate apparatus can be obtained.

Sometimes the saline is not retained.   This may be due to a too rapid inflow of the fluid, or to its being at the wrong temperature.   In other cases the lower bowel must be cleared out with a simple enema before toleration to the inflow is established.   If this method proves impracticable, subcutaneous infusion must be employed, and may require to be repeated. At times the continued flow of saline into the subcutaneous tissue may be useful, but a watch must be kept on this method, otherwise the tissues become quite " water-logged."

It has been found in practice that much saline can be absorbed by the rectum, if the apparatus is introduced at regular intervals and kept in position only for a short time. This it may sometimes be necessary to commence during the performance of the operation. Injections of sterilised saline into the axilla through the anterior axillary folds may be substituted. When the low condition of the patient is part of the primary " peritonism," some reaction from it may be expected after a wait of a few hours, but if a collapse is due to the action of toxins on the heart muscle, marking the approach of the final stage, it is wrong to wait. Every moment increases the amount of poison absorbed, and by so much lessens the chances of recovery.

It must not be forgotten that the ultimate course of the case is greatly influenced by attention to details in the treatment after operation.

In stout patients where the abdominal wall is very thick, especially if rapid operation is called for (and it usually is), or if the surgeon is short-handed, the incision is better placed though the linea semilunaris. It may be more liable to a hernia later, but this consideration must not be allowed to weigh against the satisfactory performance of the operation : time is such an important element in these cases that a quick operator will gain a success when the slower one will fail. The length of any incision should be one which will admit the hand of the operator.

The pelvic organs in the female should always be examined.

Drainage tubes may be removed in two or three days unless the discharge at this time continues profuse or the temperature has not come down. At any time it is better to shorten the original tubes rather than put smaller ones in.

It is not usually advisable to give anything by the mouth in the first six hours after operation ; the absorption of saline into the circulation relieves the sensation of thirst and increases the dilution and rapidity of excretion of toxic products. On this account there is no doubt that the steady introduction of fluid into the system by one means or another is of great value after operation in cases of peritonitis.

At this stage the question of giving an " anti-toxic serum " arises ; the infective process in most cases of appendicitis is due to the bacillus coli ; and an " anti "-serum to this organism has been prepared. I have employed it in a number of cases, but cannot say that it appeared to materially alter the course of the disease when comparison is made with instances not so treated. The serum should be injected into a pectoral or gluteal muscle ; a dose of 20 c.c. is given immediately after the operation, and this may be repeated at intervals of twenty-four hours for two or three days. Joint pains and fleeting rashes not infrequently follow this administration. It is well to have a vaccine prepared from the fluid removed at the operation, for it is often of value when the progress of the case is not as satisfactory as could be wished. Especially when the temperature keeps above normal, although there is no pus pent up anywhere, and discharge from the wound goes on without evident cause.

For the relief of the pain and discomfort still present after the operation an injection of morphine may be given, if a good night's rest is not otherwise to be obtained ; but on account of its action on the bowel the dose should not be repeated.

After every operation some vomiting is to be expected, and for the first twenty-four to thirty-six hours no definite treatment is called for to combat it ; if, however, it continues longer, becomes more frequent or offensive, an attempt to check it must be made. The slighter cases may be stopped by the administration of a dose of $\frac{1}{32}$ gr. cocaine in an ounce of water at intervals of an hour ; sometimes minim doses of tincture of iodine are successful. If these measures fail, and the patient is much distressed, the stomach should be washed out with dilute sodium bicarbonate solution ; this will at any rate give rest for some hours and probably allow of the proper administration of a purgative, which will materially benefit the condition.

In the more persistent cases the prognosis becomes very grave, as either a general toxæmia, secondary intestinal obstruction or acute dilatation of the stomach is present.

An attempt to obtain an action of the bowels should be made on the second day following the operation. I usually give a 3 to 5 gr. dose of calomel, followed after four hours by ℥ij doses of magnesium sulphate or other saline purgative at hour intervals till an action is obtained ; in obstinate cases I have found a $\frac{1}{16}$ gr. of elaterin very useful, the value of which was first demonstrated to me by Dr. John Harold. The diet for the first few days should be fluid in character ; if no adverse symptoms are present by the third or fourth day, small amounts of chicken cream and fish may be given, and at the end of a week the patient will be on practically a full diet, if it is fancied.

Meteorism, sometimes very intense, associated with a feeling of great abdominal discomfort, appears in some cases. Indicating as it does a paralysis of the muscular coats of the intestine, its persistence will always give cause for anxiety ; a turpentine enema (℥i—℥ij turpentine in ℥x of acacia emulsion) or the action of one of the above-mentioned purgatives may relieve the condition. If these fail, and the passage of a long rubber rectal tube proves equally ineffective, three or four subcutaneous injections of eserine salicylate ($\frac{1}{100}$ gr.) may be given, though in my experience it is of small value in those obstinate cases which are due to more or less complete intestinal stasis, when the necessity of a second operation must be considered. Pituitary extract is now used by many (1 c.c.), repeated hourly for three or four doses. If the obstruction is caused by an intense local peritonitis little can be gained by such interference ; in cases where it is due to mechanical kinking or strangulation of the bowel, operation will afford relief.

The wound will require at least a daily change of sterile dry gauze for some time ; if the discharge is copious and offensive, gauze soaked in 1 in 1000 lysol or in 1 in 80 carbolic is to be preferred. Any local tension must at once be relieved by the removal of skin sutures. Cellulitis or sloughing of the abdominal wall may require more radical measures such as incisions and the frequent application of hot dressings, but if the wound has been well guarded during the operation the local infection will be slight if any.

All degrees of faecal fistula may develop in the wound[1]

---

[1] See " Diseases of the Appendix," 2nd ed., p. 282.

from the second or third day to the eighth ; they may be due to the giving of the sutures in the cæcum at the point of removal of the appendix or to a sloughing of part of the bowel wall where involved in the inflammation.   They tend to spontaneous healing in practically all cases ; the diet in these circumstances should be readily digestible or such as to leave little débris ; violent purging should be avoided ; the dressings must be frequently changed, and an outside pad of carbolised tow, wood-wool, or peat moss will confine the offensive odour and prove an economy.

The onset of black vomit is never a satisfactory symptom, for it indicates a severe degree of toxæmia, and must cause considerable anxiety to those in charge.   Other signs of toxæmia are present, frequently associated with constipation and distension of the abdomen.   Washing out of the stomach, with the administration of turpentine enemata may prove very useful.   Should turpentine fail, the administration of a pint of molasses or common treacle, or yeast, will not infrequently cause an action of the bowels and a rapid general improvement.   It is advisable to protect the skin by means of ointment, and of these Wallace's ointment, vaseline or zinc are most useful.

A serious amount of cardiac weakness leading to rapid pulse, breathlessness, and dropsy of the legs may develop during convalescence, due to the toxæmia, of which we have already spoken ; it requires energetic treatment with digitalis, strychnine, and other cardiac stimulants, diet, etc., and careful nursing, over a period which may be prolonged, and demands much patience, even when the wound (usually in an adult) has done well.

Should there be dilatation of the stomach as a complication, the state of the patient may give well-founded cause for alarm. Improvement follows gastric lavage, position, enemata, etc. If washing out is not tolerated, it is sometimes possible to make the patient wash the stomach out himself.   He should be given a large quantity of warm water and induced to reject it again.   In a case which I saw with Dr. Noyes, of Worthing, the patient did this most successfully.[1]

---

[1] See *Lancet*, Vol. I., 1914, March 21.

LOCALISED SUPPURATION.

Appendicular Abscess.

Localised suppuration is much more common than is generally believed ; inflammation of the appendix, being of a septic nature, frequently terminates in suppuration, and one of the dangers of the disease is the latent character which some of the abscesses assume. Sometimes pus is found about an appendix long after the temperature has become normal and all pain and tenderness gone. As a rule, however, some thickening may be felt in the region of the appendix or an abnormal resistance to pressure. If an attack of appendicitis of more than average severity has been experienced, and a swelling has formed in the iliac fossa, there is usually suppuration present, but a sudden fall in the temperature, which had continued high, and improvement in the general condition, may indicate the escape of the pus into the bowel.

In other cases, after the temperature has become normal, or almost normal, it rises again, and with that there is an increase in the size and tenderness of any inflammatory mass, the position of which varies with that of the individual appendix. There are localised suppurations secondary to disease of the appendix which are found in other parts of the body, but these are treated of elsewhere. If, however, the local signs of abscess are not found in the iliac fossa or loin, a vaginal or rectal examination should be made (Fig. 17).

The rigidity of the lower part of the right rectus usually persists, but no longer conceals the swelling beneath ; indeed, the muscle is often pushed forward. This swelling is tender, especially where most prominent, but fluctuation is rarely found unless the case has gone so far that the abdominal wall is being penetrated or the purulent collection unusually large. Percussion over it shows a change from the normal, and where the parietal peritoneum has become adherent the note is evidently dull ; should the abscess contain gas then hyper-resonance will be found, with some dulness varying with the position of the patient.

When the abscess has been permitted to penetrate the abdominal wall, there will be redness and œdema of the skin, with bulging, fluctuation, and possibly a tympanitic area when gas has accumulated.

Occasionally the thigh is flexed, everted and abducted, and as a child with an abscess walks badly and complains of pain when examined, such are occasionally sent to hospital with the diagnosis of "hip disease."

In the diagnosis of some cases a blood count is of great importance, and is referred to on p. 151.

A good instance of a retroperitoneal abscess of large size which it was difficult to diagnose, as for a long time it was concealed, is shown by a case seen with Dr. Wilson Stoker.

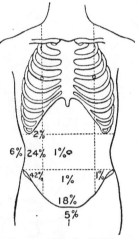

FIG. 17.—Clinical Diagram with the regional percentages of Appendix Abscesses (from Surgical Diseases of the Appendix Vermiformis, etc., 2nd ed.).

The patient, an unmarried girl of 23, became ill and feverish in June, 1908, and this condition became worse in August. There was no vomiting and no local pain, but a general weakness with fever. Dr. Stoker, who was consulted towards the end of August, had her carefully nursed, and in September a swelling was found by him in the lower abdomen. The fever was of a hectic type, and night sweats with loss of flesh occurred. She had had two similar attacks of fever, the first when 7 years of age and the second seven years before the present illness. The periods were painful and irregular. On September 17, the lower abdomen appeared somewhat fuller than normal, and there was resistance to pressure. On percussion no very markedly dull area was present, but under the lower part of the left rectus the note was tympanitic as if from a gaseous abscess ; it was not tender, and the upper limits of the swelling were fairly defined and higher on the right side. Exploration on the 20th showed the pelvis covered in as by a cloth with a yellowish-white membrane, and the only thing recognisable was the sigmoid flexure, which passed down in its usual position. The small intestines were displaced upwards and to the left. The uterus, ovaries, bladder, etc., were quite hidden, and the appendix was also concealed. Incision gave release to a large quantity of yellow pus without characteristic odour. A drainage tube was put in. Considerable shock followed, from which she recovered in a few hours.

A sinus formed and would not heal, so in June, 1909, the appendix was excised. There had been some fæcal discharge for a few days and a bullet probe passed in for several inches. The appendix was turned round an enlarged and cystic ovary, and was much thickened, strictured, and adherent.   She made a satisfactory recovery.

When these abscesses are watched from the commencement there is as a rule little difficulty in ascribing them to their right source (Fig. 18). But when seen for the first time some days after the onset of an illness' there are other conditions which must be remembered which may cause similar appearances. Of these may be mentioned— (1) Pyo-salpinx ; (2) inflamed or suppurating ovarian cyst ; (3) acute pyo - nephrosis ; (4) tuberculosis of the peritoneum ; (5) actinomycosis ; (6) abscess secondary to malignant disease of the bowel ; (7) malignant disease of the cæcum or ascending colon.

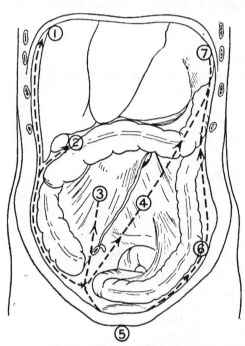

Fig. 18.—Diagram of the paths of Peritoneal Infection in relation to Appendicitis. The primary form is in the right iliac fossa. 1. Right-sided subdiaphragmatic abscess. 2. Right-sided subhepatic abscess. 3. Right-sided ante-renal abscess. 4. Left-sided ante-renal abscess. 5. Pelvic abscess. 6. Abscess in the left iliac fossa. 7. Left-sided subdiaphragmatic abscess. Between 4 and 7, a left-sided subhepatic abscess may be found. Between 6 and 7, a subsplenic abscess may occur. (From " Surgical Diseases of the Appendix, etc.," 2nd ed.)

In Pyo-nephrosis the tumour is in the right loin and is distinctly outlined. It has projected gradually from the kidney region, moves on deep inspiration. Occasionally a calculus can be seen with the X-rays. There may have been renal colic with pus in the urine.

Inflamed or Suppurating Ovarian Cyst.—The change in the cyst may arise in various ways, frequently from twisted pedicle, and is difficult to diagnose when seen after a few days'

illness, should the cyst be entirely intrapelvic. In the beginning
of the illness a swelling would be found of a size too large for
any recent inflammatory condition to have reached ; later
it may still retain its definite outline. Where it is above the
pelvic brim it has probably been recognised before the onset
of the inflammation.

In Pyo-salpinx there is a tumour present on vaginal examination, possibly on both sides, though the side which is causing
the trouble is the more tender. There may be a history of
dysmenorrhœa, menorrhagia, backaches, vaginal discharge,
and possibly feverish attacks. I have known a patient certified
and treated for tuberculosis when suffering from this disease
before the pyo-salpinx ruptured.

Abscess secondary to malignant disease of the bowel may be
due to the giving way of a stercoral ulcer, which has formed
secondarily to a carcinoma of the lower part of the large
intestine or rectum. It is a very serious complication, and in a
stout subject might be mistaken at its commencement for an
attack of appendicitis. There is usually a history of obstruction, obstinate constipation, or diarrhœa for some time before
the complication shows on the right side of the abdomen.

Occasionally a Growth in the Cæcum undergoes a change,
possibly from necrosis of tissue, and suppuration takes place
around it ; it is a very distressing complication, because an
incurable fæcal fistula forms after the pus is evacuated. Here
again it is possible to get a history of illness with the presence
of a localised swelling before complaint was made of the more
acute condition.

The resemblance between an appendix abscess and a tumour
may be very close. A case seen with Dr. Arthur Browne is
a good example of this difficulty.

A man of 50, stout and previously healthy, had an attack of abdominal
pain and vomiting five weeks before. The pain was severe and in the
right iliac fossa. For about three weeks a definite swelling had been
noticed, tender on pressure, and painful when he was moving about.
He had not felt ill enough to keep altogether in bed, and occasionally
walked about the room. There was a hard swelling, the size of a large
fist, with rounded outline on the right side of the abdomen, between the
umbilicus and anterior superior spine, dull on percussion, very tender,
but without fluctuation and movable on the deeper parts. It came
forward and, at the outer margin of the rectus muscle, was adherent to
the abdominal wall. The temperature was normal. About eighteen

months before he had had an attack of pain on the right side of the abdomen but it was not of long duration, and no swelling had been noticed. The operation was done in two stages—(1) incision of abscess ; (2) removal of appendix twelve days later. The appendix, which was large with very thick walls, was adherent to the parietal peritoneum under the right rectus. The abdominal wall was very thick from fat deposit and the muscles and fasciæ very much degenerated.

In these cases the previous history is very important, and as a rule a new growth is more prominent, clearly outlined, and less tender. Still the diagnosis will occasionally be very difficult in fat patients.

I have elsewhere[1] published the account of a case of large Colloid Growth of the Ascending Colon

in which there had been an attack of appendicitis for which a female patient had been treated in a provincial hospital, and dismissed when the inflammatory symptoms had subsided. She was aged 59. The growth was excised and an ileocolostomy performed, from which great benefit was obtained, the woman being in good health when seen several months later. Here there was a large swelling left when she had recovered from the acute illness, the importance of which was not recognised as there was no obstruction of the bowels. The growth probably obstructed the appendix.

Hyperplastic Tuberculosis of the cæcum is a chronic disease, and at first presents no evidence of swelling ; later this may be found in the iliac fossa, or even above the iliac crest, but as time advances it surely becomes evident, whilst there are increasing signs of tuberculosis in other parts, especially the lungs. The tumour is more or less cylindrical, somewhat nodular, and rather fixed ; it may be tender. It is of slow development, and irregular abdominal pains merge into the symptoms of obstruction. Excision is indicated if the general state of the patient permits.

In Actinomycosis a swelling forms and increases gradually with a brawny infiltration of the tissues, followed by the formation of sinuses, the purulent discharge from which contains granules of a yellow colour and hyphæ, which show clearly the nature of the disease. Some amelioration may be obtained by repeated incisions and the administration of potassium iodide.

The vast majority of abscesses of the appendix diminish in

[1] " Surgical Diseases of the Appendix, etc.," p. 273.

size and become absorbed or disappear by discharge into the bowel, probably through the appendix ; therefore it is unnecessary to interfere, unless (1) the abscess has become chronic ; (2) increases in size ; (3) gives rise to much pain. Operation should then be performed whether there is reason to think it has become adherent to the parietal peritoneum or not. A rapidly increasing abscess is a source of danger.

When an abscess is pointing, having made its way through the muscular wall of the abdomen, a simple incision is all that is required, with provision for drainage.

If the pus is covered by peritoneum in the iliac fossa, the McBurney operation by separation of muscular fibres should be done, the first incision being made parallel with the fibres of the external oblique. If the covering omentum or intestine is adherent to the wall, all that is then necessary is to pass the finger in between this coil of gut or omentum limiting it and the parietal peritoneum downwards towards the appendix. The pus will then come away easily. If the abscess is not adherent, a strip of gauze should be passed around with the end of a blunt-pointed pair of scissors and the abscess opened in a similar way with the finger. In both a large tube should be inserted. In the latter the gauze plug may be removed in thirty-six hours.

A pelvic abscess may be opened after displacement of the rectus muscle inwards and ligature of the deep epigastric vessels, but it is usually best to open it through the rectum in the male and young female, or through the vagina in the married woman.

The patient having been placed in the lithotomy position, and a duck-bill speculum introduced into the rectum, a longitudinal incision is made over the most prominent part, dividing the mucous membrane ; the deeper parts are then opened up with a director, along which a closed pair of forceps is passed, opened and withdrawn. This will suffice to make an opening large enough for the escape of pus and the necessary drainage. After the evacuation of the pus and cleansing of the parts as much as possible, a strip of antiseptic gauze is introduced and left in the opening for forty-eight hours, when it probably comes away during an action of the bowel.

Where the abscess is opened through the vagina, it is best to

shave the vulva and douche the vagina with sterilised saline.
The cervix uteri is seized with a vulsellum, which is given to an

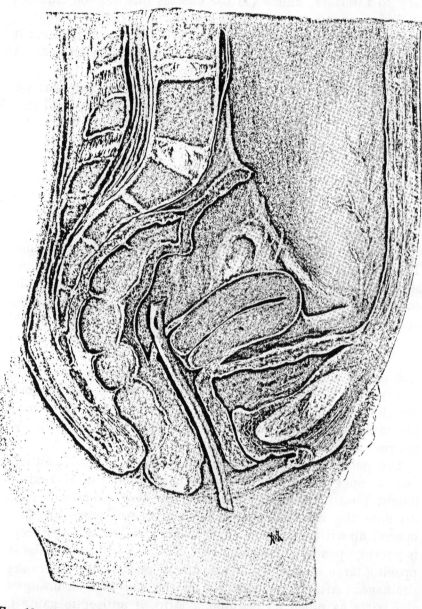

FIG. 19.—Sagittal Section of a female body, with a rubber tube inserted
in the Vagina and through the Posterior Fornix to illustrate the
vaginal drainage of the Pouch of Douglas (from " Surgical Diseases
of the Appendix Vermiformis, etc." 2nd ed.).

assistant. The parts are well retracted and an incision made behind the cervix with the point of the knife directed upwards and towards the posterior surface of the uterus (Fig. 19). It is advisable to go deeper than into the rectal wall as the vagina is the thicker. The pus is then evacuated in a similar manner, the finger introduced to make the opening large enough for a good-sized tube. This should be long enough to project from the vulva, gauze is carefully packed round the tube in the vagina, and an external pad applied with a **T** bandage. The gauze is changed every day and the vagina douched, but the tube is not disturbed for a week or so, when it may be removed if the condition is satisfactory. Recovery may be delayed by some pelvic cellulitis, in which case there will be an irregular temperature for some time.

If the abscess rises directly from the pelvis and the suprapubic position is chosen for drainage, the position of the bladder must be defined, and operation only done when that viscus is empty and out of the way, as shown by the insertion of an instrument into it. It is sometimes held up by the abscess and cannot fall into position when emptied ; it then lies well above the pubes and would be in danger.

I think it is rarely permissible to attempt to take away the appendix when the abscess is opened, and that a much better result in a large series of cases of varying severity will be obtained if it is removed when the inflammatory mischief has quieted down.[1] It must be removed if you wish to make the patient safe.

Sudden Diffusion of the Pus from Rupture of an Abscess into the Peritoneum.

A most serious condition may arise through the bursting of an appendix abscess into the peritoneal cavity, and formerly, in the experience of most, this accident was a fatal one. In appendix suppuration there is an attempt made by nature to localise the pus ; occasionally for some reason this is only successful for a time, and there is a further extension of the pus and involvement of more of the peritoneum. This takes place slowly and is not accompanied by the definite signs

[1] See " Surgical Diseases of the Appendix Vermiformis and their Complications," 2nd ed.

which we have spoken of as "peritonism." A very different clinical picture is presented by the patient in whom an abscess containing a large amount of pus has suddenly burst, distributing its septic contents throughout the abdomen.

Examples of this complication which were treated within two days are instructive, and have been selected as most typical.

A ward maid at a fever hospital, aged 19, was admitted ✳ on November 3, 1904. Her illness commenced with pain in the right iliac region seven days before admission. She was obliged to go to bed, but resumed work on the following day and did her usual duties as well as she could until about fifteen hours before she came into hospital, when a sudden acute pain attacked her and she was obliged to return to bed. There had been diarrhœa for two or three days. When I saw her with Dr. Hector Mackenzie she was propped up in bed, her nostrils were working rapidly, and she was breathing with some difficulty. Her face was dusky and anxious-looking, she was restless, but quite clear in her mind, and able to answer questions. The respiration was 32, thoracic and shallow, the tongue furred and dirty, the pulse 100, and temperature 100·6°. The lower abdomen was distended and did not move at all on respiration ; the upper half moved moderately. On palpation there was a marked resistance in the lower half of the abdomen, especially over the right iliac fossa, where there was a definite swelling. There was great tenderness here ; the abdomen was generally tender. On percussion extensive dulness was found in both flanks, but not in the middle line. The liver dulness was obliterated. At the operation an abscess was found to have given way on its pelvic aspect, and the pelvis was filled with offensive, semi-purulent fluid, which was generally diffused throughout the lower part of the abdominal cavity. Lavage with warm saline solution was carried out, and drainage through the openings made in the abdominal wall. The patient made a good recovery, and later on the appendix was removed.

Another case which presented similar symptoms, and also ended in recovery, was that of a man aged 33 years, who was sent to the hospital by Mr. Hallam, and admitted the day following the admission of the patient whose case I have just recorded.✳

The patient had had an attack of pain in the abdomen on October 31, chiefly on the right side, but did not give up his work. During the night of November 3 an attack of intense pain was experienced, and he came to the hospital in the morning sixteen hours later. When examined he was found to be perspiring freely, his face was pale and anxious-looking, respirations were shallow and diaphragmatic. An attempt to breathe deeply caused him much pain in the abdomen. The pulse was 104, temperature 101·2°. There was no vomiting, the bowels were confined, the abdomen did not move on respiration, and was very tender on examination, especially in the right iliac region and in the loins. There was dulness in the flanks and the liver dulness was obscured. The abdominal muscles were rigid, this rigidity being most marked on the right side. In the right iliac fossa there was an ill-defined swelling. At the operation two incisions were made, one through the right rectus muscle and the other through the middle line below the umbilicus. Offensive, semi-purulent fluid was generally diffused throughout the peritoneum ; the intestines looked very congested and œdematous ; the abscess had ruptured to its outer side. Lavage with saline fluid of a temperature of 110° was thoroughly performed, the hepatic and splenic regions being carefully irrigated. Drainage was employed from both wounds. These were healed by December 17, and later on the appendix was removed.

In this case, as in the former, suppuration had followed perforation of the appendix beyond a stricture. It will be noted that in both these cases there was a definite fixed swelling in the iliac fossa, in addition to the free fluid, the history of a recent abdominal pain which subsided to some extent, then a sudden and alarming return of pain and vomiting.

OTHER ABDOMINAL SUPPURATIONS.

HEPATIC ABSCESS.

It is not often that we see the large abscesses of the liver which used to come under observation some years ago. They were frequently so very large that the patient was not only reduced to a skeleton by the accompanying fever, night sweats, and possibly diarrhœa, but he had little chance of surviving the shock and subsequent drain which the release of such a large amount of pus and closing of such a large cavity entailed on his resources. I have seen such abscesses full of thick chocolate-coloured pus opened, and the result has been a hæmorrhage into the cavity in some or a high hectic fever which proved fatal in a short time in others.

The training of the members of our profession, whether civil or in the Services, is so much improved, and their ability as operators so high, that these cases no longer progress to such a dangerous extent. They are wisely treated in the colonies and not sent home for treatment, with the possibility of serious complications during a voyage of uncertain duration.

Mr. Cantlie has suggested that hepatic abscesses should be treated by means of trocar and cannula followed by siphon drainage ; he gives excellent reasons for the operation which he advocates, but I do not know of any statistics which enable us to compare his method with those in general use.   It would be well if he could give his exact results.   The majority of surgeons, I take it, are more comfortable as to the results of operation for such abscesses if they feel that there is nothing to interfere with the free escape of the pus through an opening which they consider more adequate.

The early evacuation of these abscesses is to be desired, as it is in the case of abscesses in other parts of the body.   The majority are situated in the upper and back part of the right lobe of the liver, but there are no reasons why suppuration should not commence in any part.   Those which begin within the liver, or which are in the most common situation, may possibly be permitted to attain a size large enough to enable them to be searched for with a probability of success.   Those which develop on the anterior surface should be opened quite early, and a long illness cut short.   We no longer have that fear of the peritoneum, which formerly acted as a deterrent to operation before the wall of the abscess was adherent to the parietal peritoneum.   A plug of gauze can be placed to shut off the peritoneal cavity and the operation expeditiously concluded at one sitting.   It is not necessary to use sutures.   The cavity does not require to be scraped out neither does it need syringing ; both may cause hæmorrhage.

G. H., an ex-soldier, aged 35, was admitted ⨯ on June 6, 1905.

He stated that on May 30, about 9 a.m., he had a sudden attack of vomiting: he had no breakfast that morning.   On June the 1st he had a dull aching pain in the lower part of the back on the right side, extending in front to about 2 inches below the margin of the ribs and 2½ inches from the middle line.   He vomited several times during May 30 and 31, and June 1.   He had been feverish.

This patient had been previously under the care of Dr. Mackenzie in 1904, from November 8 to December 31, and on November 11 an abscess of the liver which had been causing symptoms for ten days was opened and drained.   The abscess was a small one containing greenish pus, which was sterile on examination in the clinical laboratory.

The surface of the liver was dark-red in colour, and the abscess was not bulging, nor the liver adherent, but the area underneath which the pus had collected was softened.   The point of a pair of artery forceps was pushed into it, the forceps opened, withdrawn, and replaced by a rubber tube.

The man had been in India, Malta and South Africa, and had suffered from dysentery in 1897, and on more than one occasion since. He had also had enteric in South Africa.

On his second admission the man looked ill and his breathing was hurried. Deep inspiration caused sharp pain. There was the scar of the previous operation in the right hypochondrium. The liver edge could not be felt because of the extreme resistance of the right rectus, much tenderness was complained of, on even light pressure, over this area. There was no friction to be heard. A dragging pain was caused when he turned on the left side, and he was usually found lying on the right. The liver dulness extended vertically downwards to 1 inch below the rib margin, from the fifth rib. Pulse, 80; respiration, 44; temperature, 100·2°. There was nothing abnormal found in other parts.

His symptoms did not improve. On June 10 he was unable to sleep because of pain. On the 14th an incision was made through the right rectus ; on passing the finger along the anterior surface of the liver, an area of bulging was found towards the summit, the upper part of which was soft, whilst the part at the base of the projection was unduly resistant. This area was isolated with gauze packing, a trochar put into the swelling, along which a pair of forceps was passed and exit given to about 3 oz. of yellow pus. A drainage tube was placed in this and the area shut off from the general peritoneal cavity with a strip of gauze. The temperature became normal at once ; in three days' time there was hardly any discharge, and the wound had healed ten days after the operation.

This abscess was nearer the middle line and less accessible than the former one.

PERIGASTRIC AND SUBDIAPHRAGMATIC ABSCESS.

Perigastric Abscess.

In cases of localised suppuration secondary to perforation of a gastric ulcer, the opening is usually a small one and the abscess forms gradually. There is a history of gastric ulcer, with an increase of any pre-existing epigastric tenderness and pain ; swelling in the stomach region, which increases from day to day, and a feverish attack. Although we do not find any of the food contents of the stomach in these abscesses, the smell of the evacuated fluid is so characteristic that no one can have any doubt of its origin when the pus is released. It is often impossible to find the perforation. There is sometimes bulging, fluctuation, and the presence of free gas in these abscesses. The smaller abscesses are rarely diagnosed and have not infrequently proved fatal from secondary rupture, whilst the larger collections are likely to cause death from exhaustion, filling as they may do the upper abdomen. When these abscesses spread downwards they more generally run along the left side of the spine, and along the side of the descending colon, than behind the peritoneum.

In one case treated with Dr. S. West at the Royal Free Hospital that was the course taken, and the abscess had attained a large size at the time it was opened in the left iliac fossa. The patient, a woman, recovered.

The possibility of a need for counter-openings must be considered and a careful watch kept for signs of involvement of the pleura.

An abstract of a case described in a communication to the St. Thomas's Hospital Reports is of interest[1] :—

A married woman of 26, admitted ✳ October 23, 1902. She had been confined on August 6, and about seventeen days later began to complain of pain in the lower chest, which extended down to the front part of the abdomen. This was very severe, generally came on after taking food, and frequently caused vomiting, which gave great relief. On admission there was a swelling in the umbilical region which was rounded and smooth. Above it was a very hard nodular mass the size of an orange, which appeared fixed and did not move well with respiration. Continuous with this, but deeper in the abdomen, was a smooth rounded mass, which extended 1½ inches below the umbilicus from the middle line to the line of the right nipple. This also appeared fixed. The rounded prominence in the epigastric region was recognised as a dilated stomach, the greater curvature of which reached 2½ inches below the umbilicus, and to the left nearly to the middle line. The lesser curvature was just below the most prominent part of the tumour. Peristalsis was poorly marked. The swelling was extremely painful on pressure, and she complained of a more or less continuous aching at all times.

On November 5 the epigastric swelling had increased in size, but the temperature was normal. On the 8th the pain had become acute, and was not relieved by vomiting. The temperature was again elevated. On November 11, 24 oz. of pus were evacuated through a median epigastric incision. The fluid was first of a yellowish watery appearance, and then pus-like matter escaped, afterwards blood-stained fluid. The cavity was situated in front of the stomach under the liver, being shut off by adhesions of the omentum to the abdominal wall. A drainage tube was inserted. For a few days progress was good, but there was again complaint of abdominal pain, and on the 18th another fluctuating swelling was found extending down towards the left iliac fossa. An

[1] "Chronic Perforation of a Gastric Ulcer," by William H. Battle (Vol. XXXI., p. 385).

incision was made about 2½ inches above the left anterior superior spine, and a large retroperitoneal abscess opened ; it contained several ounces of sour-smelling pus. The peritoneum encircling the two openings was stitched together and a drainage tube put in. At the same time an offensive whitish slough, resembling sloughed omentum, was taken out of the higher incision. Ten days later a slough of similar character was removed from the lower incision, evidently derived from the cellular tissue. About December 1 she began to pass clay-coloured stools, and the discharge from the lower wound stained the dressings green and yellow ; it continued for a few days, and then ceased. Rectal feeding was commenced after the second operation and continued for ten days, but she was permitted to take some fluid nourishment by the mouth. Recovery was complete.

It was noticed that the patient had an unusual amount of tenderness about the epigastric swelling when she was admitted, but until the occurrence of the sharp attack of pain on November 8 there was nothing very marked to indicate a complication of the kind which ensued.

In some cases perigastric abscess is formed more rapidly. In nearly all much illness may be saved by early incision. Should the pus make its way behind the stomach, or have originated in an ulcer placed on its posterior wall, especially if the perforation is large, the process of suppuration may be very tedious and even fatal. Pin-point perforations are responsible for a large number of these abscesses. Care has to be taken when the peritoneum is opened lest the stomach wall (if it is adherent) be mistaken for the wall of an abscess.

Subdiaphragmatic Abscess.

A localised collection of pus which is in contact with the under surface of the diaphragm. When perforation or suppuration occurs in connection with the stomach, duodenum, liver and bile passages, pancreas and spleen, the pus will probably have some relationship to the under surface of the diaphragm. Suppuration may also extend from the lower part of the abdomen. The late Mr. Barnard analysed the causes in 76 consecutive cases which occurred at the London Hospital : 21 were due to perforation of gastric ulcer, 12 to appendicitis. Leith, who collected 212 cases, says that 74 were due to gastric ulcer and 20 to appendicitis. The proportion given by the former is probably the more correct. To the affections of the organs mentioned are included, in Mr. Barnard's list, parturition, pyæmia, splenic infarct, extension of thoracic disease, acute periostitis of transverse process of lumbar vertebra,[1] resection operations, typhoid, pyo-salpinx, ruptured gut, congenital cystic kidney, and injury.

There will usually be a history of some cause such as gastric ulcer for the formation of an abscess in the upper abdomen— pain, relieved by vomiting and increased by taking food ; hæmatemesis. An attack of dysentery, typhoid, malaria. The onset may be sudden or quite insidious and pain is the first symptom. Vomiting is very common, especially in cases

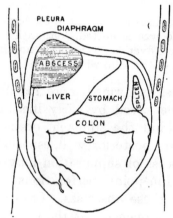

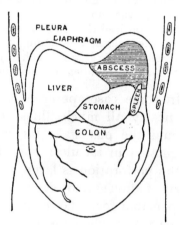

Fig. 20.—Diagram of the Anatomical Relations of a Right-sided Subdiaphragmatic Abscess (from "Surgical Diseases of the Appendix, etc.," 2nd ed.).

Fig. 21.—Diagram of the Anatomical Relations of a Left-sided Subdiaphragmatic Abscess (from "Surgical Diseases of the Appendix, etc.," 2nd ed.).

where perforation has occurred. Amongst the general symptoms is pyrexia, which varies much in severity, is frequently accompanied by sweating at night, and gastro-intestinal disturbance. Rigors are of bad prognosis. Leucocytosis was found in all the cases in Barnard's series which were examined for it.

As regards the abdominal signs and symptoms. In most there is an abdominal swelling caused by the purulent collection, or the bulged liver substance over a tropical abscess. It does not move on inspiration, and varies according to the particular anatomical variety present. There may be bulging

[1] See also Major Maddock, *British Medical Journal*, Vol. I., 1914, p. 852.

and fluctuation with dulness on percussion, unless gas is present, when an area of tympanitic resonance will be found, varying with the position of the patient. The parts bounding the abscess towards the abdomen will be tender and dull. A peritoneal rub has been heard.

When the pus is between the liver and diaphragm, the liver, being adherent at the margin of the abscess, does not descend on inspiration.

Changes at the bases of the lungs may indicate extension of inflammation through the diaphragm, or a compression of the lung. Barnard records the presence of basal signs on the opposite side in two cases of perigastric abscess. The measurement of the affected side is often increased, whilst bulging may be easily seen, or the intercostals are pressed outwards and the tissues feel œdematous over these muscles.

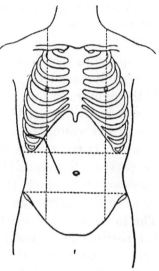

Subphrenic abscesses should be treated as such collections are treated in other parts of the abdomen ; if they are left to become very large the chances of recovery are much diminished ; still it is surprising how rapidly a young patient may improve even after months of delay, when the abscess has been emptied and drained. In 23 out of

FIG. 22.—Clinical Diagram of Incision for exploring the Right Subdiaphragmatic Region (from " Surgical Diseases of he Appendix, etc.," 2nd ed.

Barnard's 76 cases the abscess ruptured—into a bronchus, 4 ; right pleura, 2 ; left pleura, 3 ; peritoneum, 1 ; stomach, 8 ; intestine, 2 ; colon, 1 ; through the skin, 2.

In the diagnosis of these abscesses X-rays are useful if the state of the patient makes it possible to apply them and there is any obscurity in the case. The use of an exploring needle is not advocated ; it may be a very dangerous weapon and very misleading : there is more than one case on record where the needle failed to find the pus, and others where it caused a fatal result.

The subphrenic abscess may be satisfactorily treated by one of two methods—

(1) Exposure and drainage from the front when the abscess tends to pass in that direction. If the abscess has not reached the margin of the ribs, but is situated between the upper and anterior part of the liver and the diaphragm but is not under the line of incision, the peritoneum is packed off, a finger passed upwards into the abscess and replaced by a large rubber tube. The abscess is washed out gently with saline solution, and a layer of fresh gauze placed to prevent escape of any pus into the general peritoneum. This can be removed in thirty-six hours.

(2) If the abscess is behind and above the liver or above the spleen, a section of a rib (the ninth is probably the most commonly selected) should be made and the pleura opened. If the diaphragm, which is often œdematous, is adherent to the pleura, an incision of $1\frac{1}{2}$ to 2 inches should be made in the middle line of the wound, and the upper margin of this sutured to the pleura. If the pleura is not adherent, a line of sutures should be passed all round, shutting off the pleural cavity. Whilst these sutures, which may be continuous, are passed it is well to have the diaphragm which is exposed held up with forceps. The incision is carried through to the surface of the liver ; if the peritoneum is not adherent, then a plug should be passed and packed into the lower part of this space before further exploration is carried out. The forefinger is then passed along the surface of the liver in the direction in which the abscess is supposed to be, a bullet probe being substituted if nothing is found. Where there is a probability that the suppuration is in the liver, whether tropical abscess or suppurating hydatid, a trochar and canula is passed into it, the opening enlarged, and a drainage tube inserted. In any operation of this kind it is well to make certain that the peritoneum is quite shut off before the incision is closed.

Drainage will be required for some time, and the surgeon must not be hurried into shortening the tube or diminishing its size.

Suppuration in the splenic region is usually secondary to an attack of appendicitis with spreading inflammation of the peritoneum some time after an operation has been satisfactorily performed for the arrest of the mischief so far as the lower part of the abdomen is concerned. Captain F. E. Wilson, I.M.S., has recently drawn attention to perisplenic suppuration in cases of malaria with cachexia ; he gives three instances in which he opened such abscesses. He writes :[1]

"The points on which I rely in making a diagnosis in such cases are : (1) Continuance of fever under thorough quinine treatment and after the disappearance of all forms of the parasite from the peripheral blood ; (2) local evidences of softening, pain, or adherence to the abdominal parietes ; and (3) leucocytosis. What probably occurs in the spleen is the necrosis of areas of hypertrophied splenic tissue, this being followed by infection from the blood-stream. Unfortunately I have not had the laboratory facilities at my disposal to determine the infecting organism in each instance."

Suppurative Perisigmoiditis in Childhood.

Professor Ransohoff has published in the "Annals of Surgery"[2] two cases of perisigmoiditis in children which went on to suppuration.

The first was a child of 6 with a seven days' history of anorexia and constipation. Strong purgatives were given and the sixth day sharp abdominal pain ensued, with repeated vomiting, rise of temperature, and meteorism. The abdominal muscles were rigid, bowels distended, with persistent fever and leucocytosis. In three days' time an infiltration was found in the left side of pelvis, and on operation an abscess was opened ; this was closely connected with a patch of necrosis in the wall of the sigmoid. This was inverted, fixed with sutures, and covered with omentum. Drainage and recovery in three weeks. In a second child, aged 9 months, there was an abscess in the meso-sigmoid. This child had been suffering from entero-colitis for some months, fever, diarrhœa with occasional passage of blood, and great rectal tenesmus.

The exact causation in these cases must remain doubtful ; it was suggested that there might have been a diverticulum of the sigmoid, but such is unknown in children. An alternative diagnosis before operation was left-sided abscess due to appendix disease. No foreign body was found.

Concealed Abscesses.

It is not necessary to enter into a description of the other varieties of abscess which are seen in the abdomen : there is nothing that requires special mention ; the principles of treat-

[1] *Lancet*, 1913, p. 1913.
[2] 1913, Vol. II., p. 218.

ment should be carried out as indicated in what has been said about other abscesses. Those in the kidney region may be mistaken for suppuration due to appendix disease, but this will be ascertained at the operation, for the odour of the pus is characteristic.

At the Children's Hospital, Shadwell, it was not unusual to see cases in which abscesses were pointing, or already discharging, at the umbilicus ; these were usually regarded as probably tuberculous in origin : there is no doubt that in many instances they are caused by the pneumococcus, and in such the prognosis is good.

There are, however, many instances of concealed abscess met with in practice, the position of which is not easily ascertained, nor the cause discovered, when they have been found and successfully treated. Some of these are residual abscesses following on suppurative appendicitis ; some are of tuberculous origin ; others originate in the pelvis the result of tubal disease ; whilst others have their origin in the liver, or possibly in connection with a malignant growth which is of itself too small to give localising symptoms. Pain is not a characteristic symptom, but the patient becomes feverish, listless, loses weight and strength ; his complexion is pale and muddy. The tongue is furred, the bowels constipated ; he has no appetite, and sleeps badly ; whilst in the morning his clothing is wet with perspiration. The pulse is increased in frequency, but there is nothing abnormal found on examination of lungs or abdomen. Examination of the pelvis in women may show evidence of suppuration about the uterus, but there may be nothing abnormal discovered. Typhoid fever is suspected, but the tests for that and tubercle are negative. The blood is examined and leucocytosis is found, indicating the presence of suppuration somewhere ; the difficulty is to locate the abscess. The surgeon may suspect that it is in the subphrenic region by exclusion of other places as a result of examination and the history of the particular case, but it may still be impossible to point to any one localising sign. Here the X-rays may be of use, and comparison of the measurements on the two sides of the chest should be made.

The following cases will illustrate this part of our subject. In the first, under the care of Dr. Box, it was thought that the patient might have had appendicitis as a cause for the disease, though this was not proved.

The patient, a youth of 18, was admitted on August 11, and left on November 15, 1911. He gave a history of pain in the abdomen on August 1 and complained of headaches, and for three days before that had epistaxis on and off. The pains were short and sharp in character. He walked about for four or five days ; his doctor then sent him to bed and afterwards to hospital.

On admission he had a temperature of 102·4° and a pulse of 104 ; and nothing could be discovered on examination of the abdomen, nor of any region of the body. The temperature continued at 102° to 103° every night until the end of August, and all the tests for paratyphoid, typhoid, tubercle, and syphilis were negative. The pains in the abdomen disappeared. On the 26th it was reported that the percentage of polynuclears was 73·25 and that of small lymphocytes 19·75.

Examination with the X-rays on September 29. " Right side of diaphragm moves less than left. Some opacity of right base seen on screen examination." There is an area of definite tenderness on pressure over the lower ribs on the right side behind. Four days later he was complaining of pain there. Area of liver dulness increased. During the greater part of September the temperature was better, and from the 13th to the 24th it did not rise above normal. After this, however, it became high again, and with the symptoms which now developed, increased pain and tenderness in the hepatic region, there was no doubt of a collection of pus under the diaphragm, and on October 4 this was opened by a transpleural operation with resection of part of a rib. The diaphragm was incised and the peritoneum opened ; at this point it was not adherent, so a gauze plug was inserted shutting off the peritoneal cavity below. The finger passed upwards between the liver and diaphragm entered a large abscess cavity. A drainage tube was inserted and the gauze plug left *in situ*. The bacteriological examination showed the presence of the *staphylococcus aureus*. Recovery was now rapid.

In a second case there could be no doubt that the operation clearly proved the hepatic abscess to have been the cause of the symptoms.

A patient, aged 29, was seen on August 4, 1904, at Brighton with Mr. W. H. Bowring and Drs. Hobhouse and Sanderson. When on a voyage some eighteen months previously he had suffered from an attack of dysentery, but had apparently completely recovered from the illness and its consequences until April, when he complained of pain in the right shoulder and feverishness. These feverish attacks have continued since, without any long intermissions, but signs of any local trouble have been slight, excepting for two attacks of pain of rather sharp character, which in one instance was followed by jaundice of short duration. The patient had been under observation and treatment since April, and the temperature had shown a very marked range from 105° at night to 98° and even 97° in the morning.   If kept strictly to his bed, the temperature would become normal, only to resume the previous course on his return to a more active life.   On July 24 the gall-bladder and ducts were explored by a surgeon who had suggested the possibility of a gall-stone impaction in the cystic duct.   Nothing abnormal had been found, however, and the progress of the case had been but temporarily interrupted.

On August 3 a localised dulness had shown itself at the right base, and on the insertion of a trochar and canula, clear fluid had come away. This dull area was recent and not of large extent.   There had been some tenderness along the ninth interspace since the tapping.

The patient was a tall man, much emaciated.   He had a rapid pulse, the tone of which was not good.   It was explained to him that there was an abscess of the liver, between the posterior aspect of that organ and the diaphragm, and that it was necessary to open it through the chest wall.

Part of the ninth rib on the right side was excised, the pleura sutured to the diaphragm, and the incision carried through that muscle.   Several large veins were visible in it, and it was somewhat œdematous and adherent to the liver.   A trochar was passed into the liver, upwards and inwards and pus found.   The opening into the abscess was enlarged, and about 15 oz. of yellow pus evacuated.   Two drainage tubes were inserted.   The added drain from the abscess was too much for the patient, who died exhausted a few days afterwards.

In the case of a young lady of 16, who had been under treatment for some weeks for typhoid fever, the cause of the symptoms was a tuberculous pyo-salpinx.

I was asked to operate by Dr. Mackenzie, who had seen the patient in consultation.   The distended tube extended upwards into the posterior part of the left iliac fossa and fluctuated.   She had fever and was much emaciated.   Operation confirmed his diagnosis ; the swelling was very adherent and difficult to separate, being very closely attached to the upper part of the rectum, and although no opening could be found at the time of operation, in view of the density of the adhesions and difficulty of separation, it was considered advisable to put in a drainage tube.   A fæcal fistula formed but closed in a few days, and the patient recovered.   Some years later she married and has had children.   There has been no further manifestation of tubercle.

Another abscess, the cause for which was obscure, whilst the localisation of the pus was difficult, was the following :—

R. W. R., a man of 33, was admitted ✱ on July 12 and left September 10, 1913.

Patient, who was formerly in the army, left China six years ago. Whilst there he had malaria and an attack of jaundice, but not dysentery.   He also contracted syphilis, for which he underwent two years' treatment.

Six weeks ago, when apparently in good health, he had a sudden attack of pain in the epigastrium, which doubled him up. This lasted for five hours. Next day he returned to work and continued his occupation for another week, but at the end of that time felt so weak that he saw a doctor, who sent him to bed, where he was kept for a fortnight. He has had some breathlessness on exertion, slight cough, and pain over the liver, where he has noticed some swelling.

A sallow-complexioned man with pyorrhœa. There is swelling over the liver region, especially laterally. The hepatic dulness extends from the fourth rib to about 3 inches below the costal margin and well beyond the middle line to the left. No tenderness : no complaint of pain. Behind over the right lung there is dulness almost to the apex, and the breath sounds are almost inaudible. Temperature, 98° ; pulse, 108.

On July 30 it was noted that there was considerable swelling. The result of the hydatid complement fixation test was returned as negative. The X-ray examination showed fluid in the right pleura. On this day the abscess was opened by transpleural incision from behind after excision of 3 inches of the ninth rib. The pleura was sutured to the diaphragm round an area through which a trochar was passed and then an incision made. Thin purulent fluid was evacuated to the extent of several pints ; it was not offensive. The report of the clinical laboratory on this fluid was "few pus cells, much débris, no organisms seen. No evidence of hydatid disease."

Before operation the highest temperature record was 99°, and an examination of the blood gave the following :—

Polynuclear neutrophils	.	.	.	. 57	per cent.
,, eosinophils	.	.	.	. 7	,, ,,
Small lymphocytes	.	.	.	. 21	,, ,,
Large lymphocytes	.	.	.	. 6·5	,, ,,
Large hyaline cells	.	.	.	. 7·5	,, ,,
Coarsely granular basophilic cells	.	.	. 1·0	,, ,,

PART III

PERFORATION OF ULCERS OF THE DIGESTIVE TRACT

In considering the perforation of ulcers of the digestive tract that give rise to the " acute abdomen " I do not propose to include those which take place at the site of a malignant growth, but only those which are known as " simple," the sudden giving way of an ulcer of the stomach or bowel into the general peritoneal cavity.

GASTRIC ULCERS.

In the autumn of 1894 Sir Alfred Pearce Gould opened a discussion at Bristol on the surgical treatment of simple ulcer of the stomach and duodenum and typhoid ulceration of the ileum and colon. The influence of this debate in Great Britain did a great deal to encourage surgeons in their treatment of these emergencies, and defined the steps of the operation which are essential when one of these ulcers has perforated. There is no doubt the profession has been much indebted to that eminent surgeon for the manner in which he brought forward this subject. At that time the introducer of the discussion only knew of seven cases of successful operation for the closure of the perforation in a gastric ulcer. At the present time the diagnosis and main principles of treatment are so well understood that no surprise is expressed when recovery follows operation. Success is often attained.

The first operation for perforation of a gastric ulcer in St. Thomas's Hospital was done in 1892. This was not successful, but in August, 1896, a success was obtained for the first time. Forty-nine cases had been submitted to operation up to 1904, the ulcer being treated by suture and the peritoneum washed out : 58·1 per cent. recovered. The average time in the successful cases t at had elapsed between perforation and operation was 23 hours ; in the fatal cases 32·6 hours.

The results of operation in the second half of the period mentioned are better than in the first. Cases are recognised and sent into hospital earlier, and operation is more quickly and surely performed.

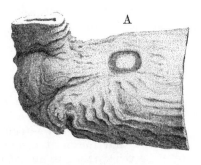

During the year 1910 the operative mortality after suture of perforated gastric ulcers was three out of fourteen, or 21 per cent. In all the anterior surface was affected, and the perforation was closed with sutures. The cause of death in the three cases

FIG. 23.—Acute Perforation of a Gastric Ulcer (A) (St. Thomas's Hospital Museum).

which did not recover was peritonitis, perisplenic abscess, and gastric hæmorrhage. Three cases which were admitted

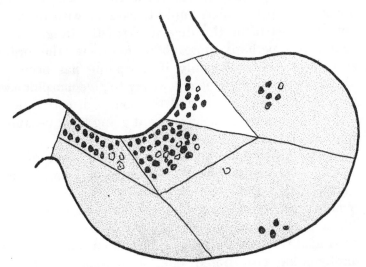

FIG. 24.—Stomach Perforations. Diagram to illustrate most common positions of Perforation. The dark circles indicate Anterior, and the clear circles Posterior, Perforations.

too late for operation died from general peritonitis. 1903–1912 inclusive, 116 cases, with 70 cures and 46 deaths.

In these perforations (most commonly occurring in women·

under 30 years of age) the symptoms which are grouped under the term " peritonism " are usually very marked, the sudden onset of pain causing signs of distress which are unmistakable. There is considerable variation as regards the amount of shock ; sometimes it is so excessive that nothing can save the patient. Shock is followed by collapse, and the patient may die in a few hours without response to medical treatment.

In the autumn of 1905 a girl was admitted ✗ with a history of sudden seizure of pain in the region of the stomach so severe that she screamed out, and had to be carried home from the tram from which she had just alighted.   When seen at the hospital half an hour later the diagnosis of gastric perforation was confirmed, but the state of shock was so profound that the most vigorous treatment, including saline infusion into the veins, failed to overcome this, and the patient died within six hours.   She was quite unconscious, made no resistance to abdominal examination. nor did she complain of pain.   There was a large perforation about the size of a penny in the anterior wall of the stomach near the pylorus.   A curious fact, noted at the necropsy, was the presence of extensive gaseous emphysema of the body a few hours after death.

As a rule the patient rallies from the shock, and other symptoms develop which resemble those met with in perforations of other parts of the digestive tract.   In gastric and duodenal cases, perhaps more than in others, the previous history is important, especially if morphine has been given recently to relieve pain.   It is not wrong to give morphine when the diagnosis has been made and the course of action decided upon, but there must be no subsequent going back because the patient " appears better."

In a large percentage there is vomiting soon after the perforation has occurred, but the absence of vomiting is not against the diagnosis of perforation.

Probably there is no form of the acute abdomen in which there is a greater amount of fluid to be found free in the peritoneum.   At operation, only a few hours after the onset of symptoms has been noted, one has been surprised to find the flanks and pelvis quite full of a thin greenish fluid, acid and sour-smelling.   This statement applies to cases in which the stomach was comparatively empty at the time, as well as to those in which the perforation occurred soon after a large meal.   Much of it is doubtless of a protective character, thrown out from the peritoneum covering the bowels and omentum in response to the irritation of the acid contents of the stomach.   In this respect it resembles very closely the condition which obtains soon after the sudden rupture of the wall of an abscess, hydatid or other cyst, where the escaped fluid floods the peritoneum.

Rigidity of the recti muscles in the upper part of the abdomen will be present, with great tenderness in the epigastric region.

In any case where there is a difficulty in diagnosis between a perforated gastric ulcer and an acute diffuse peritonitis secondary to a gangrenous appendix, the presence of much free fluid, as determined by percussion within a few hours after the commencement of symptoms, should compel a strong leaning towards the stomach as the site of the lesion which has caused the illness.   A tympanitic note over the liver region in an abdomen which is not distended may be an important additional proof, and is not infrequently observed in gastric perforations soon after the sudden onset of pain.   Its absence, however, must not be regarded as a reason for postponing operation in a case otherwise calling for it.   It was not present in the following instance of large perforation, in which the accident occurred although the patient was under exceptionally advantageous conditions, the stomach having had rest for two days.

A groom, aged 45, was admitted ✶ on September 30, 1904, with symptoms of gastric ulcer.   The history of the case was that he had often been sick in 1902 and 1903.   Vomiting occurred about half an hour after food, and the vomited material was very acid.   In January, 1904, he vomited a large amount of blood, which was quite black ; this vomiting recurred a few days later.   In July he had a similar attack of hæmatemesis.

When admitted he was suffering a good deal from pain in the epigastric region, and was obliged to lie on the left side.   The abdomen was normal in appearance, and with the exception of tenderness in the epigastrium was without evidence of disease.   He was sometimes unable to keep down milk.

During the next few days he complained at times of the severe pain, and hot fomentations were required for his relief.   Vomiting also occurred at intervals.   On October 22 it was decided to put him on rectal feeding and give nothing by the mouth. ·

At 2 a.m. on the 24th he had a severe attack of pain, perspired very freely, and his pulse rose to 120.

When seen with Dr. Mackenzie twelve hours later he was evidently suffering acutely.   Lying on his back, with head and shoulders raised, he looked pale, agitated, and intensely anxious, whilst his face and fore-head were covered with sweat. His respirations were hurried, painful, shallow, and irregular, the pulse rapid, and he complained much of pain in the abdomen ; he was unable to take a deep breath on account of the pain, and on examination of the abdomen it did not move much with respiration. It was generally tender, rigid, and rather distended. The liver dulness had not disappeared ; there was dulness in both flanks, also across the lower abdomen above the pubes. He had vomited. The temperature was 100·6°.

Operation was performed as soon as possible. On opening the peritoneum there was a flow of greenish thin sour-smelling fluid. The stomach was somewhat adherent to the under surface of the liver, and when they were separated by the finger there was a gush of free gas. The finger was passed to the pyloric region at once because of the diag-nosis of perforation of ulcer in that situation, made by Dr. Mackenzie. A sharply-cut ulcer, large enough to admit the forefinger, was found on the anterior surface of the pyloric end of the stomach. The stomach wall round this perforation was much thickened. The hole was closed with interrupted sutures. The peritoneal cavity appeared to be filled with the greenish fluid, there being large collections in the pelvis, the flanks, the subhepatic and splenic regions. A counter-opening was made above the pubes and the abdomen thoroughly washed out with normal saline. The intestines were not much distended.

The deposit of lymph was limited to the parts around the perforation. Normal saline to the amount of two pints was passed into the median basilic vein during the operation, as the pulse became very feeble and rapid. The stomach was a good deal dilated. The upper wound was closed and a glass drain placed in the lower one. Recovery was slow but satisfactory, and he left on December 7, 1904, for his home in Devonshire. The induration surrounding the ulcer compelled the infolding of an unusual amount of stomach wall.

I do not think authors of text-books, when writing of the diagnosis of gastric perforations, have paid sufficient attention to the valuable information to be obtained by percussion. In nearly every case the amount of free fluid present is con-siderable, and it can be detected quite early, accumulating in the flanks. It should not be possible for any case of acute abdominal pain to be introduced to the surgeon with the peritoneum full of fluid and no statement of its presence made. This excess of fluid helps us to place out of court such con-ditions as pneumonia, diaphragmatic pleurisy, thrombosis of the superior mesenteric vein, various kinds of poisoning, and acute dilatation of the stomach. There are four or five states of the acute abdomen in which we get an excess of fluid—perforated gastric (or duodenal) ulcer, rupture of an abscess (usually appendicular), rupture of extrauterine fœtation, ruptured pyo-salpinx, or the rupture of a large cyst. As a rare occurrence it is seen after the rupture of a large empyema of the appendix. A case in which there is reason to suspect gastric perforation, but about which you are not sure, should be carefully examined for the signs of free fluid, not only at the time when first seen, but every hour afterwards, for there are few emergencies that better repay prompt surgical attention.

Contrast with the case just described the following and the importance of what I have said will be evident :—

A nurse, aged 20, was admitted on November 28, 1913, having been sent up by Dr. Lock, of Uxbridge, for perforated gastric ulcer.

She had suffered from very bad indigestion at intervals during the past three months, and, having been on night duty, was in bed on the 26th in the afternoon, when she had a sudden severe pain in the epigastrium. She was very sick. The pain was better on the 27th and 28th, but she still had tenderness.

A somewhat chlorotic woman with flushed cheeks, and without any sign of anxiety. A pulse of 124, and respirations, 28 ; temperature, 100°. She complained of some pain in the abdomen, but of no great severity, and the sickness had not recurred. Her general condition was good. The abdomen was somewhat distended, generally tender, but not very markedly so, yet the muscles were rigid, and there was shifting dulness in the flanks. The tongue was furred and the bowels confined. There was a difference of opinion as to the absence of liver dulness, but the diagnosis was " a small perforation of the anterior wall of the stomach and considerable effusion in the peritoneum." It was somewhat difficult to convince the patient that she required immediate operation, because she did not feel very ill.

It was not easy to find the perforation, for no gas or fluid escaped during the search, and it was only by examination of a small patch of lymph with a small probe that it could be found ; even then it was not possible to force fluid through it from within the stomach by any kind of pressure. This opening was in a patch of thickening about the size of a florin to the left of the middle line near the lesser curvature and was covered in by interrupted Lembert sutures. The fluid in the general peritoneal cavity was purulent, especially in the pelvis, and generally diffused, but contained no traces of food. It was washed away with sterilised saline, through a drain in a suprapubic opening. The upper opening was closed ; a drainage tube was left in Douglas's pouch. Uninterrupted recovery.

The operation for perforation of a gastric ulcer may be divided into three parts :—

(1) The abdominal incisions ; (2) the finding and treatment of the ulcer ; (3) the cleansing of the peritoneum.

In preparation for the operation it may be necessary to do a great deal to combat the shock and bring the patient into a condition to bear the required manipulation. The usual preparation of the skin with iodine is advisable, and the surgeon must remember to have the hair of the abdomen and suprapubic region shaved. This part of the preparation is apt to be overlooked. The upper incision is made first, should be about 4 inches or more in length, and is made in the epigastrium, from the left costo-xiphoid angle downwards to the left of the middle line. Before the peritoneum is opened it may bulge irregularly into the wound from the gas which has collected behind it, which bubbles up when this layer is incised. There may be none if the case is an early one and the perforation small. The amount of fluid is very variable, usually of a mawkish smell from gastric juice, and acid in reaction ; there are frequently particles of half-digested food in it, according to the size of the perforation, the character of the last meal, and the time which has elapsed since it was taken. In cases where there is much fluid it is a good plan to pass the hand through the upper wound to the under surface of the hypogastric region, cut down on it, and place a tube in the pelvis ; the fluid can then run away under an aseptic pad whilst the necessary manipulation of the stomach is being carried on.

As the perforation is most commonly on the anterior surface near the lesser curvature, this is the part which should be examined in the first place. The stomach should be firmly but gently pulled downwards, whilst the fluid is mopped away as it comes from the opening, that already in the peritoneum being kept back and partly absorbed with wide strips of gauze. Sometimes the opening is temporarily blocked by a particle of food, but as a rule there is an increasing flow of fluid with bubbles of gas as a result of the increased tension when it is pulled upon.

If the opening is small or concealed by lymph, a more careful search may be necessary, but the injection of air into the stomach by means of an œsophageal tube as an aid to localisation is not either advisable or necessary. Abnormal redness of the surface, the presence of a patch of lymph, or the discovery of a hard plaque of tissue, when the perforation

is small, may indicate it.   Any recent adhesions between the
stomach and liver should be separated and folds opened out.
If the stomach is much dilated, filling up the epigastric region,
it should be emptied, either through the perforation or through
an œsphageal tube.   If distended intestine causes difficulty
it may be punctured with a trochar or the point of a knife and
the puncture closed with a stitch.   The sutures to close the

perforation should be of
silk, interrupted, sero-
muscular, and passed
after the method of
Lembert.   If escaping
contents cause embar-
rassment a stitch or two
may be inserted across
the opening.   As a rule
No. 1 silk is satisfactory
for the sutures, but if the
stomach wall is softened
No. 2 should be used.   I
have found a single row
of these sufficient, but
they should penetrate as
deeply as the submucous
layer and extend well
beyond the perforation.
As a rule they should be
passed from side to side,
especially in the region
of the pylorus, to avoid
narrowing of the outlet.
All should be inserted

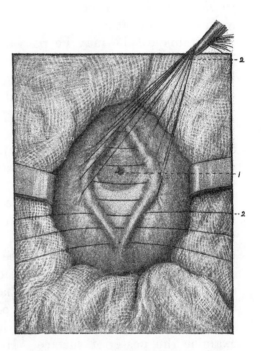

Fig. 25.—Perforation of Gastric Ulcer.
Insertion of sutures where there is
much thickening of the base (1).
Sutures bringing a ridge of sero-
muscular tissue across the ulcer without tension.

before they are tied, and if there is any doubt of their hold on the
stomach wall reinforcing sutures should be put over them.   In
small perforations a continuous Lembert suture may be used ;
whenever this is feasible the suturing should be performed
with the viscus outside the wound, resting on sterilised gauze
moistened with warm saline.   When the perforation is in a
fixed part, suturing must be done with the stomach *in situ ;*
here the wound must be well opened out with retractors, and

it may be found necessary to cut the left rectus, although this should not be lightly done. Where there is an opening in an indurated area which will not hold stitches you must bring a fold of stomach over it from the cardiac side and suture that securely to the parts beyond the induration.

When the condition of the patient, the position of the ulcer, or the large area of induration makes it impossible to close the perforation as advised, there are various courses open to the operator.

A drainage tube may be passed down to the opening and gauze packing placed round it for some thirty-six hours. It may be possible to cover the opening by suturing some omentum over it, or the liver may be utilised in this manner.

A gastro-jejunostomy may be performed to diminish the leakage from the wound, but it must be remembered that although the amount in the upper abdomen may seem small, there may be a considerable quantity of fluid in the pelvis.

So far I have spoken of the perforation of ulcers on the anterior surface of the stomach, for perforation is most commonly met with as a complication of these anterior ones. The posterior rarely perforate into a free portion of the peritoneum, owing to the tendency of adhesions to form between the surface of the stomach and the pancreas. If the history of the case points to a perforation, and none can be found on the anterior surface or along the lesser curvature, you must examine the posterior surface. Here there will probably be little fluid present in front of the stomach when the abdomen is opened, but search may reveal small bubbles of gas under the peritoneum as it leaves the greater curvature of the stomach. This perforation can be attacked through—(1) the gastro-hepatic omentum, which readily yields and gives direct access to the area usually affected, or (2) by tearing through the gastro-colic omentum. The route chosen will depend on the difficulties of the individual case and the position of the ulcer ; in many the route above the stomach will give the easier access. The finger pressing on the anterior wall readily brings the lesion into view.

The following is a case of perforation of an ulcer on the posterior surface of the stomach.

M. J., aged 25, engaged in a laundry, was admitted ☨ January 2 and left on February 10, 1911.

She gave a history of three to four years indigestion, pain and discomfort after meals. On three occasions during the past three years she has had acute attacks of pain similar to the present, and has been ill in bed for some time afterwards. During the last three weeks she has had more pain than usual and has " had the wind " badly. About 9 p.m. the day before admission the pain was so bad that it doubled her up and she had to go to bed. There was much shock. She did not vomit until the morning of admission ; and the symptoms when she came in were probably influenced by morphine, which had been given before her journey to hospital.

She was drowsy and her general expression placid ; the pupils were small. Pulse, 128 ; temperature, 101·6°. The tongue was very dry and coated. The abdomen was moving poorly, was generally distended and rigid. It was extremely tender all over. On percussion there was an area of dulness in the left flank below the spleen, which shifted on movement. Friction could be heard over the left chest in front ; liver dulness present at the side. On making an incision over the stomach a little gas escaped, but not much fluid. Nothing abnormal was seen on the anterior surface, but as fluid with flakes in it and small bubbles of gas was coming through a small hole in the gastrocolic omentum this opening was enlarged and the posterior surface explored. A perforation was found near the lesser curvature towards the pyloric end ; it was surrounded by an indurated area the size of a sixpence. It was shut in by means of two rows of silk Lembert sutures. The lesser sac was washed out as well as the general cavity, and tubes were left in, one being passed into the lesser sac, the other into Douglas's pouch. Convalescence was retarded by an attack of pneumonia in the left lung. There was some discharge of a purulent nature from the lower wound for a fortnight.

We have placed considerable stress on the need for careful suturing ; it is now necessary to emphasise the need for thorough treatment of the peritoneum. The pelvis must always be examined, for although the amount of fluid is small in the upper abdomen, there may be a considerable accumulation in the pelvis. Irrigation is required in most cases of gastric perforation, because of the partly-digested food producte which have escaped and the irritating effect of the fluid with which they are mixed. Without this it is almost impossible to get rid of the various particles which have been swept into the outlying parts of the peritoneum. The fluid used should be sterilised saline (sodium chloride ʒj., boiled water Oj.) at a temperature of 105°. If no irrigator is at hand a glass tube, or the end of an œsophagus tube, attached to indiarubber tubing (recently boiled) arranged as a syphon or attached to a funnel, will serve the purpose. Failing these an ordinary Higginson syringe worked by an assistant, whilst the surgeon performs the needful manipulation of the parts. If, however, the case is quite early and the extravasation limited, irriga- tion may be unnecessary and a limited cleansing by means of moist swabs suffice, but as a rule, in my opinion, a combina- tion of the two is required if there are many food particles in the peritoneum. Try to cleanse the peritoneum from above downwards, and make certain that the hepatic and splenic regions are cleared early ; the amount of fluid in those parts is often very large, and trouble may arise there from septic infection after the operation.

Some pints of saline will be required and irrigation should be continued until the fluid comes away clear. There is no need to dry the peritoneum ; it does good to leave clear fluid of this nature to be absorbed. The necessity for drainage depends upon the particular case : if operation has been early, and the amount of extravasation is small and limited, the abdominal wound may be closed ; in the majority of cases it will be advisable to drain.

The "Fowler position" should be adopted as soon as the patient has recovered from the anæsthetic.

Before the patient leaves the operation table a rectal injec- tion of sterilised saline with an ounce of brandy should be given, and the use of continuous saline *per rectum* should be commenced a short time afterwards.

There is no objection to the administration of sips of tepid water by the mouth, but nothing else should be given for the first forty-eight hours. If there is much complaint of pain, and the patient is very restless or unable to sleep, a sub- cutaneous injection of morphine may be given, but it is to be avoided if possible.

The treatment above advised is best calculated to prevent the more common causes of death after this accident— peritonitis, shock, subdiaphragmatic abscess. There are two complications which cannot be guarded against :— (1) Perforation of a second ulcer, stated by Finney to be present in 20 per cent. of the cases. The occurrence of a second perforation in the same ulcer when it is large.

(2) Hæmorrhage may occur from the same ulcer, or another near it.

Subacute Perforations.—By this is meant the occurrence of a very small perforation so that only a little fluid escapes, which may be walled off by adhesions. This may happen in gastric and duodenal ulcers, the pus forming around the perforation. The abscess may gradually extend if untreated and eventually attain a large size. If in connection with a duodenal perforation, bile may appear in the discharges. Should they rupture into the general peritoneal cavity, the result will probably be fatal, as it is almost impossible to find, or isolate, the leaking point (see *Perigastric Abscess*, p. 141).

PERFORATIONS OF DUODENAL ULCERS.

These ulcers are far less frequently met with than the gastric, and it is not always possible to diagnose the one from the other. They are far more common in males over 30 than in females, but Mr. J. W. Struthers[1] had to operate for this perforation under the age of 20 in two instances, and only 1 in 27 was a female. Osler says they may be distinguished by the following definite characters :—

" (*a*) Sudden intestinal hæmorrhage in an apparently healthy person, which tends to recur and produce a profound anæmia. Hæmorrhage from the stomach may precede or accompany the melæna. (*b*) Pain in the right hypochondriac region, coming on two or three hours after eating. (*c*) Gastric crises of extreme violence, during which the hæmorrhage is more apt to occur. Certainly the occurrence of sudden intestinal hæmorrhage, with gastralgic attacks, is extremely suggestive of duodenal ulcer."

Unfortunately, in many cases, there is no history of local pain preceding the attack.

It is advisable to speak of this variety of perforation separately from the gastric, because it is often difficult to distinguish perforations of these ulcers from acute disease of the appendix with peritonitis, especially if the appendix is situated to the outer side of the cæcum, or has never attained its proper position in the iliac region.

When the perforation is that of an ulcer of the stomach, the symptoms are those of a general peritoneal invasion ; when

[1] Edinburgh Medico-Chirurgical Society, *Lancet*, Vol. II., 1912, p. 1371.

the perforation is in the duodenum, the escaping fluid, which rarely contains solid particles, flows down the right side, external to the colon, into the pelvis. In these cases, therefore, the resemblance of the attack to one of acute perforative appendicitis is very close, and a mistake in diagnosis has been made by the most experienced. Mr. Struthers,[1] in relating his series of 27 cases, says that in three of them the pain was referred chiefly to the right iliac fossa, and the maximum tenderness and resistance was below the umbilicus on the right side, but the temperature and pulse-rate were not markedly raised.

Moynihan states that in 51 cases collected by him a correct diagnosis was only made in two, whereas the primary incision was made over the appendix in 19.

At the time of operation the appendix may be found surrounded by an area of inflamed peritoneum, and may be itself so inflamed that the surgeon is misled. It would be well, therefore, always to examine the duodenum in its first part, when disease of the appendix is not manifested by gross naked-eye change, such as gangrene or perforation.

Do not forget to examine the pelvis for extravasated fluid ; failure to do so in any case of perforation may prove fatal, whether the ulcer be of the stomach (anterior or posterior surface) or other part of the digestive tract.

The following case is typical :—

A cabman, aged 39, was admitted ✕ on June 13, 1907, complaining of much pain in the abdomen. He had suffered from pain in the epigastrium for ten years, coming on about an hour after food ; also from a feeling of distension and flatulence, but had never had any vomiting. The attacks had come " off and on." Six weeks before admission he had noticed that his motions were black. At midnight on June 12 he had taken a glass of beer, the drinking of which was followed immediately by violent pain in the abdomen. This was especially severe over the pubes. He vomited one and a half hours afterwards, was in great pain all night, and had constant aching pain in the right shoulder.

On admission he was in a condition of collapse, with a pulse of 140 and temperature of 99°. There was marked tenderness all over, but more especially down the right side, and dulness in both flanks. The muscles of the abdomen were very tense. Sixteen and a half hours after perforation an epigastric incision gave exit to a gush of fluid and gas, whilst another incision over the hypogastric region gave freedom

[1] Edinburgh Medico-Chirurgical Society, *Lancet,* Vol. I., 1912, p. 1371.

to much more. The ulcer was found in the first part of the duodenum. Saline infusion was required during the operation, and had to be repeated later in the day. On June 29 a subdiaphragmatic abscess was opened, after resection of part of a rib. He left hospital quite well on July 31.

There was the sudden onset of abdominal pain (which is usually most severe above and to the right of the umbilicus), with marked shock, followed by vomiting. He had had no latent interval, but the symptoms which precede the onset of a peritonitis were definite. Bile-stained fluid may be found in these cases, and the sutures (of No. 1 silk) should be put in by Lembert's method in the axis of the canal. A limited irrigation should be employed, a drainage tube placed in the pelvis, and saline commenced at once, by the usual method of administration *per rectum*. Mr. Struthers does not consider irrigation required, but advocates drainage for the first twenty-four hours or more. As it is advisable to put a drainage tube into the pelvis, no harm is done by making the preliminary incision in the lower abdomen to examine the appendix. A diagnosis of intestinal obstruction has been made, but the rigidity, fixation and tenderness (especially evident on the right side), and the incompleteness of the constipation may serve to prevent this error in most instances.

The advisability of performing a gastro-enterostomy must be considered whenever operation for perforated gastric or duodenal ulcer is performed, but the number of cases in which this addition to the gravity of the other operation can be made is limited. To do it in some would be to ensure the death of the patient, and there are few in which it can be said to be required " there and then " to save life. A secondary operation can be performed with safety later, should symptoms demand it. It is the ulcer of, or near, the pylorus which is most likely to lead to contraction, but the suturing of a perforation should never diminish the passage to such an extent as to render a gastro-enterostomy a matter of urgency.

At the present day there is perhaps a tendency to do too much, for the surgeon naturally wishes to place his patient in the best position for complete recovery, and that without further operation. Much will depend on the condition of the patient, the duration of the illness, and the way in which the anæsthetic is tolerated.

Should the surgeon think it right to perform a gastro-
enterostomy the anterior method will be the one chosen. It
can be quickly performed and does not involve much disturbance of parts. The anastomosis should be made towards the
pyloric end, and near the greater curvature of the stomach.
Let the communication between them be fully two inches in
length, and about 18 inches from the commencement of the

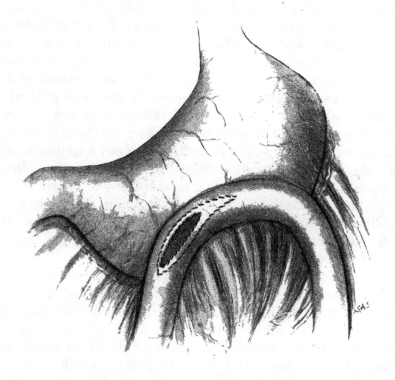

FIG. 26.—To Illustrate the Relations between Jejunum and Stomach
in the Operation of Anterior Gastro-Enterostomy.

jejunum. The clamps should be applied obliquely so that the
opening slopes from the left downwards to the right, and it is
advisable to apply the outer suture for some distance above
the inner row to prevent kinking of the loop, although the
application of one or two extra sutures to hold the left
extremity of the curve of the loop in position will answer the
same purpose. This anastomosis is performed in a manner
similar to that described under entero-anastomosis (p. 280).

It is not necessary to impress upon the reader the value of

muscular rigidity in the acute abdomen as a proof that a grave lesion has occurred within. This rigidity is a very important sign of perforation, the abdomen being often literally as hard as a board, and in the diagnosis from other acute states it must be specially looked for and its variation in different areas noted.

The acute diseases which are likely to be mistaken for perforations of the stomach and duodenum are mainly the following :—

(1) *Acute pancreatitis* resembles perforation of a gastric or duodenal ulcer very closely at times ; there is the same onset, with severe pain, vomiting, and collapse. If this is soon followed by exudation into the peritoneal cavity of a large quantity of fluid the resemblance is very great. Usually, however, the pain remains very intense in the upper abdomen, dulness on percussion is patchy, and there is a general superficial tenderness without very marked rigidity. A rise of temperature is frequent. The patient is usually a male, stout and over middle age.

As showing the difficulty occasionally encountered the following case may be quoted :—

A motor-cab driver, aged 33, was sitting on his cab outside one of the large cricket grounds waiting for a fare, when he was suddenly taken with a severe pain in the upper abdomen and vomited. He was subject to indigestion and had taken food shortly before. He was a stout man. On admission twenty-four hours later he was evidently very ill, suffering from severe pain and tenderness in the epigastric region ; had a pulse-rate 68, laboured respiration, and temperature 97°. The abdomen was moving badly, and there was abnormal resistance to pressure ; in addition there was slight dulness in the flanks.

Operation was performed shortly after admission, but the fluid, of which there was a large quantity, was blood-stained, and after a search fat necrosis of the omentum was found. The abdomen was washed out, and a drainage tube packed off with gauze was passed down to the pancreas through an opening in the gastro-colic omentum. He was relieved of his pain, but died suddenly the fifth day of illness, with temperature 103°, rapid cardiac failure and delirium.

No tumour could be felt before operation. Cammidge's reaction was positive.

(2) *Acute Intestinal Obstruction.*—Here there is vomiting which continues, complete constipation, and paroxysmal pain, with a peristalsis which can be seen or felt. Distension

soon comes on, but between the paroxysms of pain there is no rigidity.

In the sudden onset of gall-stone obstruction due to a large stone in the duodenum, there may be difficulty for a time, for the pain is high up and not accompanied with intestinal peristalsis. There is no free fluid.

(3) *Ruptured Extra-uterine Gestation.*—The following case will illustrate clearly the difficulty sometimes caused by this mischance.

E. S., a married woman aged 31, was admitted ✶ on December 1, 1913, and left St. Thomas's Hospital January 2, 1914. She had suffered from indigestion for many years, with pains coming on about fifteen minutes after taking food. She had never brought up any blood. It was between seven and eight weeks past the last period. At 7 a.m. on the day of admission she was seized with violent pains in and across the abdomen, chiefly in the epigastrium. These pains were of a shooting character and reached right up to the shoulder region behind. She was sick twice during the day, and the pains became worse every hour. The woman looked ill, but not distressed ; the cheeks were pale, but the lips not blanched. Her pulse was small, 108 ; respirations, 36 ; temperature, 98·2°. She still complained of pain in the abdomen. This was distended, did not move well on respiration, and there was general but not very marked rigidity. She had diffuse tenderness, especially on the left side of the abdomen, where there appeared to be some greater distension. There was greater resistance to palpation in the left loin, but no tumour. On percussion there was dulness in both flanks, but this was more marked on the left side, and extended into the splenic region, and also across above the pubes. The tongue was furred ; breath offensive ; bowels not open. She complained of great thirst, but was not particularly restless. There was no vaginal discharge ; but the uterus was larger than normal.

Dr. Wilson Stoker was present at the operation, which took place about midnight. An incision was made in the lower abdomen to the left of the mid-line and the rectus muscle displaced to the left. The pelvis and lower abdomen were full of blood, and large clots were removed from the pelvis. The tubes on both sides were quickly lifted and examined, but showed no evidence of disease or change of any kind. The uterus was somewhat enlarged, and just beyond the attachment of the left Fallopian tube was a depression which would admit the tip of a forefinger, from which arterial blood was trickling into the pelvis ; this was removed with the tube and ovary after ligature of the attachments close to the uterus. The blood continued to come from above after the pelvis had been emptied, and there was a large quantity about the spleen which had not clotted and looked quite fresh. With this large amount in the upper abdomen where, according to the patient, she had first felt pain, it was considered advisable to make certain that there was no source for the bleeding in the stomach region. An incision was quickly made in the middle line above the umbilicus, and although there was much blood and blood-clots still about the spleen, nothing was found in addition to the small opening in the Fallopian tube to account for it. During this epigastric examination the pulse failed and it was necessary to rapidly close both incisions with interrupted sutures of strong fishgut. There was no time to wash away all the blood which had accumulated, but some saline was left in the peritoneum, which was drained through both wounds. The blood seemed to have penetrated everywhere. Sterilised saline was passed into the median basilic vein during the operation, and, although very little blood escaped from the ruptured tube, after the abdomen was opened she seemed to rapidly fail as blood which had previously got into the peritoneum was removed.

The foot of the bed was raised, the limbs bandaged with flannel, and warm water-bottles applied. Saline *per rectum* with some brandy was given. The pulse gradually improved and she made good progress. A vaginal discharge appeared in a day or two and required treatment. Little came away from the drainage tubes, which were soon removed, but the temperature was irregularly raised for nearly three weeks.

(4) *Acute Appendicitis.*—The usual symptoms of an acute attack of appendicitis have already been given somewhat freely, so it is unnecessary to refer fully to this part of the subject again.

A history of previous attacks with pain in the usual situation, and accompanied by fever, would indicate that there has been a diseased appendix, but the variety which is most likely to simulate the perforation of a gastric ulcer is that of a first attack with gangrene secondary to a concretion in an adult, in which there has been an unsuccessful attempt to localise the pus. Even here the amount of fever would probably contra-indicate gastric perforation. The age of the patient and the position of greatest tenderness and greatest degree of muscular rigidity are helpful, yet it is possible that the appendix has never descended into the iliac fossa but is still subhepatic.

When it is a first attack of appendicitis, there is also a history of gastric ulcer, a distinct statement that the pain began in the epigastric region, and much free fluid, the diagnosis is impossible.

E. W., a married woman, aged 33, was admitted on February 20 and left for a convalescent home on April 9, 1914.

On February 18 she was suddenly seized with severe pain in the epigastric region when lying in bed in the early morning. She vomited, and the vomiting was repeated three times, whilst the pain did not greatly improve and was also bad in the right lower abdomen. The bowels had acted after an enema.

For two years she had suffered from pain in the upper part of the abdomen, coming on about half an hour after meals and followed by sickness, which relieved it. There had also been hæmatemesis on occasions.

When first seen she was in a condition of collapse and required stimulation to restore her. She looked very ill. The abdomen was motionless on respiration, not much distended, but rigid áll over, more especially on the right side, with marked general tenderness. There was considerable dulness in the flanks and on the right side this extended up to the liver. The temperature was 102° and pulse 96 (small).

As there was the history of gastric ulcer, and the pain commenced in the gastric region, whilst with general rigidity and tenderness there was much fluid, it was decided to explore the stomach for possible perforation. On opening the peritoneum very little fluid was seen; the anterior surface of the stomach was normal, but as a hard patch could be felt on the posterior surface below the lesser curvature, this was examined by turning the stomach up. Through an opening below the greater curvature the congested base of an ulcer the size of a sixpenny bit was exposed, but there was no perforation. It was covered in with some Lembert sutures, but the posterior sac was empty. Exploration in the gall-bladder region gave exit to a large quantity of watery-looking pus with some flakes of lymph, but without offensive odour. The hand passed into the appendix region did not find any induration, but the pelvis was full of pus, which passed into the left flank. The intestines were not distended and the pelvic organs were normal. Although there was no thickening in the region of the cæcum, it was possible to feel some irregularity of surface, and exploration made through a suprapubic drainage incision (extended for this purpose) showed a gangrenous appendix which had given way. This was about 3½ inches long and gangrenous in the distal two-thirds. A ligature was applied, but the peritoneum was not sutured over it. Dr. Gardner reported that the *bacillus pyocyaneus* was the principal organism present in the pus removed. Operation relieved her pain and she looked much better next day. On March 10 a note was made to the effect that the temperature had continued high (about 102° in the evening) with a pulse of about 100 to 120. Suppuration had occurred in both incisions, and an investigation of the pus showed the *bacillus pyocyaneus*. A vaccine was made and given on February 25 and again on March 2, with a slight effect on both occasions. On March 8 the lower wound began to discharge more freely. There was evidence of pleuritic effusion at the left base.

A fortnight later there was still some fever, although the wounds had closed for some time and nothing abnormal could be found anywhere, except at the left base. No signs of mischief remained at the end of another week.

(5) *Hysteria.*—An attack of hysteria may simulate perforation sufficiently near to mislead. At p. 233 is the account of

the case of a young nurse who was operated on for epigastric pain and vomiting, supposed to be due to perforation. In a later simulation we found no rigidity of muscles, a moderate pulse-rate, and a smiling face, although she had " great agony " and vomiting. Dr. Beddard has recorded somewhat similar attacks in chlorotic women, in two of whom operation had been performed twice.

(6) *Perforation of the gall-bladder* closely simulates perforation of gastric and duodenal ulcer. Here there will probably be a history of gall-stone colic, sometimes with jaundice. The tenderness would be in the region of the gall-bladder, and incision would be required over that part. I have known an acute biliary colic due to gall-stones in a young chlorotic female resemble perforation very closely at its onset.

(7) In *lead-colic* there would be other symptoms of lead poisoning, and may be a history of previous attacks, but the first attack, as also the first of the gastric *crises* of tabes dorsalis, might present some difficulty.

(8) Rarer conditions which require mention but need not be particularly discussed are acute dilatation of the stomach, thrombosis of the mesenteric vessels, irritant poisoning, and pneumonia. Of these the only one which requires a special notice is the last ; we have already referred to it in speaking of the resemblance of acute pulmonary inflammation to an attack of acute appendicitis. An illustration of this close resemblance may be given.

. A. S., aged 20, admitted ✳ February 8 and left March 12, 1913. The day before he was feeling bad with general pains about the body, vomited, and could not breathe properly. He gave a history of a month's dyspepsia, and complained of acute pain in the abdomen which had commenced ten hours before. He had been treated for an attack of appendicitis ten years before. He looked very ill, his lips were white, and he appeared almost collapsed. He complained of right-sided abdominal pain ; had a pulse 130, and temperature 103·8° ; respirations, 20.

The abdomen was quite motionless on respiration. The recti on both sides were very rigid. On palpation tenderness was present, confined to the right side ; in the upper abdomen it was very pronounced, whilst there was some slight tenderness in the right iliac fossa. Nothing could be felt in the abdomen on account of its extreme rigidity and tenderness. There was no distension or abnormal dulness. The respiratory movements were almost entirely thoracic and rather shallow.

Some pain was complained of on the right side of the abdomen on deep inspiration. No abnormal signs were present anywhere over the lungs.

An epigastric incision was made and both surfaces of the stomach examined. The appendix was then removed, it was kinked, but showed no other evidence of disease. A large round worm could be felt in the small intestine. There was no free fluid in pelvis or in flanks, but a small quantity was found between the stomach and anterior wall of the abdomen. On the following day he still had some pain in the abdomen, but had passed a fair night. The pulse had improved. At 11.30 it had changed and was now 160, but improved after injection of camphor and rectal saline. At 3.30 p.m. the pulse was 146 and respirations 44, and he coughed up some rusty sputum. At 11.30 p.m. : " there are now definite signs of inflammation at the lower part of the right lung posteriorly."

On the 24th he succeeded in bursting open the wounds as a result of his violent coughing, and it was necessary to resuture.

Both lungs became affected, but no further abdominal complication ensued. The temperature became normal on the twelfth day.

PERFORATIONS OF GASTRO-JEJUNAL AND JEJUNAL ULCERS.

The knowledge that an ulceration of the jejunum is one of the causes of the acute abdomen which must be considered by the surgeon of the present day was due in the first place to Brauns. In 1899 he met with a case in which an ulcer of that part of the small intestine perforated and produced a fatal peritonitis eleven months after a gastro-jejunostomy for pyloric stenosis in a man aged 25. In this instance the operation had been by the posterior method, and the ulcer was found at the necropsy. Since that time there have been recorded many cases in which ulceration of the jejunum has required surgical treatment, and in all of them the operation of gastro-enterostomy had been performed for the relief of some form of gastric ulceration, or a result of it. From a clinical point of view they may be divided into two classes—the chronic and the acute perforative. In the former we are most likely to get an ulcer which will produce local symptoms before perforation into the peritoneum, if it does perforate ; in the latter no warning is given, but if the patient has previously had a perforation of a stomach ulcer he thinks that a similar accident has occurred again. I have purposely refrained from using the term " peptic " as applied to these ulcers, for it is not proved that they are *all* of them due to hyperacidity of the gastric juice ; indeed, in more than one the state of the gastric juice has been definitely described as normal.   The appearance in three out of the four perforations of this kind that have been under my personal notice was similar to that of some acute perforated gastric or duodenal ulcers.   They also resembled the ulcer in two cases of perforation of the ileum during the course of typhoid fever,[1] to which I shall refer later (see p. 182) ;   the naked-eye appearances were quite similar.   Some of these ulcers are probably due to an acute bacterial invasion, but I do not think the term " peptic " should be used.   It is an interesting fact, however, that they are only met with after the operation of gastro-jejunostomy, and chiefly after the anterior operation—for example, out of some 77 cases 52 followed anterior gastro-jejunostomy.[2]   In the paper here referred to a collection of 100 cases has been made.

The most startling complication of jejunal ulcer is acute perforation when the patient is apparently quite well in health, and in this, as in other complications, it resembles simple ulcers of the other parts of the digestive tract.   This accident happened in 21 patients, but inasmuch as in two of them it occurred twice at considerable intervals, 23 instances are now known.   Operation performed at the earliest opportunity was successful in saving life on nine occasions (Goepel, 2 [3] ; Hybrinette, 1 [4] ;   Maylard, 2 [5] ;   Battle, 4).   This improved record of results for operation makes it appear that operation for that accident has rendered it less dangerous than the slow extension of an ulcer which is shut off from the peritoneum by means of adhesions.   The formation of a localised abscess is known to follow at times, and may lead to an intestinal fistula, but it may be necessary to operate for the local ulceration, on account of the troublesome symptoms which it causes. This has involved resection of the ulcerated bowel, the jejunal end being placed into the stomach and the duodenal end into the side of the jejunum lower down.

The cases which have been under my treatment are as follows :—

[1] *Lancet*, 1903, Vol. II., p. 863.
[2] *Universal Medical Record*, Moynihan, January, 1912.
[3] " Kongress bericht," 1902, p. 10.
[4] *Revue de Chirurgie*, 1906, p. 30.
[5] *Lancet*, 1910, Vol. I.

A clerk, aged 30, was admitted July 15, 1904, for acute abdominal
distress.   He stated that about four hours before admission he had been
seized with violent pain in the abdomen, vomiting and hiccough.

On admission the abdomen was moderately distended and did not
move on respiration.   A rounded prominence was visible in the epigastrium, and immediately below this another and smaller prominence,
the latter being situated immediately above the umbilicus.   Distension
was most marked in the epigastric and umbilical regions, and there was
obvious fulness of the flanks.   There was no hyperæsthesia of the skin,
but considerable, yet not intense, tenderness.   No definite tumour
could be felt.   The resonance was impaired in both flanks, but no fluid
thrill could be felt, nor was the dulness a shifting one.   Elsewhere the
note was of a tympanitic character, this being especially marked in the
epigastric region.   The liver dulness was obliterated, the note over the
region of the liver being decidedly tympanitic.   The general condition
of the patient was good.   Temperature, 98°; pulse, 100; respirations, 20.

The presence of a scar in the abdominal wall caused questions to be
asked about previous operation, and the following history was obtained,
some of which was subsequently verified.   He had suffered from
indigestion after he became 16 years old, and three years before was
much troubled with vomiting from a quarter of an hour to two hours
after food, and on one or two occasions he brought up blood.   Twenty-
two months previously he had undergone an operation in Birmingham,
for pyloric obstruction after gastric ulcer.   Anterior gastro-enterostomy
was performed, a Murphy's button being used to approximate the
parts.   His progress after this operation was uninterruptedly good
until March 4, 1904, when he was seized with pain in the abdomen, and
had to go into the hospital again for "obstruction"; at this operation
the Murphy's button was removed.

At the operation, which was performed about five hours after the
commencement of the symptoms of perforation, an incision was made
to the left of the middle line above the umbilicus through the rectus
sheath, the muscle being displaced outwards.   There was a rush of gas
when the peritoneum was opened and a greatly distended coil of bowel
presented; this was punctured to diminish its size and gain more room
and emptied of much gas.   The opening was closed with Lembert silk
sutures and the coil returned.   The stomach, which was much distended,
was drawn into the wound; the point of attachment of the small
intestine to the gastric wall was defined, and a small round perforating
ulcer, about ⅛ inch in diameter, located in the anterior part of the
jejunum at a distance 1¼ inch from the point of attachment of the
latter to the stomach.   The stomach and the upper part of the jejunum
were as far as possible emptied of gas through the ulcer, and this was
then turned in with a single row of Lembert sutures.   The coils of
jejunum in the immediate neighbourhood of the perforation were greatly
distended, thickened, and of a dull red colour.   A small amount of free
purulent fluid was present in the abdominal cavity, with patches of
lymph on the intestinal coils.   A second incision was made in the

middle line above the pubes and the peritoneal cavity thoroughly irrigated with normal saline solution.   A Keith's drainage tube was then inserted into the pelvis through the lower incision, and the upper wound closed.   The man's general condition at the end of the opeiation was satisfactory.

There is not much to record in the after progress of the case.   He was sick three times during the night following the operation, bringing up each time large quantities of greenish fluid.   In the morning a turpentine enema was administered with a very good result.   Sulphate of magnesium (two teaspoonfuls) was given every four hours.   The abdomen was very slightly distended and not very tender, it moved to some extent with respiration, though not freely.   Pulse, 104 ; respirations, 20.

The bowels acted on the following day, the abdominal distension subsided, he became much more comfortable, and towards night the sickness ceased.   The Keith's tube was replaced by a rubber one of smaller size, there being very little discharge.   Two days later this was removed altogether.   He left the hospital on August 8, having completely recovered.

The second case was a very interesting one, being almost unique from the course of the various conditions for which operation was required.

An unmarried woman, aged 37, was admitted ✳ on March 25, 1903,[1] with symptoms of perforated gastric ulcer, which had commenced four and a half hours before.   Operation was performed at 11.15 p.m., and an ulcer near the pylorus and on the anterior surface was found and sutured, the peritoneal cavity washed out and the pelvis drained.   At the operation it was noted that there was already a good deal of narrowing of the pylorus.   She left hospital on May 12 and continued well until October, after which gastric pains recurred.   She was readmitted in April, 1904, and anterior-gastro-jejunostomy performed.   The stomach was dilated, the lower border reaching the level of the umbilicus. The pylorus was much constricted.   The operation was on the 8th, and she left hospital on April 28.

She regarded herself as cured until May 5, 1905, when she was again sent to the hospital by Dr. J. Scott Battams.

About six hours before admission she had a severe attack of pain, especially on the right side of the abdomen, with vomiting.   The bowels had acted twice that day.

In the ward the abdomen did not appear distended and moved freely on respiration.   The resonance was normal in all parts.   Pulse, 72 ; temperature, normal.   There was slight tenderness all over the abdomen, more evident above and to the left of the umbilicus.

She vomited two or three times during the night.   On the morning of the 6th the temperature had been up to 99·4°, and a distended coil of small intestine was seen above and to the left of the umbilicus.   There

---

[1] .Transactions R. Soc. Med., June, 1909.

was tenderness as before, but it was more marked over the distended coil.

When seen by me at 2 p.m. the condition was much as above described, but the distension of the small intestine in the umbilical region was greater, and there was visible peristalsis.

Operation was performed twenty-three hours after the first onset of pain, the abdomen being opened through the left rectus sheath about an inch from the middle line. A red and distended coil of small intestine presented which, traced upwards, led to the old gastro-enterostomy junction ; from this a greatly distended coil passed downwards, on the anterior aspect of which, 1⅓ inch from the line of junction, was a rounded opening from which gas and intestinal contents were escaping. The coils near were inflamed, œdematous and distended, there being lymph on the surfaces near the perforation. A knife was introduced through the ulcer and a cut made upwards, so that the line of junction between the stomach and intestine could be explored ; the finger passed easily into the stomach and then into the jejunum beyond the line of junction. There had been no contraction of the opening. After the distended coils had been emptied, the incision was closed with Lembert silk sutures and the intestine washed with sterilised saline. A second incision was now made in the middle line above the pubes through the old scar and the pelvis emptied of a small amount of purulent fluid, which was not of offensive odour. It was cleansed with sterilised saline, and both wounds sutured, without drainage. Shock was counteracted by the administration of half a pint of saline *per rectum* every two hours. The patient recovered and left a month later.

She came again for operation[1] in 1906 on account of symptoms which she herself diagnosed as due to "perforation." She had not been feeling very well for a fortnight, but there had been nothing very definite. There was, however, some pain in the abdomen on March 12 which she could not localise. At 9 a.m. on the 14th she had felt a sudden increase in pain, which was now in the upper part of the abdomen, and she vomited.

At 3 p.m. she was lying on her back, with eyes slightly sunken, but not at all anxious-looking. Her pulse was 85 and temperature 100·6°. The abdomen was moving fairly on respiration. On examination it was tender, especially to the left of the umbilicus, and still more so near the lower end of the scar representing the site of the previous operation for perforated jejunal ulcer. In that region the muscular rigidity was most marked, and there was distinct swelling. There was impaired resonance towards the left flank. No visible peristalsis ; the liver dulness was not changed.

Incision was made through the left rectus sheath and the muscle displaced inwards. A thin purulent fluid was present on opening the peritoneum ; and a coil of distended small intestine of a dull red colour, having some patches of lymph on its surface, presented immediately under the opening. Two or three patches of yellow lymph were especially evident on the line of junction of the stomach and small intestine ;

[1] Clin. Soc. Trans., Vol. XL., p. 250.

one of them, of rounded shape, covered the ulcer, which had perforated, and the probe passed directly through it into the gut.   It was about ⅛ inch below the line of junction on the jejunum, and about the size of a crow quill.   The tissues around it were indurated.   A suture was put across it, and this was infolded with a row of interrupted Lembert silk sutures.   The pelvis was cleansed from purulent fluid and lymph through a second incision.   Both openings were closed and healed without difficulty, and she left on April 12.   No adhesions were found within the peritoneal cavity at this operation, and when she was shown at the Clinical Society some months later there was no ventral hernia.

The fourth perforation was in a patient under my observation in 1910.

He was a man of 35 who had undergone an operation in 1907 by a surgeon in Glasgow for a perforated gastric ulcer, and two months later a gastro-enterostomy by the anterior method, with entero-anastomosis, for the relief of pyloric obstruction.   He had enjoyed good health until the morning of August 26.   That morning about half-past 8, when having his breakfast, he had been seized with a sudden pain in the upper part of his abdomen in the splenic region and had felt sick.   He had not, however, vomited.   Feeling himself that his symptoms were something like those whch he had experienced at the time of perforation of the gastric ulcer, he immediately sent for a medical man, Dr. Currie, who recognised that something serious had taken place.   He called in a surgeon, who, in consultation, considered that the condition was a temporary one of colic and that the patient would soon improve.   He did not advise operation.   So strongly did Dr. Currie feel that some perforation had taken place that he thought it well to get another opinion. When first seen by Dr. Currie there was comparatively little dulness in the region of the stomach to the left side, where most of the pain was, but by 11.30, three hours after the commencement of symptoms, a dull area was evidently extending from this spot, and from the great tenderness whch existed down the left side of the abdomen and the rigidity of the left rectus, it was considered that fluid was escaping and gradually diffusing itself along this side of the abdomen towards the pelvis.   I thought at the consultation that the patient had a perforated jejunal ulcer because the symptoms were similar to those in the other cases which had come under my notice, and from the fact that he had undergone the two operations mentioned.   Operation in this case was performed at 1 o'clock, as soon as he could be got into a surgical home. There was some free fluid, thin and without odour, on the left side of the abdomen, running down to the pelvis.   A perforation was found at the junction of a coil of intestine with the anterior wall of the stomach, being on the intestinal portion of the junction.   There was induration round this perforation, and the coil of intestine, which came up to the stomach and formed the loop, was a good deal distended and much congested.   The opening itself was comparatively small and was only defined on pressure of the intestine so as to force gas through it   It was closed with silk sutures, the left side of the abdomen thoroughly cleansed, some fluid mopped from the pelvis, and the wound closed without drainage. The patient made a good recovery. The amount of fluid in this case was comparatively small and of a greenish colour, without odour, but gave definite evidence of its presence and extension downwards, firstly by the increase in the dull area noticed by Dr. Currie, and secondly by the spread of the tenderness. The operation was performed so soon after perforation that no lymph had formed, and I consider that the case reflects very great credit on Dr. Currie.

There are various points in these cases which are worth recapitulating :—

(1) The ulcers gave no intimation of their presence until perforation occurred.

(2) The symptoms were very much like those resulting from an obstruction by a band, there being localised distension and, in one instance, peristalsis of the bowel near the perfora-tion.

(3) The distension of the bowel when exposed was found to be considerable, but it was relieved by forcing the contained gas through the perforation, after which, manipulation was easy. It was not easy to find the perforation in all.

(4) In no case was it necessary to excise the ulcer.

(5) In two instances a counter-opening was required for the satisfactory cleansing of the pelvis, but both wounds were closed without drainage in the second case.

The proportion of recorded cases of simple ulcer of the jejunum to the cases of gastro-enterostomy appears very much against the anterior method of operation ; but this tells as an argument less forcibly than would appear, because it is very probable that the anterior operation has been per-formed more frequently than the posterior. I formerly considered that the anterior operation possessed advantages which were likely to make it the more favoured operation of the two in a general way, and that the danger of the formation of this kind of ulcer was so slight that it might be neglected in considering the question. The introduction of the posterior " no loop " operation by the Mayos has, however, given us even better results, which in my opinion constitute it the best of the numerous methods before the profession. Since the account of it was published, I have invariably performed the posterior operation in cases requiring gastro-jejunostomy, if the state of the parts involved permitted.

PERFORATIONS OF THE SMALL INTESTINE MET WITH DURING THE COURSE OF AN ATTACK OF TYPHOID FEVER.

Although the fatal character of a perforated typhoid ulcer was fully recognised long before 1884, it was only during that year that Professor Leyden suggested operation for it and, during the same year, that Professor Miculicz operated for the first time.

This group differs from most of the others which we have been considering, inasmuch as " the acute abdomen " develops during the course of an illness which may have already severely tried the strength and endurance of the patient. It has been calculated by Dr. Hector Mackenzie that 3·3 per cent. of all cases of typhoid fever (Buizard gives 3·73 per cent.) die from this complication ; and, further, that 69·6 per cent. of them occur during the second, third, or fourth weeks of the illness. His lecture in the *Lancet* of September 26, 1903, is both interesting and instructive and will well repay perusal.

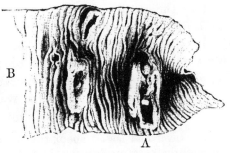

FIG. 27.—Perforation of Typhoid Ulcer, A. Other Ulcers are shown, B. St. Thomas's Hospital Museum.

Dr. E. W. Goodall found perforation in 35·9 per cent. of fatal cases at the Homerton Fever Hospital, and of the total number of cases only two recovered—one after operation, the other after doubtful perforation. Perforation may occur in the ambulatory form of typhoid or before the patient has felt ill enough to go to bed, but it is very rare before the ninth or tenth day of the disease. It is most frequent towards the end of the third week.

" Peritonism," the result of a perforation of the ileum, is often not very marked, and unless some such series of rules as those suggested for the nurse by Osler in cases of typhoid be enforced its occurrence may be overlooked. As a rule these patients are under skilled observation ; therefore there is a chance for them which is not afforded many of those in our other groups. They are watched from the beginning, and

N 2

preparation should be made for operation at the earliest moment if there is any serious change in the abdominal symptoms.

Whilst in ambulatory cases and cases of a mild nature the symptoms are definite, they may be ill-marked in a man who is in a condition approaching the typhoid state.

Then again the contents of the ileum in this disease are frequently scanty, and the perforation may not allow of the immediate escape of much fluid ; at all events, the sensitive peritoneum is not flooded at once with a highly irritating acid compound, the amount of which rapidly increases from minute to minute, as in perforation of the stomach.

The account of two cases on which I operated at the request of my colleague, Dr. Hector Mackenzie, will show to some extent the conditions which may be met with when the general state of the patients is favourable.

In the first, perforation occurred on the tenth day of the first relapse, and symptoms of perforation had been noted twelve hours before the operation, which took place on December 4, 1901, when he was under treatment for the fever. The history was as follows :—

The fever had lasted about thirty days ; there was then a period of normal temperature lasting eight days, followed by a relapse, and on the tenth day of this he complained of a sudden and severe pain in the abdomen which woke him up. After an action of his bowels he went to sleep again and slept for nearly two hours, being again awakened by the pain. He did not vomit until seven hours after the commencement of symptoms.

He was a man aged 22. At the time of operation he had pain, distension, shifting dulness in the flanks, extreme tenderness in the right iliac fossa, and a complete absence of dulness in the liver region. The pulse was 95 ; respirations, 26 ; temperature, 102·4°. The temperature fell rapidly to 97° after operation, but soon rose again.

At 10.30 a.m. incision in the median line below the umbilicus showed a collection of thin yellowish fluid under the peritoneum, with some lymph on this surface of the small intestine. Coming from the upper angle of the wound was a thin tongue of omentum adherent at its extremity to a coil of the small bowel, which appeared paler and more contracted than the other coils around. On pulling on this piece of omentum the portion of intestine to which it adhered rotated and showed a perforation from which the same kind of fluid was coming. This perforation was rounded and sharply cut, measuring about ½ inch across. A silk suture was placed across this opening to draw the edges together, and the ulcer invaginated with Lembert silk sutures (size No. 00). The lower abdomen was washed out with sterilised saline and a drain left in the lower angle of the wound. On February 22, 1902, an abscess was opened which was under the right rectus, which appeared to have resulted from an indiscretion in diet. The pus from this abscess was sterile.

The second case was in some respects similar.

A man aged 28 was admitted on July 7, 1902. On June 30, after a heavy day's work, he had been suddenly taken ill with pains, some shooting across the forehead and others of a stabbing character in the back. On July 2 he was at work, but had to return home. On the morning of the 3rd he awoke feeling very chilly, shivered and then sweated profusely, and the pains continued during the day. On the 4th he had several rigors and vomited after food. On the 5th he was able to go out and see his doctor. On the 7th, when going to the hospital, he became giddy and fell. He was a well-developed man, with flushed perspiring face, and slightly sunken eyes. The abdomen was well covered and moved well. There was slight distension in the left iliac fossa, which, as well as the epigastrium, was slightly tender to pressure. No spots ; spleen felt ; tongue dry and brown ; chest normal. Pulse, 80 ; respirations, 36. Bowels confined. The Widal reaction was absent on the 8th. For the first four days the temperature varied from 100° to 103°. On the morning of the 11th it was noted : " Pain in the epigastric region on coughing, where there is some tenderness on pressure. Tongue cleaner. Bowels well opened after enema. Temperature 100·6° ; pulse 68, good tension ; respirations, 26." At 1.30 p.m. there was a sudden onset of abdominal pain, referred principally to the region of the umbilicus, but also to the right iliac region. Vomiting occurred soon after the onset of pain. He was seen at 2.15 p.m. ; and then the abdomen moved poorly on respiration, the right side being especially rigid, resistant and tender to palpation. The pulse was 84 and the temperature 102·6°. At 4.30 p.m. he looked much worse. His expression was anxious, and eyes sunken. He lay with the knees drawn up, and complained much of the abdominal pain, which was most severe about the umbilicus, and was aggravated by coughing or drawing a deep breath. The abdomen, which did not move with respiration, was held rigidly. The resistance and tenderness were very marked, especially in the right iliac region. There was no dulness in the flanks and the liver dulness was not encroached on. The pulse was now 104, and smaller than before, but the temperature was unaltered. Operation was performed at 7.15 p.m., five and three-quarter hours after the onset of the acute pain. The anæsthetic was ether, preceded by gas. A 4-inch median incision below the umbilicus was made, and some thin, light yellow pus-like fluid containing some small yellowish masses, without fæcal smell, was seen between the nearest coils of intestine. On tracing a coil downwards towards the cæcal valve there was soon found a round, clean-edged perforation about ¼ inch in diameter, with a slough adherent to it on its inner side. The opening was closed with Lembert sutures. After the lower abdomen had been washed out the abdomen was closed without drainage. The patient's condition at the end of the operation was good. On the 14th the Widal reaction, which had been negative before the operation, was now positive. The abdominal wound did not close satisfactorily for some time, and he only left on September 10. This man was readmitted on September 18 of the same year for periostitis of the femur. He was readmitted on January 3, 1903, for abdominal pain, which had come on after a slip when he was carrying a sack of coals. This was very severe, and was probably the result of rupture of some adhesions. Next year he came under observation again for abscess of the thigh, which closed under treatment. The pus contained typhoid bacilli, and the bone was bared but not necrosed.

I may mention here, as a curious addition to this history, that the thigh wound reopened after he left the hospital, and as recently as December, 1904, the pus contained typhoid bacilli on bacteriological examination. It is sad to relate that his wife, who dressed his wound for him, caught typhoid about August, 1910, and died soon after admission to the hospital as a result of the severity of the attack.

Influence of Perforation of Typhoid Ulcer on the Temperature.

The chart (Fig. 28) illustrates the rapid fall to 96·8°, rebound to 102·8° on evening of operation ; then a gradual return to the previous run of temperatures until, on the seventh day after the perforation, the records were much the same as before it. This patient had a second relapse in January and a third in February of the following year, but recovered.

In both instances the ulcers were single and of a punched-out character, with surrounding healthy tissue, and did not suggest that they resulted from the spread of the necrotic process seen in the Peyer's patch of an ordinary typhoid patient.

There may be more than one perforation, but as a rule (in 88 per cent.) it is solitary and small. The incision should therefore be made near the middle line, rather than over the iliac fossa.

Messieurs Dujarier and Matthiew[1] state that it is found in the last 60 centimetres of the lower end of the ileum in 93·51 per cent., and it is almost always on the free border of the gut.

Another perforation may sometimes be found co-existing

[1] *Le Journal Medical Français*, October, 1912, p. 426.

with the one in the ileum, and this may be in any part of the digestive tract below the diaphragm.

The amount of shock was not excessive in either patient whose case has been related. The rate of the pulse in the first case was increased in frequency from 68 to 84, forty-five minutes after the perforation, and to 104 three hours afterwards. In the second it was more constant at about. 95 for from two to ten hours after the onset of acute symptoms.

In neither instance was there any history of shivering, which is described by Dr. Goodall as an initial symptom in at least 26 per cent. of his cases.

The diagnosis of these perforations in the course of enteric fever is not always easily made. Patients suffering from this disease frequently complain of abdominal pain. This has occasionally been so severe that an exploratory operation has been performed, but without any lesion being found to account for the symptom.

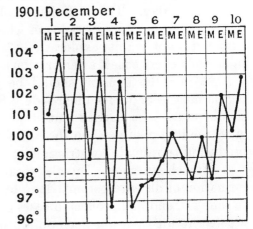

FIG. 28.—The Temperature after Perforation and Operation for Typhoid Perforation. Perforation during relapse (tenth day), 10.20 p.m., December 3; operation, 10.30 a.m., December 4. (Case p. 180.)

The signs on which chief reliance should be placed in making a diagnosis are local pain and tenderness, with rigidity and fixation of the abdominal muscles and disappearance of the liver dulness.

If there is a doubt about the presence of a perforation it might be well to percuss the hepatic region on each examination. A gradual diminution in the normal liver dulness would be very significant. In one of our patients the latter sign was not evident five and three-quarter hours after the perforation had occurred, and you must not wait for it.

A sudden drop in the temperature in the absence of

hæmorrhage is suspicious, but there may be no change in this respect for some time.

Rarely peritonitis develops during the progress of typhoid fever and no evidence of perforation has been found, whilst in some instances this inflammation has evidently preceded the symptoms of perforation, for which an operation has been undertaken.

I do not think there is now any real difference of opinion amongst surgeons regarding the necessity for operation in cases of perforation occurring in the course of typhoid fever. It is hard to believe that there is any amongst physicians of the present day. The fact that exploration has not revealed a perforation in every instance in which the abdomen has been explored is not against exploration ; a fatal ending is assured in practically every case if a perforation is not treated by operation.

As a rule the incision should be made through the right rectus muscle or to its inner side. Suture of the perforation should always be carried out if possible ; this undoubtedly gives the best results when the bowel will hold sutures without producing too much constriction of its lumen.

A French surgeon, Duval, speaks rather highly of the formation of an enterostomy done by bringing the perforation to the skin, and in 22 collected cases gives 10 cures to 12 deaths, a better result than has been obtained by any other method.

Owing to the mortality of enterostomy for other conditions, I can but think that the surgeon should be very loth to perform this operation in a disease like typhoid, as it must interfere so seriously with nutrition.

In a limited number of cases excision of the area involved might be necessary, but, as you will quite understand, such an operation is a severe one, more than most typhoid patients could possibly undergo with any prospect of survival.

Professor Buizard gives a summary of 664 operations :—

Cures, 182 (27·41 per cent.) ; deaths, 482 (72·59 per cent.).

Examination of his statistics shows that the improvement continues as regards results of operation for typhoid perforation, and the mortality diminishes yearly.

Taking five-yearly periods :—

1884—1889, 90 per cent. ; 1889—1894, 86·36 per

cent. ; 1894—1899, 75·63 per cent. ; 1899—1904, 69·7 per cent. ; 1904—1909, 64·63 per cent.

From a study of cases operated on we learn that recovery may follow—

(1) In spite of the desperate condition of the patient ;

(2) In spite of the supervention of complications necessitating other operative assistance ;

(3) In spite of one or more relapses of the fever.

Operation, to be successful, must be early. You must not wait too long for recovery from collapse. Armstrong says that in ten operations performed during the first twelve hours there were four recoveries ; but that in ten done during the second twelve hours success was only once obtained. All those died which were operated on twenty-four hours or more after the onset.

Ashurst states that two out of 31 cases recovered in the third twelve hours, and 18 out of 55 when more than thirty-six hours had passed.

A curious clinical observation has been recorded by Dr. Poynton,[1] who discovered much fluid in the peritoneum of a typhoid patient in the early stages of the disease.

The attack was acute, and Widal's reaction had proved negative. An operation was performed, as it was thought it might be a case of acute perforation of the appendix. On opening the abdomen no disease of the appendix or perforation of the bowel was found. The whole of the peritoneum appeared to be much congested, no lymph was present, but a considerable quantity of almost clear fluid escaped through the incision. The wound was closed, and the patient recovered, after a typical attack of typhoid fever. The *bacillus typhosus* was found in the fluid.

This finding of a large quantity of fluid in the peritoneum of a typhoid patient is very unusual, but its possible occurrence is a thing to be remembered, as a somewhat similar condition was found in a patient subjected to an operation for typhoid perforation by Mr. Gordon Watson.

A female aged 11—the twenty-sixth day of the disease. Operation about an hour after the first symptom. Dulness in flanks when first examined, and "the abdomen absolutely full of fluid " when opened. Ulcer 18 inches from the valve ; closed with suture. Peritoneum everywhere injected, but quite glossy.

[1] Transactions of the Medical Society, London.

It is evident that this effusion had been present before the signs of perforation were manifested. The septic fluid from the bowel would therefore be considerably diluted directly it entered the peritoneum.

Tuberculous Ulcer of the Small Intestine.

The occasional perforation of a solitary tuberculous ulcer of the small intestine is sometimes encountered in an operation for peritonitis, the nature of the ulceration being proved by microscopical examination after removal by excision. In some of the cases there is no history preceding the perforative symptoms, and nothing can be found at the operation pointing to the causation of the disease. Cruise [1] gives an account of thirteen instances of intestinal perforation found in 475 necropsies on patients who had died from chronic pulmonary tuberculosis. Ten of these were complete, into the general peritoneal cavity, and in the majority the symptoms were characteristic, commencing with sudden violent pain and shock. The shock may be quickly fatal, or an acute peritonitis may develop. Cruise says that in five the symptoms were most indefinite, two having absolutely no abdominal symptoms; he came to the conclusion that perforation of the intestines occurs most commonly in chronic tuberculosis in from 1 to 5 per cent. of the cases. It is never possible to diagnose with certainty a partial perforation, and the existence of a local abscess due to perforation can only be diagnosed when the mass can be felt.

In any case, when the symptoms and history point to a perforative peritonitis, special attention should be given to the ileo-cæcal region, for here we find not only the perforation in cases of latent typhoid, but also in tuberculosis. If the perforation is not found close to the cæcum, follow the small intestine upwards, and go slowly, looking for any change from the normal and for the presence of fluid, which may be seen flowing from the direction of the opening.

If nothing is found in the small intestine, examine the sigmoid. Professor Léjars [2] mentions a case in which he closed a fistula remaining from an enterostomy for acute obstruction,

---

[1] *American Journal of the Med. Soc.*, 1911.
[2] " Urgent Surgery," p. 544.

and two days afterwards the patient died from acute peritonitis due to perforation of a solitary tuberculous plaque low down in the sigmoid. It is in this region that perforations of intestinal diverticula are found.

Mr. Lionel Norbury showed a patient before the Clinical Section of the Royal Society of Medicine[1] for whom he had operated for perforated tuberculous ulcer of the small intestine, and I am indebted to him for the accompanying illustration (Fig. 29).

The patient was a man aged 39, who gave a history of occasional attacks of epigastric pain. He was admitted eight hours after the onset of an acute abdominal pain, chiefly felt in the lower abdomen, which doubled him up; he vomited later. On examination, after admission to St. Thomas's Hospital, there was tenderness and rigidity of abdomen, chiefly in the lower half. Temperature, 100°; pulse, 100; respirations, 20. Abdomen otherwise normal. Operation nine

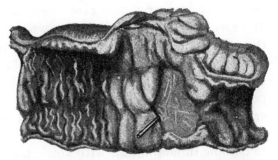

F.C.C.

FIG. 29.—Perforation of Tuberculous Ulcer of the Small Intestine. Probe placed in the opening. Mr. Norbury's case.

hours after onset of symptoms. There was a small amount of free fluid and lymph in the abdominal cavity, but no free gas. The appendix and stomach were normal. A hard swelling was found which involved the small intestine 2 feet from the cæcum; this narrowed the lumen of the bowel considerably, and there was a small perforation in the wall of the bowel in this situation. Four inches of the ileum with the ulcer were resected, and an end-to-end anastomosis performed. Dry sponging of the pelvis and closure of the wound without drainage. The patient recovered without any adverse symptoms. Microscopical examination proved the ulcer to be tuberculous, but no other evidence of intra-abdominal tubercle could be found at the time of operation.

The state of the parts around an ulcer such as this does not permit of the simple application of sutures; it is necessary to excise and then perform anastomosis, in order to obtain the best result. The surgeon will, however, be guided by the

[1] See Vol. IV., 1911, No. 3, p. 50.

local condition and general state of the patient ; he might find it impossible to do more than place a tube in the intestine, attach it to the abdominal wall, and drain the peritoneum.

THE PERFORATION OF DIVERTICULA OF THE LARGE BOWEL.

During recent years the attention of the profession has been drawn to the formation of diverticula mostly in the sigmoid colon.   These diverticula are of varying size and number, and changes which take place in them are responsible for some of the cases of the acute abdomen which require surgical treatment.   The larger number of them are in stout males over 50 years of age.   Dr. Telling has written a very full account of this disease, for which the profession is much indebted to him. He points out that as the diverticulum increases in size it becomes atrophied, until there is frequently only a layer of peritoneum between perhaps a hard dried lump of fæcal matter or a foreign body and the general peritoneal cavity.   It will be readily understood, therefore, that such patients will be liable to chronic inflammation with thickening and other changes to which the appendix vermiformis is liable, there being a very close resemblance between one of these pouches, placed as it frequently is in an appendix epiploica, and the appendix.   It is also evident that the result of anything like a perforation into the general peritoneal cavity will be a very serious thing for the patient.   Nothing but early operation will be of avail to prevent a rapidly fatal ending, these perforations taking place at a time of life when the power of resistance is not always at its best.   An abstract from a paper published by Mr. Gordon Taylor [1] will illustrate the clinical character of such a case, and indicate the treatment which it demands.

The patient, a man aged 57 years, markedly obese, after a four-mile walk in the morning was suddenly seized with very severe pain in the abdomen while taking his mid-day meal.   He became somewhat collapsed, and required help to reach his bedroom.   Almost immediately after the onset of the pain, which was accompanied by vomiting, a loose motion was passed.   About seven hours after the commencement of the attack the patient was lying on his left side with his knees drawn up on the abdomen.   There was great tenderness on pressure over the

[1] *Lancet*, 1911, Vol. I., p. 495.

left iliac fossa, and most marked cutaneous hyperæsthesia was present in this region ; the rest of the belly wall was soft. The liver dulness was normal, and there was no evidence of free fluid in the abdominal cavity ; the temperature was subnormal and the pulse was 100. The symptoms strongly suggested appendicitis and the possibility of a left-sided appendix was considered.

There is generally a history of pain commencing on the left side of the abdomen, and as most of the pouches develop in the sigmoid this is to be expected, and that region, in a doubtful case, should be examined first. In the paper from which the above case is taken another is described, in which the pouch was situated in the ascending colon.

The patient, a man of 70, did not get medical advice until a week had passed, and at that time his condition was desperate from diffuse peritonitis.

When considering the localised suppurations which are met with in the abdomen we referred to these diverticula ; their presence probably explains many conditions which were formerly obscure. The cases of successful operation for this perforation are not very numerous, but, with the improvement which has taken place in our recognition of the causes and treatment of peritonitis, the list will doubtless increase, as early operation becomes recognised by the profession at large as the only satisfactory treatment.

PERFORATION OF STERCORAL ULCERS.

As recently as 1896 the late Mr. Grieg Smith wrote about stercoral ulcer : " Although no special description of this disease has, so far as the writer knows, been written, and although it is not of frequent occurrence nor of great import-ance, yet its undoubted existence and real gravity may justify its being classed under a separate heading." He then mentions a few instances of intra-abdominal abscess, in which a foreign body was found, but admits that some of them were most probably due to disease of the appendix. He writes : " The condition as I have met with it is simply a diffuse subperitoneal cellulitis," and he evidently regarded it as always dependent on the irritation of a foreign body.

Sir J. Bland-Sutton has given examples of fæcal abscess, associated with small but sharp foreign bodies, in the large intestine ; and Dr. H. D. Rolleston, in a paper on " Pericolitis Sinistra," gives instances in which ulceration developed in a diverticulum of the colon, and produced suppuration around. These ulcerations were not, however, like the variety which is under consideration here, but come under the heading of " Abscess Secondary to Diverticula. of the Large Bowel."

Stercoral ulcers behave much in the same way as ulcers in other parts of the digestive tract ; they may perforate suddenly and produce general peritonitis, or extend gradually and give rise to a localised intraperitoneal abscess. When it is recognised that they are usually secondary to a condition which of itself is seriously threatening the patient's life, it will be appreciated why they prove so fatal. The patient, who is most frequently suffering from chronic intestinal obstruction, caused by carcinoma of the large intestine low down, appears to have his last chance of recovery taken away if a stercoral ulcer, perforating suddenly, floods the peritoneum with the very septic contents of the bowel above the obstruction. In a patient already weakened and distressed by the obstruction, this additional attack is usually more than can be successfully combated, and proves fatal in a few hours.

In May, 1912, I saw a young and strong-looking man with Dr. A. E. Godfrey, of Finchley, for a swelling of the liver which we considered to be secondary to a carcinoma of the large bowel, which was producing few symptoms beyond constipation. We advised the patient to have nothing done in the way of operation unless more urgent symptoms developed. A day or two later another medical man was called in by a relative. He gave the patient a small white powder (? calomel), and within four hours after taking this acute peritonitis with collapse developed suddenly and death occurred within twenty-four hours. I have no doubt that a latent stercoral ulcer had burst probably as the result of a violent purgative.

When any one the subject of chronic intestinal obstruction of a mechanical kind complains of sudden increase in abdominal pain and has a rise of temperature, not necessarily a very high one, the possibility of the giving way of a stercoral ulcer must be remembered. This possibility is increased if there is, in addition, an excessive sensitiveness to palpation, previously absent, but perforation may give no immediate sign of its occurrence, as in the following instance :—

Some years ago I was asked by the late Mr. C. Mortimer Lewis, then of Steyning, to see a lady with him, who had carcinoma of the rectum. She was over 80 years of age, and had only sent for him that morning because her bowels had not acted for a week. He examined the abdomen, found it much distended and tympanitic, whilst the rectum was completely blocked by a carcinomatous growth. When we saw her together a few hours later she was much the same, but without any vomiting. Her temperature had been 100°, the pulse was good, but the tongue was brown and dry. Incision was made to perform colostomy in the left iliac region, but when the peritoneum was opened it was found to be flooded with black liquid fæcal matter, which was still escaping freely from two ragged openings in the immensely distended sigmoid flexure. These openings (with thin and irregular edges) were situated one above the other in the anterior part of the bowel, which passed down behind the middle line of the abdomen. Pints of this offensive fluid came away before it was possible to secure the sigmoid flexure to the abdominal wall. The peritoneum was cleansed as well as possible, but the patient did not rally from the operation.

In this case it is possible that the bowel had given way in the morning, when the patient sent for her medical adviser. Up to that time she had for some days gone on, taking dose after dose of medicine without relief, whilst the immense accumulation of fæcal matter above the constriction had caused excessive stretching and local injury to the bowel, which had ended in acute bacterial necrosis. The necessary removal from the bed to the operating table may have given rise to a further escape and diffusion in the peritoneum.

Treatment of this most unfortunate complication should be directed to the cleansing of the peritoneum, the insertion of a Paul's tube in the opening from which the fæcal matter is escaping, and the suturing of the damaged bowel to the part of the abdominal wall most easily reached. Strain on the wall of the bowel, usually softened and easily torn, must be avoided. By this means the opening will serve as a colostomy opening and the obstruction be relieved. The difficulty in cleansing satisfactorily the fouled peritoneum will render the prospect of recovery doubtful. Yet success may occasionally be obtained.

On March 27, 1901, I saw a patient in consultation with Dr. S. Faulconer Wright, of Lee. He was 71 years of age, and stated that he had always been healthy until the 21st of that month, when for the first time he experienced abdominal pain. This was accompanied by vomiting and constipation. Since that time the pain had continued with occasional vomiting, and the bowels had not acted.   The abdomen was much distended and tympanitic, the note around the umbilicus being high pitched.   There was no diminution of the liver dulness, and no evidence of free fluid in the peritoneum.   The tenderness was not extreme, but he winced when touched.   His general condition was fair, and the temperature was normal.   An incision was made in the middle line below the umbilicus, and when the peritoneum was opened free gas escaped, and fluid fæcal matter was seen covering the intestine in the region of the cæcum and extending into the pelvis.   This had come, and was still escaping, from a stercoral ulcer on the anterior surface of the distended cæcum, which had recently given way.   It was large enough to admit the little finger, and its outline was somewhat irregular, with a thinned edge.   Into this a Paul's tube was passed and secured, the cæcum being sutured to an incision in the right iliac region.   After the bowel and peritoneum had been cleansed as thoroughly as possible, a long drainage tube was passed into the pelvis and the median wound was sutured.   The small intestine was generally adherent, coil to coil, and fixed in the posterior part of the abdomen, evidently the result of an old attack of peritonitis, the cause for which was not ascertained.

Under the skilful management of Dr. Wright the patient recovered, and was able to go daily to the City to business for several years afterwards, when he died from an attack of bronchitis.   The artificial anus never closed completely, and gradually, as time went on, this opening became more important, until hardly any fæcal matter found its exit by the natural anus.   The patient wore a flat, circular indiarubber bag, containing a large flat sponge, fitting accurately to the abdomen over the artificial anus.   The dieting had to be very carefully arranged, on account of occasional stoppages, which, when they occurred, caused considerable pain, only relieved by the escape of fæcal matter by the artificial opening.   His general health was afterwards excellent.   What the nature of the obstruction was in this case it is impossible to say ; the fouling of the peritoneum and the condition of the patient made it inadvisable to explore.   The complication of perforation was such a serious one that the clear indication was to deal with that, more especially as its treatment was calculated to give relief to the obstruction which was responsible for it.   The cleansing of the peritoneum was no doubt aided by the limitation of the fouled area in consequence of the old intestinal adhesions.   The after history of the case is instructive, inasmuch as the obstruction often recurred, and a " safety-valve " action permitted of relief on each occasion.   It was thought at the time of operation that the obstruction was caused by a ring carcinoma of the sigmoid flexure, the growth of which is sometimes very slow ; anyway, the case is a most instructive and encouraging one.

It may perhaps be possible to suture the perforations, and afterwards make an artificial anus in a more favourable part of the large bowel.

PERFORATION OF STERCORAL ULCERATION ASSOCIATED WITH OBSTRUCTION OF THE LARGE BOWEL.—A case was admitted on

March 18, 1913, and successfully operated on by Mr. Stewart Rouquette.

G. C., a man of 61, complained of pain on the right side of the abdomen for six weeks, but three days before it was worse and he was doubled up by it. He had vomited and was evidently suffering from obstruction. The abdomen moved well on respiration ; was more or less tympanitic on percussion ; rather tender in the right lower half, with some rigidity of the rectus. Temperature, 99·8° ; pulse, 64. Nothing could be felt *per rectum*, and the bowels were not acting. Mr. Rouquette, who made an incision through the right rectus muscle, found free gas in the peritoneal cavity which had escaped through two openings in the anterior part of the cæcum. The cæcum was much distended, the openings small, with thin edges ; very little fæcal matter had escaped. The wall of the cæcum around the openings appeared normal. The openings were closed with silk sutures. The appendix was removed. A carcinoma of the upper rectum was found, and a colostomy performed on the left side.

The right incision permitted a discharge with fæcal odour for about seven days, but the patient left on April 24 in a very fair condition with the colostomy wound acting quite satisfactorily.

It appeared probable that the cæcum had given way during removal from bed to theatre.

" Stercoral ulcer " is one of the most serious complications of chronic intestinal obstruction, even when the peritonitis pro- duced is purely local in its character. If there is an ill-defined area of dulness in the cæcal region, with tenderness and a sense of resistance, whilst rectal examination shows an apparent thickening on the right side of the pelvis, this complication should be suspected. Fluctuation may be found if the case is seen at a later stage. Should the patient be fat and nervous the diagnosis may be very difficult ; even with the assistance afforded by the administration of an anæsthetic it may be hard to say that there is much wrong with the side really affected. There is nothing like the definite induration which is found in a case of localised inflammation or suppuration secondary to a disease of the appendix which it resembles closely in some other respects. It comes on in a person suffering from intestinal disturbance ; the pain is in the right iliac fossa, and is accom- panied by increased distension of the abdomen and a rise of temperature. Tenderness is more marked in the right iliac fossa than in other parts of the abdomen. Yet there are differences—a stercoral ulcer, giving rise to a localised extravasa- tion and abscess, is specially met with in elderly females who give a history of chronic constipation, recently more obstinate, and associated with "wind in the stomach." The rise of temperature is not great, and the area of tenderness is not so easily localised as in appendicitis.

The collection of fluid fæces which forms in the peritoneum has a tendency to spread laterally, for it is not easily localised, as it escapes readily, and it may be the operator will find it up to or beyond the middle line should he make an exploratory median incision to find out the exact site of the obstruction when there is a doubt. Whether he thus discovers it by accident, or makes direct or intentional incision into the abscess, a counter-opening and the insertion of a large drainage tube will generally be required. If the opening in the cæcum be found, a tube should be passed into this, so that the contents of the bowel, which rapidly come away, may be conducted beyond the abscess cavity. These contents, pus mixed with fluid fæcal matter, are extremely offensive, more so than most abdominal collections of a purulent character, and that is saying a great deal.

Under the best conditions the prognosis is bad ; the discharge of large quantities of fæcal matter, with an increasing admixture of pus, causes much local irritation, and may end in rapid exhaustion. Should the inflammation subside and an artificial anus form, it is not placed in a convenient position, and may lead to all the disadvantages of an opening on the right side—that is, if the obstruction becomes complete. The case under the care of Dr. Wright suggests the possibility of a more satisfactory course of events, the opening acting as a safety valve when required by the temporary stoppage beyond, and causing but little inconvenience in the intervals. Another danger in these perforations is the tracking upwards of the pus and the formation of a large collection in the sub-hepatic or sub-phrenic regions ; a second incision would be required for the better drainage of this extension, but exhaustion from the discharge would not unlikely prove fatal. It will be evident that recovery from these collections will take some time, during which the original cause of the trouble—probably a malignant growth—is increasing in size and becoming more difficult to treat radically.

The establishment of a short circuit between the small

bowel and the large beyond the stricture would be the ideal operation, but it is not often that the septic state of the abdomen allows this to be done.   You cannot do it at the first operation when the condition of the patient is bad and the complication a very serious one, perhaps of considerable and ill-defined extent.   Later the result of a prolonged septic discharge makes it very unlikely that the sutures required would hold after the junction had been effected ; but you must judge each case on its merits.

Messieurs Challiet and Thomasset [1] say that when the large bowel gives from softening of its coats in cases of obstruction, the rupture is found at the junction of the ascending colon and cæcum to the outer side of the longitudinal band.   The second variety, or gangrenous perforation, is found in the left portion of the colon ; it is generally solitary, of small size, with gangrenous eroded edges.

[1] *Arch. Gen. de Chir.*, 1911.

PART IV

ACUTE CONDITIONS HAVING THEIR ORIGIN IN THE FEMALE GENERATIVE ORGANS

SALPINGITIS. PYO-SALPINX. EXTRA-UTERINE GESTATION.

SEVERAL conditions of the female generative organs may be rightly considered under the heading of the " acute abdomen " : The spread of an infection through the Fallopian tubes, the rupture of a pyo-salpinx, the giving way of the sac of an ectopic gestation, necrosis of a subperitoneal uterine fibroid or the twisting of its pedicle ; also accidents attending the growth of an ovarian cyst.

(1) *Infection through the Tubes, etc.*—An acute, urgent, and occasionally fatal illness is sometimes produced by the spread of a gonococcic inflammation from below. The tubes not having been occluded by a pre-existing inflammation, it is possible to see purulent fluid coming from one or both of them when they are lifted for examination.

This was the case in a young married woman seen with Dr. Fitzgerald. Acute abdominal symptoms had commenced three days before and the patient was very ill with quick pulse, abdominal pain, and distension. She had suffered from a vaginal discharge for three weeks. At the operation there was purulent peritonitis in the pelvis, with acutely inflamed tubes. The pelvis was cleansed and a drainage tube put in afterwards. Both tubes had to be removed, but part of one ovary was left. She made a satisfactory recovery. The origin of the disease and its nature were easily proved.

If the symptoms are severe and cause anxiety, in these cases it is better to operate, for, although the inflammatory condition settles down in most, a chronic disease of the tubes will remain and repeated inflammatory attacks be the rule. There are many more lives crippled and spoilt by chronic salpingitis than is usually acknowledged. It is not advisable to remove the ovaries, nor is it always necessary to remove both tubes.

In other infections by bacilli, such as puerperal, streptococcal, or influenzal, the symptoms will be similar and require prompt treatment.

In puerperal peritonitis the most active of the organisms present is the *streptococcus pyogenes*, which finds entrance through some breach of surface in the genital tract or passes directly by way of the Fallopian tubes, the infection being only too commonly conveyed in the first place by the attendant at the confinement. If it finds access to the pelvis by way of the Fallopian tubes, a peritonitis of great intensity quickly commences; luckily the nature of " child-bed fever " is generally recognised, and the precautions now taken render the disease a comparatively rare one.

The invasion of the system by the streptococci in this disease is usually marked by an attack of shivering, or a rigor and rapid rise of temperature, with much increased pulse-rate. Any discharge which may be present becomes offensive. There is abdominal pain in the hypogastric region of varying severity, sometimes vomiting and usually offensive diarrhœa.

Tenderness in the hypogastric region spreads and is sometimes very acute. The abdomen becomes distended ; rigors recur ; the temperature becomes of a pyæmic type, there is profuse sweating and complete anorexia ; the diarrhœa is troublesome ; delirium is present at night ; and evidences of secondary mischief in the lungs, pleura or pericardium or other remote parts develop, and the patient dies exhausted. Dulness may be found in the flanks as a result of the collection of free fluid in the peritoneal cavity or a considerable exudation in the subperitoneal cellular tissue, especially if the inflammation has spread by way of the lymphatics.

The treatment should be in the first place to disinfect the uterus and vagina, to take away remaining débris of placenta and decomposing clots, to remove infective fluid which has accumulated in the pelvis, and possibly in the flanks, and to provide good pelvic drainage.

It is wise to begin the administration of anti-streptococcic serum at once (the usual stock " polyvalent " preparation) and continue this treatment with a vaccine prepared from fluid removed from the peritoneum at the operation.

In cases where the uterus has been ruptured, perforated, or is extensively infiltrated, it may be advisable to remove it.

These cases are always most serious, and require energetic treatment from the commencement. They are not all of them of the fulminating variety, but it is important that the milder cases should be treated with decision. In performing the needful dressings after operation, and in douching, etc., the attendant should use sterilised rubber gloves.

A careful watch must be kept for the development of secondary abscesses, which should be evacuated as soon as they are found. If possible a local anæsthetic should be used, or gas and oxygen ; they must not be permitted to attain any size.

(2) *Rupture of a Pyo-salpinx.*—The following case will illustrate this accident. It is the account of a patient admitted for acute abdominal symptoms. It will be noted that there is a certain amount of similarity between the symptoms caused by a ruptured pyo-salpinx and those due to a ruptured ectopic gestation.

L. S., aged 21 years, was admitted ✶ February 20, 1906, early in the afternoon. The history was that she had been suddenly seized with abdominal pain during the night of the 19th. This pain had been very severe in the upper part of the abdomen, and she had vomited. She had had a meal of pork during the previous evening. At 4 o'clock in the morning a medical man was sent for, who gave her some medicine, which she could not keep down. In her previous history there was an account of indigestion of indefinite character some years ago. There had been profuse vaginal discharge for some months, and the menstrual period was a fortnight overdue. There had been no action of the bowels for two days.

When seen with Dr. H. Mackenzie late in the afternoon the patient was lying on her back, looking very ill and anæmic, and seemed collapsed, drowsy, and apathetic. There was a small circular flush on each cheek. The skin was dry. The respirations were somewhat quickened (24), and the pulse was 110. The temperature was 101·4°. She complained of pain in the abdomen, which was found to be moving quite well in the upper half, but was less mobile than usual in the lower part. On palpation there was much complaint of tenderness, especially in the left iliac region and right up towards the liver. Nothing abnormal was found ; the abdominal wall was quite without rigidity, and offered no resistance to palpation. On percussion the note over the whole abdomen, including the liver, was normal. At 5.30 abdominal exploration was carried out ; an incision was first made in the epigastric region, and the stomach and duodenum examined. The hand was then passed downwards to the iliac fossa and appendix region and onwards to the pelvic organs. A tumour was felt to the left of the uterus. This was recognised as a pyo-salpinx, and it was thought that a rupture of this would account for the condition. A second incision was made in the middle line above the pubes, and when the peritoneum was opened, thin, somewhat viscid, odourless pus was found, extending from the pelvis into the flanks. The intestines were packed off with strips of sterilised gauze, and the pyo-salpinx was removed after the application of three (No. 4) silk ligatures. There was no inflammation of the peritoneal coat of the intestine, and no lymph was seen. The area of infection was cleansed with moistened sponges, and drainage was provided by a rubber tube and a strip of gauze. The right ovary was somewhat fixed by adhesions, which were freed, but it appeared to be healthy, as did also the tube on that side. The upper wound was sutured in layers by Mr. Bletsoe, the house surgeon, whilst the pelvic condition was being treated. The pyo-salpinx formed a tumour of the size of a hen's egg, the walls of the Fallopian tube were much thickened, and there had been a rupture not far from the ostium abdominale, which itself had been closed by adhesion to the broad ligament. The ovary formed part of the inflammatory mass removed, and could only be distinguished on dissection. The plug was removed on the 24th; there was a small amount of clear discharge. The bowels had acted twice. The pulse was 76 and the temperature was normal. Pain was quite relieved. She progressed satisfactorily, and left hospital on March 13.

Pyo-salpinx is recognised as the most important condition giving rise to peritonitis having its origin in the pelvis, repeated localised attacks being common. As a source of diffuse spreading peritonitis it is less frequent, for the thickened tube does not often rupture as it did in this case and allow the purulent contents to become diffused. There can be little doubt that the gonococcus is extensively spread by the rupture of a tube, and although Dr. Dudgeon[1] and Mr. Sargent conclude that it possesses a slight pathogenicity when introduced into the peritoneal cavity, it does produce a peritonitis which may be ultimately fatal. We must endeavour to operate before peritonitis becomes extensive. The prognosis is thereby immensely improved, and the duration and severity of the illness diminished.

None of those who saw the extent to which purulent diffusion had taken place in this patient doubted that general peritonitis must have ensued had operation been delayed. It was the aspect of severe illness, with the history, which induced Dr. H. Mackenzie to suggest the desirability of exploration, for local signs of the gravity of the attack were absent. There was no trace of protective rigidity of muscle, whilst the tenderness

[1] " The Bacteriology of Peritonitis," p. 53.

found was not in any way remarkable. Nothing indicated the probable origin of the symptoms, and although the epigastric region was explored this was in deference to the former history of indigestion, with a recent heavy meal, rather than to any idea that stomach ulceration had really given way, for there were no localising signs. I have stated that the appendages on the right side appeared to be healthy, and were therefore not removed. It was probably right to leave them ; but the result of so doing, in a case formerly under my care, in which a pyo-salpinx had given rise to intestinal obstruction, has made me less confident of this than I might otherwise have been. The appendages on the left side appeared normal, and were therefore left, but in the following year the patient returned with peritonitis, the result of a rupture of the remaining tube.

A woman, aged 26, was admitted ✸ January 31, 1903. She stated that she had been quite well until the 25th, when she was taken ill with pains all over her. The attack passed off, but came on more severely at 4 a.m. on the 25th, and was accompanied by severe pain in the right hip which spread all over the abdomen. On admission the abdomen was distended, did not move well on respiration, and the patient looked ill. The abdomen was not tender ; it was easy to examine, but nothing abnormal was detected on palpation. Examination *per rectum* showed nothing unusual. The temperature was 100·6°, and the pulse was 104. On February 3 she had an attack of abdominal pain with vomiting, there being visible distension of small intestine and peristalsis. The bowels acted well just before the attack. Operation was advised because it was recognised that she had recurring attacks of obstruction due to a mechanical condition, but she refused consent until February 6, when another more severe attack of pain and vomiting induced her to think more seriously of her illness.

Incision was made through the right rectus sheath and the muscle temporarily displaced. On opening the peritoneum a coil of small intestine was found to be distended and to pass down into the pelvis, which seemed unusually full. At first it appeared as if the uterus was very large and smooth-walled, but further examination showed the swelling to consist of two parts, a softer one to the right, and when the finger was passed into Douglas's pouch a groove could be felt marking a division between them. The pelvis was isolated with sponges and a large pyo-salpinx, which ruptured during the process, was brought outside, separated from its attachments, and removed. The pus was very offensive. The ovary was included in the mass removed. The left side appeared to be normal. The loop of obstructed gut was found adherent to part of the boundary wall of the pyo-salpinx which had been left behind—it was kinked from before backwards ; another loop also adhered to this part, but was not obstructed. These were freed and some omental adhesions were also separated or divided between ligatures. The pelvis and lower abdomen were washed out with warm saline solution, and a tube was left in which extended into Douglas's pouch. On the third day some distension of the stomach was present, and this was followed by a more or less general meteorism which gradually subsided under appropriate treatment, although the patient was for a time seriously ill. The tube was removed on the seventh day after operation. She left the hospital on March 14, 1903.

On October 20, 1904, the patient was readmitted with symptoms of diffuse peritonitis. She had enjoyed good health since leaving the hospital until three weeks before her return; she then had a menstrual period, followed a week later by hæmorrhage from the vagina which lasted for three or four days. This was followed by acute pain on the right side of the abdomen which spread to the left side. This pain continued for a week, and then for the three days previously to her coming up it increased considerably, and was again accompanied on the first and third days by hæmorrhage. She had vomited four times only and on the day of admission. The abdomen was slightly distended but scarcely moved with respiration. The left rectus was rigid, and the lower half of the left side. Great tenderness was complained of all over the abdomen. The flanks were resonant. The pulse was 120, and the temperature 102°. A tender swelling could be felt *per vaginam* in the left fornix. Mr. Sargent, who successfully operated, found that the pelvis contained pus, whilst a sero-purulent fluid invaded the lower abdomen. The left Fallopian tube was of the size of a thumb; its walls were much thickened and distended with pus. The ovary contained a large cyst in which was a blood clot of the size of a tangerine orange. The lower abdomen was washed out with saline solution. From the history of disturbed menstrual function it was thought that the blood clot might represent the remains of an ovarian gestation, but careful examination in the clinical laboratory did not confirm this idea.

(3) *Ectopic Gestation.*—Another part of this subject—that of ectopic gestation and its rupture as a cause of the " acute abdomen "—introduces us to additional symptoms : those caused by the increasing accumulation of blood in the peritoneum and the effect of its loss from the circulation on the general state of the patient. The rapidity with which it is poured out and the effect of this are so great that the patient may die as suddenly as if a deadly poison had been taken. Luckily, most of the victims of this accident are not so quickly overwhelmed, and time is given for attempts at a rescue. It is not my intention to enter into a discussion of extra-uterine gestation, its varieties, diagnosis, modes of ending, etc., but simply to introduce the subject as it occurs in actual practice

as a surgical emergency, so that you may be able to recognise and successfully treat it.

Of instances of the milder type when the hæmorrhage is not excessive but recurs, the following recent case may be quoted :

M. C., aged 32 ; seen in consultation with Dr. Bulger, November 7, 1913, and transferred to the hospital for operation.

Her menstrual periods had been regular until the beginning of September ; between that date and the middle of October there had been no period.   On October 14 a discharge commenced, which had persisted, of thin blood-stained fluid.   There had been slight pelvic pain from time to time for a month.   A week before there had been an exacerbation of this pain, and again on November 4, the pain causing the patient to perspire profusely.   The day before admission the pain came on again and at midnight was very intense, lasting for three hours.   This pain was in the pelvis and both groins, and there was great tenderness of the lower abdomen.   She became very faint and white-faced.

Dr. Bulger, who had been called in, diagnosed ectopic gestation with hæmorrhage, and found an enlarged uterus with fulness in Douglas's pouch.   There was also distension of the abdomen with some tenderness in the lower part.   On admission she was much the same, but had a temperature of 98·4° and a pulse of 128.

At the operation later in the day we found scattered blood-clots over the omentum, and Douglas's pouch was partly filled with black coagulated blood.   The left Fallopian tube was very congested and dilated, especially near the fimbriated extremity.   Here there had been a rupture of the tube and hæmorrhage was still proceeding.   A piece of amnion was found in the removed clot.   The other side was normal. The tube and ovary were removed.   The peritoneum was sutured with catgut, the sheath of the rectus with silk, and the skin with fishgut.   Convalescence was interrupted by a troublesome attack of cellulitis.

Of the more severe cases of hæmorrhage I have selected one of rupture of a sac situated in the wall of the uterus in which symptoms were very urgent and the state of the patient somewhat desperate.   It is a rare position for the sac to occupy, but there is no means of ascertaining this before the abdomen is opened, and the indications for operation are the same as in examples of the much commoner rupture of a tubal gestation.

A married woman, aged 35 years, was admitted ⚹ April 23, 1903. Her history was as follows :—She was treated in a London hospital nine years before for " peritonitis " after a confinement.   She had had five children.   The youngest was eighteen months old.   The last menstrual period was six weeks previously ; one should have come on about a week before admission. She had always suffered from leucorrhœa, but during the past few weeks this had been worse than ever. About a month previously she began to suffer from attacks of vomiting which came on especially after food, which she was unable to retain. There was also some indefinite pain in the abdomen. A fortnight previously she attended the out-patient department and was treated for gastritis. The abdominal pain got worse, and at 4 o'clock on the day of admission she had a very severe attack which doubled her up and later completely prostrated her. She vomited several times and became very cold, pale, and collapsed. During the afternoon she fainted. She was brought to the hospital thirteen hours after the onset of the severe pain. On admission she was blanched, emaciated, and in a state of collapse. The abdomen was held rather rigidly, and was generally tender, especially in the lower part. In the left iliac region there was a rounded elastic swelling, and there appeared to be fluid in the lower part of the abdomen, and to a less extent in the flanks. The pulse was 120 and feeble, the respirations 26, sighing, and the temperature was 97·2°. At 8 p.m. a median incision in the lower abdomen about 4 inches in length was made, and the dark colour of the blood could be seen before the peritoneum was incised. When the abdominal cavity was opened there was an immediate gush of blood mixed with clots, and the hand was at once passed to the uterus and tubes. The left one was enlarged, and so was brought to the surface. The enlargement was found, however, to be due to a hydro-salpinx, so the uterus and right tube were drawn up for inspection. The former was ruptured at a point on the fundus to the inner side of the place where the right tube joined it. It was larger than normal ; the opening was about 1½ inches in length and placed transversely. From it there protruded a fluffy mass of delicate moss-like tissue which filled the opening and bulged over the edges. This was evidently placental tissue. From this place there was a constant oozing of blood. This tissue was removed with a curette and the cavity from which it came scraped out. The opening was then closed with a continuous Lembert suture. This arrested all bleeding. The left tube was then removed. The intestines appeared pale, almost bloodless, and contracted. The peritoneal cavity was carefully cleansed of clots and free blood by saline irrigation and gentle sponging, after which the abdomen was closed. Four pints of saline infusion were injected into the left median basilic vein during the operation with evident benefit. The patient slowly recovered. On the third day she complained of abdominal distension and pain in the epigastric region due to acute dilatation of the stomach, for which the stomach tube was employed, with lavage. Some distension of the abdomen continued for about three days, but the temperature remained normal, and the pulse about 100. Convalescence was slow, and she did not leave until June 29.

In another patient the diagnosis was rendered unusually difficult, there being a diseased appendix present, also because of the history of the illness and the absence of clotting in the blood which had escaped into the peritoneum.

A woman, aged 31 years, was admitted ✕ April 14, 1904. There was history of irregular periods, and a white discharge on and off between the periods, but general good health until April 8. She was then seized with internal pain, which was so bad that on the following day she was obliged to go to bed ; it improved, but recurred severely on the 12th. It was most marked on the right side, running up to the right breast, and affected the right leg so that it was very painful to move. This pain started with the period, which was a fortnight overdue. When the discharge ceased the pain went, but came on again when the discharge returned. Almost fainting, on admission she appeared a pale, anæmic woman. The abdomen, slightly distended and tender, was difficult to examine satisfactorily, as the patient held herself very rigidly. There appeared, however, to be more dulness in the right flank than in the left. On vaginal examination the uterus was normal, freely movable, and a little retroverted ; there was no fulness in Douglas's pouch or abnormality of the uterine appendages. The tongue was furred, but the bowels were acting. The pulse was 112 and the temperature 99°. On the 18th she was again seized with pain in the right iliac region. The vaginal discharge recommenced, being of a red colour. She felt very faint. The pain passed off during the night, and on the next morning her temperature was 100·2°, and on the following evening 101°. The history, character, and duration of the pain, with the rise of temperature, made it very probable that the appendix was diseased, whilst the account of the menstrual irregularities induced Dr. W. W. H. Tate to suggest the possibility of an extrauterine gestation which was leaking into the peritoneum as a result of some rupture of the sac. On the 29th the operation by temporary displacement of the rectus was performed, and a diseased appendix removed after the application of the clamp. As free blood was present in the peritoneum when it was opened, and there was some in the pelvis, the opinion expressed by Dr. Tate was confirmed, and rapid incision in the median line low down gave access to the pelvic organs. The right tube was thickened at one part, and from the ostium abdominale hæmorrhage was still proceeding. This was ligatured and removed with the ovary. A tumour about the size and shape of a pigeon's egg was attached to the left broad ligament. This was excised, and proved to be an intra-ligamentous cyst with papillomatous growth inside it. The appendix was catarrhal, and strictured near its base. The right Fallopian tube was enlarged and thickened ; the ostium abdominale admitted a little finger, and its mucous membrane was rugose. The uterine end of the tube for a distance of 1 inch was normal ; beyond this it was dilated, and contained a large clot which was attached to the upper and posterior part of the interior. No fœtus was found. The right ovary was cystic, and contained a recent corpus luteum, besides several old ones. A pedunculated cyst containing blood-stained fluid was attached to the right broad ligament. The incisions in the abdominal wall were closed after the pelvis had been sponged and flushed with warm saline solution. A week later she complained of pain in the left side of the pelvis, and a hæmatocele gradually formed and suppurated, being opened *per vaginam* about thr e weeks after the operation. She left hospital quite recovered on June 4.

This was, then, a case of tubal abortion, the loss of blood coming from the open mouth of the tube, whilst the unusual character of the pain was explained by the condition of the appendix. There was no sudden seizure, as in the case of the patient with intramural gestation ; but the result would have been fatal ultimately, and I have quoted it as a contrast to the former example. In all operations for hæmorrhage the uterine appendages should at once be brought out of the wound and examined. No attempt to clear away blood-clot must be permitted until the source of the hæmorrhage is found and its flow arrested. No case is beyond surgical aid until actually dead. Examine both sides, for there may be a ruptured sac in each tube. As a temporary measure it is advisable to apply clamps to the uterine end of the tube and to the broad ligament beyond.

The sudden onset of an appendix suppuration may simulate the bursting of the sac of an extrauterine gestation, if menstrual irregularity and no marked rise of temperature are present. A further sudden access of symptoms due to bursting of the abscess, with collapse, simulates a similar condition with renewed hæmorrhage.

Some years ago I was called upon to go into the country at night to see a lady with an acute abdominal illness. The history was that ten days before, when the period was a week overdue, she had had a severe attack of abdominal pain, with faintness and sickness, from which she had gradually rallied. This had been regarded by her medical attendant as probably due to the rupture of an extrauterine gestation, but as she slowly improved he did not think that operative interference was called for. On the morning before I saw her she had been again suddenly seized with a similar attack of abdominal pain, and became collapsed. The condition of collapse continued when I arrived, and was extreme. The pulse was imperceptible, the temperature was subnormal, the extremities were cold, and the patient restless. On the following morning the condition was not improved, and, in fact, for four days she was so ill that it was not thought worth while to take her temperature. As a result of careful tending she recovered, so that on the seventh day after I had first seen her it was possible to open a large collection of pus which

had been known to be present in the lower abdomen for the week, and
which had not much increased in size.   There was no blood-clot in this,
and, although the appendix was not found, it was regarded as the
probable cause of the suppuration.   During the gradual closing of the
abscess an extension of it to the left of the umbilicus was especially slow
in recovering, and pus could be expressed from this part when everywhere else the condition appeared satisfactory.   In this region adhesions
formed between coils of small intestine, and I operated for acute
intestinal obstruction due to them later in the year.   Still later in the
same year an attack of appendicitis made it advisable to remove the
appendix.   A good recovery ensued.

IMPORTANT CHANGES COMPLICATING TUMOURS OF THE UTERUS
AND TUMOURS OF THE OVARIES.

We will consider in the first place some of the complications
arising from changes in ovarian growths because of their greater
prevalence :
  (1) Torsion of pedicle causing hæmorrhage into the cyst,
      acute inflammation, suppuration, or gangrene of a
      cyst.
  (2) Rupture of the cyst, due to intracystic pressure, softening
      of the wall, or injury.
  (1) In torsion of the pedicle the tumour becomes rotated to
a varying extent, and according to the amount of obstruction
to the blood supply of the cyst will be the urgency of the
symptoms.   In all cases of sudden and complete torsion
" peritonism " is present ; sometimes the pain is so severe that
the patient completely collapses.   A careful examination at
this period of the illness will often show the presence of the
tumour either in the pelvis or in the lower abdomen, or the
patient may have been treated for an abdominal swelling which
had caused little or no discomfort, and therefore the question of
operation had been postponed, if it had been considered.   If
the case is complicated by abdominal distension, then it may
be difficult to find the cause of the urgent symptoms, for the
rounded outline of the tumour will be obscured or completely
hidden.   Here there should be no hesitation before exploration
is carried out and the state of affairs adjusted, and in the more
acute cases the patient does not object, for she is suffering so
much that she cannot hide the extent of her sufferings ; moreover, the relatives can see how ill she is.

As the symptoms of " peritonism " pass off they are replaced by those of (a) hæmorrhage, (b) peritonitis, or (c) obstruction.

(a) Patients have been known to die quickly as the result of intraperitoneal hæmorrhage, as in the well-known case described by the late Sir Spencer Wells. In this the hæmorrhage had been previously into the cyst, which had burst, giving rise to an enormous extravasation in the peritoneum. In nearly all of the torsions about which we are speaking there is hæmorrhage into the tumour, but should leakage take place into the peritoneum, of a gradual character, possibly intermittent, the usual symptoms of loss of blood will become evident, with an increase of dulness in the lower abdomen and flanks.

The clinical appearance after hæmorrhage from a cyst which has become more or less filled with blood as a result of torsion of the pedicle resembles very much that presented after a ruptured ectopic gestation. The treatment is similar and the urgency as great.

(b) The vomiting may continue as the shock passes away, and the character of it change. Pain continues, with great tenderness in the lower abdomen. In addition there may be distension, with constipation and retention of flatus. It is possible in these cases that the obstruction is real and caused by the pressure of the tumour, which, owing to a shortened pedicle and increase in size, can no longer accommodate itself to ordinary intestinal movements. This is, however, not so common as in those cases where the constipation is incomplete, flatus is passed, the vomiting irregular, but rarely urgent. Here the symptoms may be those of localised peritoneal irritation with distension and a temperature, pulse, and general condition indicative of septic poisoning from some intra-abdominal source.

(c) When a suppurating cyst ruptures, well-marked peritonitis will develop and prove fatal unless operative procedure is quickly resorted to under favourable surroundings. The importance of early attention to a cyst which is causing pain and a rise of temperature following on a sudden bout of pain is therefore evident. Although after some attacks of this kind it is common to find omental adhesions at a subsequent operation, showing that recovery may follow, there is always the risk that an infection of the cyst has commenced which will terminate in gangrene, which no effort on the part of the patient or medical attendant can localise. It is very dis-heartening to find an acute peritonitis in the late stage caused by a gangrenous cyst with twisted pedicle,which is surrounded by lymph and stinking purulent fluid, where operation has been repeatedly postponed.

The history of attacks of a painful character in the lower abdomen is given in a proportion of the cases of cyst which ultimately show torsion of the pedicle, but such attacks are likely to be misinterpreted and may be due to suppuration. Vaginal examination should not be neglected.

Suppuration of Cysts secondary to Infection from the Diges-tive Tract.—A married lady of 41 was under my care in February, 1907. Her previous history was good; but for four years she had complained of pain in the lower abdomen, especially on the left side, when walking and during the catamenia, which were, however, quite regular. In July, 1906, she had an attack of diarrhœa, following pain of greater severity than usual, across the lower abdomen. Vomiting lasted for three days and she was kept in bed for a week. Some swelling was said to have been present on the left side. Three weeks afterwards she had another attack of pain and diarrhœa and was kept in bed for ten weeks. On this occasion the pain was on the right side, which was very tender. The temperature rose to 101·2° and remained there for nearly the whole of the time. She was evidently very ill.

On examination the abdomen was normal generally, but there was a complaint of tenderness in the lower part to the right of the rectus muscle. At the position of greatest tenderness a rounded swelling could be felt. The uterus was rather fixed; nothing else abnormal was discovered. At the operation a multilocular ovarian tumour the size of a cricket ball was found. It was adherent to the side of the pelvis and broad ligament, and had a short pedicle. The appendix was adherent to it, as was also a coil of small intestine. The former was removed, the small gut was separated, a denuded place being covered in with a peritoneal flap from the surface of the cyst. During its removal the cyst emptied itself of very offensive pus and altered blood. The smell of this was so very fæcal in character that the large intestine in the pelvis was searched for a possible opening, but it was uninjured. The main cyst was bound down by very firm adhesions, which required very considerable force to separate them. The solid gauze packing was removed, and the area involved cleansed with sterilised saline. Another small cyst (not adherent) the size of an egg was removed from the other side. Drainage. There was an offensive discharge for a fortnight. The wound closed in three weeks.

A suppurating ovarian cyst is not uncommonly found in cases where the appendix is removed after localised suppuration. The spread of an appendix inflammation to a cyst may produce adhesions to the surrounding parts so extensive as to render its excision quite impossible.

This was seen in a patient recently sent to me by Dr. Kinloch, of St. Albans. It was necessary to drain the cyst, because its firmly adherent walls were so thin that they separated in flakes with much hæmorrhage.

(2) Rupture of an ovarian cyst may take place quite early after its formation, as in a case brought to me by Dr. Whitehorne Cole.

An unmarried lady had consulted him for some slight symptoms of ill-health, and when leaving his house on her way home was seized with a sharp pain in the abdomen, and became so faint that she was helped to a chemist's. Here she soon recovered and on the following day was apparently quite well.

We thought that the symptoms might have been produced by rupture of a small ovarian cyst. An exploration showed that this had been the cause of her symptoms ; a ruptured ovarian cyst the size of a large egg was found on the left side and removed.

When the patient has a larger cyst the symptoms of rupture may be more acute, whilst, on the other hand, in the absence of sepsis, it may be impossible to say when the wall of the cyst gives way.

J. B., a married woman, aged 60, was admitted under the care of Dr. Cullingworth and transferred on April 27, 1903. She left May 17.

For twelve months she had noticed increase in size of abdomen, but rapid increase during two months. The pain at first was rather indefinite, but more troublesome of late, dragging and tearing in character, worse at night. She had been losing flesh lately. No vomiting, no difficulty with micturition. There was a large swelling of irregular outline in the lower abdomen ; more on the left side. It extended above the level of the umbilicus and to the costal margins laterally. There was marked vermicular movements of the intestines in front of the upper part of the swelling. There was some tenderness over the right side of the swelling. Fluctuation could not be obtained. There was resonance on percussion over the greater part of the swelling, the only area of dulness being immediately above the pubic ramus on the left side. Uterus small, and movable independently of the swelling.

When the peritoneum was opened on April 28 a large amount of yellow jelly-like material (like Brand's essence) exuded. When this had been washed away a pedunculated ovarian adenoma the size of a football was removed from the right side. In this there was a large rupture with everted edges, evidently of some duration. In the cyst with which this communicated was viscid yellow jelly, and the wall was lined with adenomata containing similar jelly, but a few of these were calcified. The cystoma was not adherent. The gelatinous material was difficult to wash away, and left the surface of the intestine quite woolly in appearance. Other structures were normal, and the wound was closed.

If the patient was known to have had a tumour there will probably be a change in its outline and evidences of free fluid which were previously wanting. If the opening is comparatively small and the leakage slow, very little urgency may be shown at first, a somewhat rapid increase in size of the abdomen being the most evident change. To this will be added a difficulty in lying with a low pillow or in moving about, and a swelling of the legs. Examination may give the physical signs of a very large cyst, for the fluid, being of high specific gravity, compresses the intestines against the spine; resonance is found over the colon on both sides and dulness elsewhere.

EXCESSIVE ABDOMINAL DISTENSION DUE TO RUPTURED OVARIAN CYST (treated successfully under adverse circumstances).—Some years ago I was asked by my friend Dr. A. J. Southey, of Colnbrook, to see a patient with him in a village not far from London who refused to leave her home and go to a hospital. She was a single woman of 30 who had noticed an abdominal enlargement for some months which had increased rather rapidly for a few weeks, so that he feared the case would have a fatal ending if he could not induce a surgeon to go and relieve her. After talking the case over it was arranged that we should meet at the house prepared to do ovariotomy if the diagnosis which appeared most probable proved correct. Mr. Carter Braine, the eminent anæsthetist, kindly agreed to accompany me. On arrival we found the patient in the front room of a row of cottages, the window of which came quite up to the pavement. The patient, who was greatly distended, had some dyspnœa, and considerable œdema of both lower extremities which extended on to the abdominal wall. The surroundings were most unfavourable for operation, there being a limited supply of linen, of soap, and only a low table that would bear her weight. The only other person in the house was a woman of the working class whose acquaintance with modern ideas of cleanliness appeared very limited. The supply of boiled water was very inadequate, but we kept this assistant engaged in preparing more.

The abdomen was very large and of rounded outline, dull all over excepting in the flanks. A fluid thrill was felt throughout.

She did not like lying on her back, and when she was under the anæsthetic it was necessary for her to be held in position whilst the incision was made. Many pints of fluid were taken away, and an ovarian tumour, one of the larger cysts of which had ruptured, was removed from the left side. Another and smaller multilocular growth was found in the pelvis, adherent to the right side and posterior aspect of the uterus ; to free this required the aid of strong scissors. The intestine remained flattened against the posterior wall of the abdomen, and the abdominal wall in front seemed very thick, heavy, and altogether too large. The remaining fluid was cleared away with gauze swabs and the incision closed. She made a good recovery. Dr. Southey gave most valuable help, and through his devotion to the welfare of the case without any consideration of his own interest, the life of this woman was preserved, for she had made up her mind that she would " die at home ! "

The air which is left in the peritoneum in such cases may take three to four weeks before it is absorbed, as was shown in a case where there were hernial sacs in the groins, which had been overdistended before operation.[1]

Occasionally the remaining tumour can be made to travel from side to side in the fluid, if the pedicle is of adequate length. Again, an infected cyst may become adherent to the bowel and discharge its contents into it. In this way a patient may progress with fair comfort for a long time, excepting for occasional inflammatory attacks in the cyst and the increase in size of the rest of the tumour.

There are two conditions affecting subperitoneal uterine fibroid which may give rise to an acute abdomen, the first is the twisting of the pedicle, the second is acute necrosis. Both are rare compared with the frequency with which the complications of ovarian tumours obtrude themselves on our notice.

TORSION OF THE PEDICLE OF A SUBPERITONEAL FIBROID OF THE UTERUS RESEMBLING ACUTE APPENDICITIS.—An unmarried woman, aged 40, was admitted for " appendicitis " on October 30 and left November 21, 1913.

So far as the patient knew, she had always been well, with the exception of troublesome constipation, until October 26, and her periods had been normal.

On that day she was suddenly attacked with pain in the lower abdomen, not more one side than the other. This pain continued all day, and in the evening she noticed that the abdomen was swollen. The pain was worse after food, but she did not vomit ; it was also increased by micturition, and there was some difficulty at the commencement of the act.

On admission the pain was chiefly on the left side, but easier. Later

[1] See Trans. Med. Soc. Lond.

in the day there was distinct tenderness on the right side, with some distension of the lower abdomen, and an ill-defined swelling to the right of the middle line.   The temperature was 100·6° and pulse 108. Vaginal examination was negative.

She was kept in bed, and the distension diminished so that a swelling in the right lower abdomen could be defined.   Its upper boundary was rounded, and the whole swelling gave the impression that it was the size of an ostrich egg and arose from the pelvis, but it was not possible to ascertain whether there was any fluctuation in it or not.   As the inflammatory symptoms were quieting down, operation was postponed until November 7.   The incision was made to the right of the middle line and the rectus displaced outwards.   The tumour was a sub-peritoneal fibroid, growing from the right posterior aspect of the fundus, the size of an orange, the pedicle of which was twisted.   This was clamped and the fibroid cut away.   The left ovary was cystic, so this and the tube were removed with the uterus by supra-vaginal amputation.   The uterus presented many fibroids of different sizes in and about the body, but the one which had been removed was the largest.   This was inflamed, and on section showed extensive hæmorrhage into its substance.   The appendix was long and contained concretions, so it was excised ; it had not been recently inflamed.   Recovery was uneventful.

After the tumour was definitely outlined on lessening of the intestinal distension, she said that she had noticed swelling there before the present attack.   There had been no menorrhagia.

When the rotation has been more gradual in its progress we may find adhesions to the surrounding parts, which in their turn as they become organised may produce obstruction of the bowels.

In 1903 Dr. Fairbairn[1] made a valuable contribution to the study of one of the varieties of necrotic change, the so-called " necrobiosis " in fibro-myomata of the uterus.   Although this is well recognised amongst gynæcologists it is not often met with, nor does it necessarily demand immediate operation. Still, there are cases in which urgent symptoms arise, commencing with an attack of acute pain in the lower abdomen.   Pain was present in 16 out of 23 cases which Dr. Fairbairn collected, and in all it was the reason for the patients seeking advice.

The following is a good example of the more acute process :—

A married woman, who was four and a half months pregnant, was admitted in 1903.   Five days before she had been suddenly seized with an attack of violent pain in the lower abdomen, and the pain and vomiting continued when she came in.   For four days a swelling had

[1] *Journal of Obstetrics and Gynæcology*, 1903.

been noticed. The abdomen was enlarged, presenting two tumours rising from the pelvis. The one on the right was the size of two fists ; that on the left was the pregnant uterus. The temperature was 99° and pulse 118.

At the operation a necrotic fibroid was removed from the anterior and right aspect of the uterus. The attachment of this tumour to the uterus was easily separated with the finger, but it was difficult to stop the bleeding from the raw surface left, as the tissues were very soft and sutures easily pulled out. Pressure with sponges soaked in hot saline solution appeared to answer most effectively. The wound was closed, and she recovered without miscarriage, although a low temperature and quick pulse continued for some days.

The attachment of the tumour to the uterus, which was pushed to the left, was in this instance very slight, and it was not possible to bring flaps completely over the raw surface. The tissues around the attachment appeared to have undergone inflammatory softening and would hold neither sutures nor ligatures.

Similar cases are referred to by Dr. Fairbairn in his paper, notably those under the care of Bland-Sutton, Doran, and Mackenradt. Bland-Sutton has pointed out the liability to mistake these cases for axial rotation of an ovarian cyst. In either case operation would be required, and therefore the mistake would not have any serious consequences. Most of the patients were pregnant and there was no history of menorrhagia.

PART V

OTHER CAUSES OF THE ACUTE ABDOMEN

At intervals one meets with cases showing acute abdominal symptoms, such that a diagnosis of one of the diseases already described may be wrongly arrived at ; yet on opening the abdomen the appendix, intestines, and stomach do not show any of the expected lesions, there is no obstruction of the bowels, and search must be made for other possible causes of the symptoms. Acute pancreatitis or acute cholecystitis are perhaps the most likely of these. Very occasionally an acute dilatation of the stomach may have given rise to the symptoms.

ACUTE HÆMORRHAGIC PANCREATITIS.

In this disease the onset is sudden and associated with severe abdominal pain, located usually in the upper abdominal and umbilical regions. The signs often suggest acute intestinal obstruction; at other times perforation of an ulcer of the stomach or duodenum, or acute bacterial invasion of the peritoneum, such as that by the streptococcus, may be suspected. A history suggesting previous inflammation of the gall-bladder or ducts is occasionally obtained. The following case is that of a patient who recovered after operation :—

A widow, aged 57, was sent to my care by Dr. G. Brebner Scott, of Brixton, for an acute abdominal illness, on February 23, 1909. At 6 o'clock on February 22 she complained of great pain in the abdomen. She said that it began on the right side and spread rapidly to the left, and also extended upwards to the right costal margin. She was sick at the same time, and could keep nothing down subsequently. Her bowels had acted naturally the previous morning.

There was no history of biliary colic or of injury, and she had been quite well until this illness. She was a well-nourished woman, who still complained (at 6 p.m. on February 23) of abdominal pain. This was now general all over the abdomen. She looked ill, had a pulse of 110, and a temperature of 101°. The abdomen was distended, generally hard to the touch, and very tender, but not specially so in the iliac fossa. On percussion there was patchy dulness, both in front and on the lateral aspects of the abdomen, but not in the flanks. No abnormal swelling could be felt, but the wall of the abdomen, which was fat, was also distended and resistant. Her tongue was dry and bowels not acting. At the operation, which was performed about twenty-four hours after the beginning of symptoms, an incision was made on the right side through the rectus muscle. When the peritoneum was opened a good deal of blood-stained fluid escaped. There was no lymph on the peritoneum, but the omentum appeared somewhat thick and infiltrated, whilst in more than one spot there was fat necrosis. The pancreas appeared harder than usual, and enlarged. The gallbladder was normal ; no stone could be felt either in it or in the biliary passages. The small intestine on the right side was distended. The peritoneum was washed out with normal saline solution and the incision was closed. She was relieved by the operation, but on the following evening her temperature rose again to 100° and pulse to 136, so the incision was reopened, the presence of fat necrosis confirmed, more fluid evacuated and a drainage tube put in. The following day Cammidge's test C was reported as positive. The patient was very ill for some days, and at one time appeared very weak, flushed and despondent. Drainage was continued until March 10, after which she gradually improved. It is not necessary to give any further details. She left hospital on April 20, having quite recovered.

A more acute case, but one which came under treatment eight hours after the commencement of symptoms, was that of

G. L., aged 39 ; admitted January 25 and left March 3, 1914. For about a fortnight he had had a feeling of slight illness, but never any abdominal pain or special symptoms. At 3 p.m. on the day of admission he had gone to bed to rest, when he was seized with violent pain in the epigastrium. This continued and he vomited till he came up five hours later. He was a big, strongly-built man who looked very ill, had a respiration of 28, pulse of 72, and temperature 97°. The abdomen moved very badly with respiration and was rigid all over with areas of well-marked dulness in the flanks, in the left iliac fossa, and in the middle line of the umbilical region. There was general tenderness and rigidity, the tenderness being most marked over the stomach region.

The man was sent in for supposed perforation of a gastric ulcer, but in discussing the case before operation we came to the conclusion that he had acute pancreatitis. About eight hours after the onset of the pain an incision was made in the epigastric region to the left of the middle line, the rectus sheath opened and the muscle displaced to the left. As soon as the peritoneum was opened there issued a quantity of thin watery blood. More of this fluid was found in the flanks and iliac fossæ, and in the lesser sac of the peritoneum.

The peritoneum over the pancreas was softened and felt rather shreddy, and it was possible to expose the gland by using a pair of dressing forceps. It felt hard, was enlarged and somewhat lobular. A tube was passed down to the gland and packed off from the peritoneum : it was in contact with the gland at its lower end, and in consequence of the size of the patient was of unusual length. A suprapubic puncture was also made and the peritoneum flushed with saline solution (temperature 110°). There was a suspicion of fat necrosis about the duodenum, but nothing definite. Fatty material came away in the irrigating fluid. Tubes were left in both wounds.

Dr. Dudgeon reported : " January 30, 1914. Cammidge's reaction test C after fermentation. Negative."

For the first five days there was free drainage of serous fluid from the upper wound, but after that a thick purulent discharge from both wounds. For some days he complained of a great deal of epigastric pain, and there was fever with a pulse of 100. But his expression was good and the strength of the pulse satisfactory. The drainage tube was removed on March 4. The discharge gradually ceased, but the wounds were slow in healing.

Acute pancreatitis is most commonly seen in adults, especially males of more than 40 years of age, well-nourished and even fat ; possibly the patient is a free liver who has been in good health until seized with a sudden attack of severe abdominal pain and urgent vomiting. On examination the abdomen has been more resistant generally than it should have been, but not rigid. The epigastrium has been most tender, but there has been a diffused superficial tenderness, especially on unexpected light palpation, in other parts. The general resonance over the abdomen has been rather patchy in character, whilst the movements during respiration have been good. In all the pulse has been rapid, the temperature elevated, 101° to 103° ; there has been anxiety, and not infrequently a flushed face.

If the abdomen is opened within twenty-four hours the amount of blood-stained fluid will usually be small, but sometimes may be in sufficient amount to cause dulness in the flanks, and may be supposed to have come from the wound ; again, at this stage, it may be difficult to find any points of fat necrosis. In any case, in the adult where nothing is found in the more usual places to account for acute abdominal symptoms search should be made for these patches, which are yellowish-white in colour, and of small size (Fig. 30). If nothing is discovered to account for the state of the patient, then it may be well to put in a drainage tube for a few hours at all events, for a discharge of a red colour will soon come away, odourless at first, but later, and when in larger quantity, having a peculiar mawkish smell, which, so far as I know, resembles nothing else. There may be no evident swelling of the pancreas. Many cases will only be diagnosed when the opened peritoneum shows the presence of spots of fat necrosis in the omentum, the escape of odourless blood-stained fluid having first attracted attention.

This fluid may, however, be thought to have run into the deeper parts from a cut vessel in the wound, unless it appears flaky, and the operator is prepared to find it.

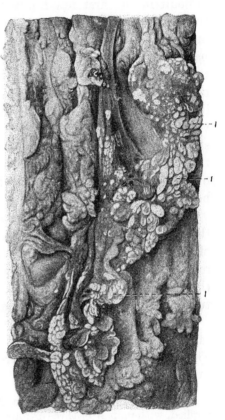

The previous history may be of the greatest importance, pointing to the presence of gall-stones or ulcer of the stomach or duodenum. Sometimes there is a history of an acute abdominal illness of doubtful causation.

The principal abdominal catastrophes with which this disease is liable to be confused are—the perforation of gastric and duodenal ulcers ; in the male the resemblance to the latter is very close, if there has been a history of former attacks of pain and there is much fluid in the peritoneum within a few hours after the

FIG. 30.—Fat Necrosis, from a Specimen in the Royal College of Surgeons Museum : 231, 1, General Pathology.

acute onset. If the vomiting continues and there is a rising temperature with patchy dulness and general hyperæsthesia of the abdomen in a stout adult with previous good health, there is less difficulty, but even then a small perforation might mislead the inexperienced, although there is a great difference in the appearance of the two patients and in the state of the lower abdomen.

In intestinal obstruction high up in the small intestine there is the same kind of initial peritonism. The symptoms are severe, vomiting troublesome, and constipation marked. There is no distension at first and but little peristaltic movement visible. If the patient is a female over middle life, without any history of gall-stone colic, the diagnosis may be difficult in the first few hours after onset, but as time passes the symptoms in this form of obstruction change, the pain is more definitely of a paroxysmal character, the site of the chief pain becomes more umbilical, whilst peristalsis is seen. In thin people a lump may be felt which is neither in the position of the gall-bladder nor of the pancreas. Distension comes on in the later stages as the gall-stone approaches the ileo-cæcal valve, and the symptoms show a considerable change as the stone is passed along. If the patient gives a history of operation for an abdominal condition, or has had an illness which might indicate the possibility of internal adhesions, this must be fully discussed.

The presence of the tumour in cases of acute distension of the gall-bladder, with its rounded outline, and the localisation of the pain and tenderness to the parts under the right upper rectus, with the rigidity of that muscle, will suffice to indicate the nature of the mischief. There may be no jaundice. A tumour is rarely felt in acute hæmorrhagic pancreatitis.

In a case seen at a later stage it may be very difficult to say that the illness is not due to an attack of acute appendicitis. This is so in hospital work more than in private. To give an example:

A deaf woman, by no means intelligent, over 50 years of age, who applied, with pain after three or four days' illness; a distended abdomen, with dulness in the flanks and general tenderness. Rapid pulse, temperature 100°, and continued vomiting. With these symptoms and signs, an inability to say where the pain began, and no history of previous illness.

Still, even in such a case as this, that of a woman admitted in December, 1913, there were signs which pointed to the appendix as the origin of the trouble

The muscular wall seemed more rigid in the right lower abdomen, the dulness was more evident in the right flank and iliac fossa, whilst the acute tenderness, indicative of spreading peritonitis, was most marked on the left. The epigastric region was without rigidity or special tenderness.

She had a general peritonitis secondary to a gangrenous appendix, and died in the following month, when convalescent after the operation, from hæmorrhage from a gastric ulcer.

These patients are not good subjects for an abdominal operation, and I believe you will get better results in most cases from simple incision with the insertion of a large drainage tube down to the pancreas with gauze packing, than from a more elaborate operation. Most of them will not stand a prolonged manipulation, with the larger amount of anæsthetic ; it is possible, however, to do much more if the patient is in fair condition and not too fat. The ideal operation is to incise the tissues over the pancreas, with due regard to the duct and main vessels, and establish a direct route for drainage, packing off the tube with gauze ; unfortunately the action of the secretion from the gland, if much escapes, on the tissues with which it comes in contact is very destructive, and if the flow is profuse you will find it difficult to prevent actual digestion of parts.

Mr. Barker[1] suggests that when the operator finds in an early case that the acute process is mainly or entirely retro-peritoneal, it will be advisable to drain the affected area by a large tube passed from the flank along a track partly made by the forefinger. In this way he may close the anterior wound without drainage, and avoid possible complications from adhesions in later life.

If the condition of the patient permits the time required for the removal of any gall-stones that may be discovered, they should be removed and the gall-bladder drained. Should a stone be present in the common duct, it should be extracted, a drainage tube passed down to the opening, and isolated by gauze. Sir Berkeley Moynihan recommends that access to the pancreas should be obtained by making an opening through the gastro-hepatic omentum ; others that the deeper opening be made through the gastro-colic omentum ; this is the more accessible route of the two, and better placed for drainage.

A stone in the common duct may be left until the state of the patient is less critical ; the drainage of the gall-bladder will effect the immediate improvement required.

[1] *Lancet*, Vol I., 1914 p. 1594.

You need not place a drain in the pelvis, for after cleansing the peritoneum, either by sponging or lavage with sterilised saline, the plugs which are placed around drainage tubes should be sufficient to prevent further escape into the general cavity of the peritoneum. Strong fishgut sutures passed through all the layers of the abdominal wall to close the wound are the best, provided they do not obstruct the rubber drains. A firm many-tailed bandage should be applied with plenty of absorbent dressing. You must trust to drainage by the anterior wound in severe cases and not prolong the operation and incur further risks by making a posterior opening.

If it is necessary to drain for a long period, a ventral hernia will certainly result, and it will be well to explain this to the friends during the course of the illness. It cannot be avoided.

The plugs should be removed after thirty-six hours, gradually, according to the amount of pain which the adhesion may cause. If the wound becomes septic the administration of gas and oxygen, and the early removal of the plugs, is indicated, and the insertion of others after a cleansing of the wound with an antiseptic solution.

ACUTE DILATATION OF THE STOMACH.

This is a rare condition, the cause of which is often doubtful ; at other times it follows an operation or injury involving the peritoneum, and it is with these that we are most concerned.

An attack starts with copious fluid vomiting, epigastric pain and distension, which becomes general ; the action of the bowels is irregular ; signs of extreme collapse are present. Towards the end of a severe case complete atony of the stomach may lead to cessation of the vomiting.

Of physical signs, the most valuable, when it is present, is succussion, but it is important to remember the possibility of the occurrence of such a condition in the acute abdomen.

Unless relieved by evacuation of the stomach contents it usually proves rapidly fatal. The extreme distension of the abdomen and generally severe condition may lead to a diagnosis of acute peritonitis, or if there is constipation intestinal obstruction may be thought to be present. A few notes of a case will bring this condition more fully before you.

On January 21, 1903, I was asked to see a girl of 15, who had been under care for two days, in consequence of an acute pulmonary affection, but there had been a sudden change in her symptoms. She was the subject of angular curvature of the dorsal spine, the result of old tuberculous disease.

On the 21st she began to vomit about 7 a.m., the vomited material being of a bilious character, and yellow in colour. The bowels acted at 8 a.m. The pain in the side of which she had complained was much better, but the constant vomiting masked all other symptoms. Temperature, 99°; pulse, 80. Nothing relieved the sickness. The abdomen was retracted, dull all over, and without tenderness on pressure. At 6 p.m. she was rather collapsed, the vomiting continued, and now she was bringing up a black, tenacious fluid. She had complained of no pain since the vomiting came on, but the abdomen was becoming distended. About 11.30 p.m., when I saw her with Dr. Bulger, the abdomen was somewhat distended but not markedly so, dull on percussion all over the front and down the left flank to Poupart's ligament. No dulness was present in right flank. A well-marked thrill of fluid could be felt in the lower part, and to the left. There was no rigidity. Her pulse was rapid, face pale and sunken, tongue black and dry, whilst there was frequent vomiting of a black, tarry fluid.

An incision in the middle line showed a greatly distended stomach, the lower margin of which passed down to the pubes ; it was bluish in appearance and flattened with very thin flaccid walls. All the intestines were empty. There was no free fluid. Distension apparently ceased at the third part of the duodenum, and no pressure could empty the contents of the stomach along this part. A tube was put in, and the opening sutured to the abdominal wall. Much black, blood-stained fluid was drained off from the stomach by this tube, and vomiting ceased ; but otherwise little relief was afforded, and the patient died on the following day apparently from exhaustion.

Here with acute symptoms we find dulness along the middle line for the first time in the acute abdomen.

As an example of the disease following an abdominal operation a case [1] may be given, as it illustrates many important points which may develop during the course of such an illness.

A woman, aged 27, came under my care from the late Dr. Heath, of St. Leonards-on-Sea, on November 7, 1901, for a swelling in the abdomen which had been noticed to be increasing for the previous nine years. On November 12 a cœliotomy was performed, the diagnosis of ovarian cyst confirmed, and a large tumour removed in the usual manner.

On the first and second days after the operation the patient's pulse was about 110, and temperature rose from 101° to 103°. The abdomen became increasingly distended ; there was no vomiting beyond that directly following the anæsthetic. A week after the operation there was

1 See *Lancet*, 1903, Vol. I., p. 1031.

evidence of slight suppuration in the abdominal wound, and some pus was evacuated with a director. There continued to be great distension of the abdomen and much discomfort.

On November 21 Dr. C. R. Box saw her with me. The epigastric area was then very prominent and a ringing coin sound could be obtained over this area and extending downwards to the iliac crests ; marked succussion was elicited on shaking the patient ; there was no vomiting. Lavage of the stomach was commenced and carried out twice daily from this time. Twenty-six days after the operation parotitis developed, associated with a septicæmic temperature and severe diarrhœa, and for some days this was uncontrollable. Antistreptococcic serum was given ; a marked rash followed two days after its administration, but it was without apparent effect on the disease. The distension of the abdomen did not appreciably diminish, and with a high temperature and the diarrhœa it continued for about three months ; much œdema of both legs and the lower part of the abdominal wall supervened. Some peristalsis in the region of the umbilicus was occasionally seen, and the stomach still showed the physical signs of dilatation.

On August 12, 1902, the gastro-intestinal functions had become practically normal, the œdema in the lower part of the body, due presumably to thrombosis of the inferior vena cava, was still present and the patient left the hospital. Seen again in January, 1903, her general health was good, though evidence of thrombosis persisted, there being some œdema of the ankles with dilatation of the veins over the lower part of the abdomen.

The subsequent history of this case is very interesting. She was readmitted under my care on November 19, 1907, for another abdominal swelling. It was stated that her general health had been good until a fortnight before, but that during that time she had suffered from pain in the stomach and swelling but no vomiting. The abdomen was a good deal distended and tense on admission, the superficial veins dilated, chiefly in the lower part, and there were numerous lineæ albicantes in the same region. A dull rounded area was present reaching almost to the umbilicus from the pelvis. This was fluctuating and tender, whilst around it the intestines were distended and tympanitic. Her temperature was slightly raised. She was kept in bed for some time in order to give the inflammatory state a chance of quieting down, but the distension did not appreciably diminish. On December 4 an incision to the left of the middle line was made, and an inflamed ovarian cyst removed. The pedicle was long and had been twisted three times from left to right. The cyst was very adherent to the omentum, but not suppurating. It was an ordinary multilocular cyst. The gut was very much distended, the sigmoid being about 5 inches in diameter when examined in the wound. It was not punctured, as the condition was regarded as temporary in character.

Much flatulent distension of the abdomen continued not involving the stomach ; many remedies were tried, but until the employment of the interrupted current late in December no definite effect appeared to have been produced by them, but the distension suddenly subsided on the 25th of that month. There was no suppuration or rise of temperature after the operation.

The unusual amount of distension of the intestines present at the time of the second admission, and the difficulty in getting rid of it after operation is especially interesting in a patient with this history. On this occasion there was no suppuration either before or after operation, yet the distension was extreme, and suggested that the nervous element was an important factor in its causation. The rapid recovery on the use of the interrupted current confirms this view. We know how marked the "reflex" effect may be sometimes of an injury to the abdomen unattended with obvious lesion, also the great distension which may ensue on the mere application of a ligature to the neck of a hernial sac in the operation for radical cure. In one patient a condition of rapid distension of the abdomen with pain, vomiting and a temperature of 103·6° ensued with a collapse which excited alarm. Appropriate remedies soon produced a change for the better and the case ran the usual aseptic course.

These cases are both of them examples of acute dilatation of the stomach but present many points of contrast. In the first the stomach had become a mere fluid-containing sac with a thin wall, which at the time of the operation was lying over the front of the intestines and gave a dull note on percussion across the middle line, an area which is resonant in all other conditions of the acute abdomen. There was most certainly no gaseous accumulation, and until quite the last stage there was no distension of the abdomen. It is difficult to account for it, unless we accept the suggestion that it was a paralysis due to some toxic condition associated with the patch of inflammation of the left lung found by Dr. Bulger, when he first saw the patient. Spinal deformity has been noticed in other cases of acute dilatation, but when not associated with the application of a plaster jacket it is difficult to understand how it could have much influence on the production of such an acute and fatal affection.

Dr. W. B. Laffer[1] collected a series of 217 reported cases, and of these 38·2 per cent. followed operations, usually one on the abdomen. The notes of the second case were published by Dr. Box and myself on account of its rarity, and as an encouragement in the treatment of such desperate conditions. We are inclined to put its occurrence down to some toxic absorption from the wound, although the amount of suppuration was neither acute nor extensive. It is probable that she owed her

[1] "Annals of Surgery," Vol. II., 1908.

recovery to the fact that her distension was general and not absolutely confined to the stomach and duodenum.

As regards the causation of acute dilatation of the stomach, the following opinion may be quoted [1] :—

"This cause we found, after experiments on the cadaver, to be the pressure exerted by the superincumbent and dilated stomach on those parts of the duodenum which lie in contact with the front and left side of the spinal column. We learned later that a somewhat similar suggestion had been made by Meyer in 1889, and by Schultz in 1890. Our hypothesis is that in the production of the train of symptoms, associated with acute dilatation of the stomach, a vicious circle came into play ; first a paralytic dilatation of the viscus occurred, and then distension, due to duodenal obstruction, induced by the weight of the superincumbent stomach."

Although the insertion of a tube after abdominal section into the stomach has been successfully tried, your main reliance should be on position, and the washing out the stomach with the stomach pump or siphon. The patient must lie on the right side with the head low.

EMBOLISM AND THROMBOSIS OF THE MESENTERIC VESSELS.

This is very rare. The results which follow obliteration of the vessels in the mesentery are the same whichever vessel becomes first affected. Gangrene of the gut invariably follows. A man between 30 and 60 years old has an abrupt onset of sudden intense pain in the abdomen, followed quickly by vomiting and collapse, peritonism is well marked. If diarrhœa is present the motions are frequent and blood-stained ; if constipation, then nothing, not even flatus, is passed. The abdomen is distended, rigid and tender. Sometimes free fluid is present. The temperature is often subnormal, the pulse rapid and of bad quality. In the second smaller group the origin is insidious and the progress varies. A diagnosis of intestinal obstruction may be made, but the true condition is only found at the post-mortem examination. Gerhardt gives the following as necessary for a diagnosis :—(1) The presence of a source for the embolus ; (2) copious intestinal hæmor-rhages, not to be explained by disease of the wall of the bowel,

[1] C. R. Box and C. S. Wallace, "Acute Dilatation of the Stomach," *Lancet*, Vol. II., 1911, p. 215.

or by impediment to the portal circulation ; (3) a rapid and marked fall of temperature ; (4) colicky pain in the abdomen ; (5) the simultaneous or previous occurrence of embolism in other parts ; (6) the occasional presence of a tumour in the abdomen, due to the infiltration of the mesentery with blood. All of these signs are not, however, present in every case.

The operative treatment consists in a resection of the part of the bowel that appears involved in the process of gangrene, and the placing of an opening in the bowel at a convenient spot above. This is done (1) because in resection of a portion of gut, the line of suture, if anastomosis of the bowel is to follow, must be in sound tissue, and it is always doubtful in these cases if the gangrene will not spread ; (2) the full operation would in most instances take too long when consideration is paid to the grave state of the patient.[1]

PERFORATIONS OF THE GALL-BLADDER AND BILE-DUCTS.

Symptoms of peritoneal involvement of variable extent arise either from perforation of the gall-bladder, or from its being in a state of phlegmonous or gangrenous inflammation. A history of previous attacks of biliary colic, perhaps associated with jaundice, may very likely be given.

The pain in typical cases will be localised in the gall-bladder region, but it may extend to the umbilicus, to the appendix region, or become generalised, in accordance with the extent of the infection. Referred pain in the right shoulder is uncommon. Confusion in diagnosis with acute appendicitis or perforation of a duodenal ulcer is likely to arise. The following is an example of the former type of case :—

On the evening of November 17, 1903, I was requested to see a patient, aged 58. Two days before he had been taken with severe paroxysmal abdominal pain accompanied with vomiting.

He had had three other attacks of abdominal pain, the first two years previously. None of them had been followed by jaundice, although the pain was always in the region of the gall-bladder, and they were regarded as biliary colic. The present attack began during the night of Saturday, the 16th, and resembled the other attacks. On the 18th he felt so much better that he went into the City to business. In the evening he came home earlier than usual, and sent for Dr. Godfrey, who found him again complaining of pain in the abdomen, with a temperature of 101°. On

[1] Moynihan, Abdominal Operations.

the following morning he was worse, and during the day he had occasional vomiting; the abdominal pain continued to be severe and gradual distension came on, whilst his expression became changed to that associated with serious abdominal disease.

When I saw him about 11 p.m. he had a greyish look and appeared distressed. There was occasional vomiting. His pulse was 84, of fair strength. The abdomen was distended and did not move well with respiration. It was tender on pressure, especially on the right side below the ribs, the area of most marked tenderness being midway between the ribs and the iliac fossa. The liver dulness was not increased, but there was some dulness below in the right flank difficult to define, as the man was very fat. The bowels had acted twice during the day. He was evidently suffering from peritonitis, but we could not decide where the origin of the trouble was. Incision over the iliac fossa showed that to be healthy, whilst there was pus along the colon coming from above where the intestine was covered with lymph. A second incision over the gall-bladder showed a recent peritonitis around it with pus, not definitely localised. The area affected was cleansed, and the gall-bladder examined. It was small, not distended, but presented a small perforation near the fundus. No stone could be felt, but the condition of the patient under the anæsthetic was bad, and it was imperative to finish the operation as soon as possible. The gall-bladder was therefore packed off with gauze, and a tube introduced above the plug down to the opening in the gall-bladder. The patient recovered and has had no acute abdominal attack since.

The cases may be very acute in their course, and early operation affords the only chance of success. The peritoneum fills rapidly sometimes from this source, and as a rule there is little in the previous history to point to the presence of gall-stones in the gall-bladder, as they are usually of large size, giving very little inconvenience to the possessor until ulceration has taken place over them and extended through into the peritoneum. Occasionally the symptoms may not be of this acute character.

It is possible to get large accumulations of fluid in the peritoneum after perforation of the gall-bladder without the production of much disturbance. This is well known where there has been a traumatic rupture of the gall-bladder or bile-duct, but a rapidly fatal peritonitis is the usual consequence when the contents of the gall-bladder have escaped through a breach of the wall in disease of that viscus, when micro-organisms are very active.

The condition of the patient will not often give the opportunity for an excision of the gall-bladder. You are usually restricted to drainage of the gall-bladder and peritoneum. Do not forget the tendency of escaped fluid to run down into the pelvis.

Perforations of the gall-bladder or bile-ducts, though by no means frequent, form an important class in the production of abdominal catastrophes. McWilliams has collected 108 cases from general medical literature.

In a series of 3,180 operations on the biliary system there were only 29 cases of perforation, or less than 1 per cent.

Dr. C. Campbell Horsfall has recorded [1] the case of a woman of 45 on whom he operated for a perforation of the common bile-duct the day after its occurrence. The patient had gall-stones. It was not possible to see the opening, but drainage was provided to the part from which bile was coming, and tubes placed in the right kidney pouch and over the pubes. He says that McWilliams collected four similar cases amongst the series of 108 perforations of the biliary passages.

(1) *Kehr.*—Female, 51 ; symptoms four days ; perforation of common duct ; cholecystectomy.

(2) *Riedel.*—Male, 56 ; symptoms three days ; perforation of common duct and gall-bladder ; cholecystotomy.

(3) *Routier.*—Female, 56 ; symptoms one day ; perforation of common duct, free bile ; cholecystotomy. Recovered.

(4) *Neupert.*—Female, 42 ; symptoms fourteen hours ; perforation of common duct at juncture with cystic duct, free bile ; cholecystectomy. Recovered.

The above five cases show in a very graphic way the importance of early operation in these cases. In two the symptoms had been in progress for four and three days respectively, and both died. The other three were operated on within thirty-six hours after perforation, and all recovered.

Occasionally the symptoms may not be of this acute character. A patient under my care in 1908 was admitted for supposed intestinal obstruction. He was a feeble old man, who had been losing flesh and strength for some time, whilst the abdomen had gradually become distended for a week or ten days before admission, during which time he had also had a little vomiting and constipation. The abdomen was distended, it contained a large quantity of fluid, and the man was emaciated and rather yellow in appearance. He appeared apathetic, had no pain, and at this time was not vomiting, but from the history it was supposed that he might have incomplete malignant obstruction of the large bowel with secondary growths about the peritoneum and in the liver. Nothing abnormal could be felt *per rectum.* His pulse was

[1] *British Medical Journal*, 1913, Vol. II., p. 118

not more than 70; his temperature was normal. An exploratory operation was done and the peritoneum found to be full of bile-stained fluid. Search was made for a possible cause of obstruction, but the intestine was nowhere distended and no growth could be felt. Some lymph was seem in the region of the gall-bladder, and amongst this lymph was an opening which led into the gall-bladder, in which there were some gall-stones. The patient did well for a few days after the operation and then rapidly sank and died.

ENTEROSPASM.

By this term is now recognised a condition in which there is a spasmodic contraction of the muscular wall of some part of the intestines ; there is no obvious structural change in the bowel, and the phenomena are usually regarded as being dependent upon some abnormal action of the nervous mechanism.

The spasm may give rise to symptoms of varying intensity, from those of chronic constipation to such as simulate acute intestinal obstruction.

Dr. Hawkins drew attention to the condition in 1906,[1] and I will give some of the conclusions he then set down.

Symptoms usually manifest themselves in patients during the active period of life ; they appear with about equal frequency in the two sexes. The individuals affected are usually of a neurotic type and often of sedentary habits.

Opportunity for direct observation of the spasm of the bowel does not often occur, but Dr. Hawkins thinks that the colon is more often affected than the small intestine. The pain in the subacute cases is sometimes localised in the right iliac region and so appendicitis may be simulated.

In one case under my care some years ago the patient, a man of 50, rather stout and very neurotic, had a swelling in the left iliac fossa, with occasional hæmorrhage from the rectum. These conditions were due to spasm of the sigmoid associated with internal hæmorrhoids.

I need here only consider the severe cases giving rise to symptoms which suggest the necessity of immediate operative interference. Sometimes the resemblance of the condition to intestinal obstruction of organic origin or even **to general** peritonitis **may** be so close that the mind of the observer is

[1] *British Medical Journal*, January 13, 1906.

left in doubt as to the right diagnosis, and exploration of the abdomen will be the only sound course to pursue.

Points which will be helpful in arriving at a decision are the presence of the trouble in highly-strung, nervous individuals, with a history of previous attacks of abdominal pain similar in character which have passed off without operation.

In a case operated on for me in St. Thomas's Hospital by Mr. L. Norbury :

The patient was a woman of 40, for whom I had removed gall-stones about two years previously. Her symptoms were those of acute intestinal obstruction, and the spasmodic contraction affected much of the small intestine. She was a typical neurotic in appearance.

I have met with the condition as a localised affection of the splenic flexure in more than one instance. Here the patients have been overworked and anxious men of over 45 years of age. Unless abdominal exploration has been carried out in any case of abdominal pain, it is impossible to say that it is of neuralgic character. I have known severe attacks of recurrent pain put right by the division of a band.

TORSION AFFECTING OTHER ABDOMINAL STRUCTURES.

Many other examples of torsion of a pedicle have been recorded in medical literature, such as the spleen, the gall-bladder, the appendix, Meckel's diverticulum, and, more frequently, tumours with a movable attachment, such as simple growths of the small intestines, cysts of the mesentery. In hydro-salpinx (or pyo-salpinx) the tube occasionally becomes twisted.

Torsion of the great omentum is a lesion to which Mr. E. M. Corner has drawn attention in the St. Thomas's Hospital Reports. It is rather more commonly met with than most of those conditions which we have mentioned in the last paragraph. Not infrequently it has been diagnosed wrongly as appendicitis, but usually there is a history of inguinal hernia on the side of the swelling or a hernia may be present. The size of the swelling, which is mostly situated under the right rectus, and the slight nature of the symptoms considering its somewhat rapid formation, are against an inflammation of the appendix. It is also more movable on the deeper structures and gives the impression of a solid mass.

An incision should be made over the inguinal region and carried upwards as high as necessary along the front of the rectus sheath, the muscle being displaced inwards and the peritoneum divided with the posterior layer of the sheath. The upper part where the twist has taken place is not very broad and is easily secured with ligatures. Early operation is desirable because of the danger resulting from gangrene of the omentum involved, but successful removal of the mass, which is sometimes as large as the adult head, has been effected after the condition has been in evidence for a long time. This has usually been during an operation for irreducible hernia. It is interesting to note that many of the subjects of omental torsion have been sufferers from attacks of abdominal pain the origin of which has been unrecognised.

VIGNARD'S CASE.—A man of 31 had attacks of pain in the right side of the abdomen for nine years. These attacks lasted four to five days, and there were four or five attacks yearly. In this patient a diagnosis of appendix abscess with inflammation spreading to a hernial sac was made.

In more than one the position of the pain with rise of temperature and presence of a swelling has led to the diagnosis of appendicitis, or partial obstruction has appeared a likely explanation of the symptoms. It is extremely likely that minor degrees of torsion are frequently present in omental herniæ.

HÆMORRHAGE FROM GASTRIC AND DUODENAL ULCERS.

Few surgeons have any doubt that operative treatment is sometimes absolutely necessary in hæmorrhage from these ulcers. It may be the only means of saving life, but the indications for its performance must be clear and definite. It is certain that in a large number of cases which have appeared to be absolutely hopeless the hæmorrhage has ceased and the patients recovered under appropriate treatment, such as complete rest in bed, the administration of morphine, saline solution given intravenously or subcutaneously, with, in addi-tion, a continuous supply *per rectum*. Nothing should be given by mouth. No visitors or business worries should be permitted.

Some of the published cases do not lead one to think that operation was really necessary, and that the patient would not have recovered without the operation. In addition it should be noted that in more than one instance no lesion has been discovered by the operator.

If, however, the character of the bleeding makes it appear that an artery has been opened up by the ulcerative process, the rules of treatment must be adhered to in the stomach as in the case of similar lesions in other parts of the body.

The need for quick and steady operative procedure will be apparent ; the surgeon must lose no time, whilst the deeper manipulations must not be hampered by an inadequate opening in the abdominal wall. The patient must be prepared as usual in abdominal cases where much shock is expected, whilst the preparations to replace some of the blood which has been lost are completed. If the loss of blood has been considerable, intravenous infusion of sterilised saline should be commenced at once and continued during the operation.

A free incision is made in the middle line to fully expose the gastric area ; the intestines must be packed off with gauze strips, and the stomach examined with the view of locating the ulcer. If nothing is found anteriorly, then it is advisable to explore the posterior surface through an opening in the gastro-colic omentum. The stomach, having been brought outside, must be partly emptied, with a trochar and canula if very full, if not very full through an incision. This incision is made through the anterior wall of the stomach parallel with the greater curvature and nearer to it than to the lesser curvature.

This stomach opening is held stretched with retractors and the interior examined in detail, commencing with the areas in which ulceration is most common. The whole of the interior should be explored when the fluid contents have been cleared away, because of the possibility of the presence of more than one ulcer. The use of any one of the various means used for arresting the hæmorrhage will depend on the size of the ulcer, its position, attachment, and the general state of the patient. These include :—

(1) Excision of the ulcer, and suture of the resulting opening.

(2) Under-running the tissues round the ulcer with catgut sutures, or applying a ligature to the artery which goes to the ulcer.

(3) Suture of the mucous membrane over the bleeding point when this is small, as in the closure of a perforation on the serous surface.

(4) Gastro-enterostomy, taking advantage of the opening already made.

Pylorectomy, which has been advised for some cases of ulceration with thickening, is seldom possible ; the operation is too severe and prolonged for cases of such urgency.

I do not advise the application of the actual cautery ; its effect on the tissues is to produce a slough, which when it separates may give rise to renewed hæmorrhage and septic trouble.

Sir Berkeley Moynihan[1] writes :

"Gastro-enterostomy, it was found, led, in all my cases, to an instant cessation of the bleeding and to the speedy and complete healing of the ulcer. The explanation of this was, it seemed to me, as follows : In all cases of hæmatemesis or melæna, the tendency to spontaneous cessation is known to be remarkable ; the cause of the continuance of the hæmorrhage in certain cases, I concluded, after an examination of several cases during operation, must be distension of the stomach." . . . "My own practice has justified my advocacy of this method ; in no case have I found reason to regret having adopted it. In all, the arrest of the hæmorrhage has been complete, and permanent."

This is a very important statement coming from such an authority.

One of my cases of gastro-jejunostomy died a few days after-wards from hæmorrhage from an ulcer in the duodenum, one of two which were present, but this was evidently because the ulcer had extended into an artery, the influence of the opera-tion being brought into play too late to arrest the process.

It may be the wiser plan, when possible, to perform the operation of gastro-enterostomy although the local trouble has also been directly treated.

In dealing with these cases it is advisable to remember that the hæmatemesis may be of hysterical origin, for such a condition is always amenable to medical treatment, and

[1] "Abdominal Operations," p. 162.

should not be submitted to operation under any circumstances. The history of the case given below not only helps to prove this, but shows in a marked degree the ills that may follow such ill-advised interference.

A nurse, aged 29, was sent to me by Dr. Frank Boxall, of Rudgwick, in September, 1902, for varicose veins of the left leg, which were causing her pain when standing. She was admitted to St. Thomas's Hospital, and Trendelenberg's operation with excision of some of the more prominent veins in the calf performed.

In her past history it was stated that she had been in another hospital a short time before for symptoms which were regarded as indicating the presence of a gastric ulcer. One night she developed acute symptoms, which were supposed to have been due to perforation of the ulcer, and an exploratory incision was made in the epigastric region by a surgeon, who found nothing but a normal state of the stomach ; there had been no perforation.

From the history this was supposed to have been hysterical. During her stay with us this opinion was confirmed by the fact that in the earlier days after her admission, when she was looking somewhat anxious in the face, she again gave an exhibition of perforation. She complained of acute pain in the epigastrium, the upper abdomen became suddenly distended, and the muscles appeared tense. There was, however, no change in her facial expression ; the pulse-rate, or temperature, and other symptoms were not in agreement with perforation ; we had also the history to go upon.

This patient left St. Thomas's about a fortnight after the operation for the varicose veins, but returned in 1904 on account of hæmatemesis. She was vomiting daily large quantities of fluid, in which there was a good deal of blood of dark colour, evenly diffused. In spite of the fact that this continued for a month without cessation, she showed no signs of anæmia, and always presented a smiling face to the world. No particular drug was given to arrest the bleeding, which was regarded as of hysterical origin. When the hæmatemesis had ceased for a few days and she had become bright and cheerful she was sent home.

In about three months' time she was sent back to the hospital with another attack of hæmatemesis of similar character, from which she recovered in from three to four weeks, and returned to her home quite well.

It was some months before anything further was heard of her, but she had not been altogether idle. It appeared that she had again developed hæmatemesis when the influence of the hospital had passed off, and this time her friends sent her to a hospital " where there was a surgeon who would operate."

Her next admission to St. Thomas's was on July 19, 1905, when she was found to have a fæcal fistula, which communicated with the transverse colon and was situated at the lower part of a scar, through which, it was stated, her stomach had been operated on. We were informed by letter that although no ulcer or cause for the hæmorrhage was found at the examination, it was thought by the surgeon that there was an ulcer in the duodenum. She said that after the operation she did very well until the tenth day, when it was found that the milk which she was taking came through into her dressings. A second operation was done and the milk no longer came through the wound, but in ten days' time fæcal matter appeared when she took medicine, and fæcal fluid came through if she had an enema administered.

The abdomen was opened in the middle line below the old scar and a lateral anastomosis of the large bowel above and below the fistula done. There were many adhesions. Recovery from this operation was quite uneventful, the fistula was allowed to close and, when she left the hospital, was about the size of an ordinary wooden match. She left at her own request.

Readmission was sought January, 1906, because she said that the escape of gas from the fistula was troublesome and caused offence to patients when she was nursing them.

There was now a fistula about the size of a cedar pencil, and as the bowels were acting well there appeared no reason why this should not be permitted to close. Accordingly a dressing was placed over it, and secured in position by means of broad strips of rubber strapping. The fistula closed to some extent, but we could not feel sure that it was not kept open in some way by mechanical means at the command of the patient. A smaller dressing was then applied, and this was covered and held in position by means of collodion. After this was applied she complained of "excruciating" pain and said that she could not possibly bear the agony of it. It was not, however, removed for a week, when the fistula had completely closed. I may perhaps mention that the fistula was found to have become distinctly larger after she had had a bath without the presence of a nurse : this was before the collodion was applied.

We were for a time under the impression that the case was now completed, but in March, 1909, she again came into the hospital during the cleaning of a charitable institution to which she had gained admission. A fæcal fistula had formed at the site of the former one, and she refused to have anything done with a view to closing it. When questioned as to the formation of this fistula she said that an abscess had come and burst, leaving the fistula behind it, but there is a possibility that it did not form in this manner. If it had been closed, and this would soon have occurred under simple treatment, for there was a free normal passage for the fæces, she would no longer have been eligible for the institution in which she had now been received.

I may add that her expression was that of a neurotic, and the diagnosis of hysteria was confirmed in many ways.

It was surely unnecessary to perform a gastrotomy for the relief of hæmatemesis in a case with this history.

Gardim [1] has given the account of a case of similar origin.

---

[1] *Clinica Moderna*, May, 1905 ; *British Medical Journal*, Epitome, August, 1905.

A girl of 22 had suffered from gastric symptoms for six years, and almost daily vomiting of blood for five months or more ; in that instance the mucous membrane of the stomach is said to have been tinged, hypertrophic and of a red colour, but there was no evident cause for the hæmorrhage. The patient was apparently cured by the operation. Gastric hæmorrhage has sometimes a purely nervous origin ; sometimes it is simply a form of vicarious menstruation, and has a relationship to the menstrual periods, as well as to emotional and constitutional disturbances and injury.

It is advisable to exclude the possibility of cirrhosis of the liver as a possible cause.

PART VI

OBSTRUCTIONS

STRANGULATION OF THE STOMACH.

THIS rare condition is only met with when the stomach has formed part of a hernial protrusion through the diaphragm into the chest. It is well illustrated by the case described, where the symptoms were entirely due to obstruction (practically total) of the stomach alone. Nothing could pass into it from the mouth, and the result was shown in the distress, frequent vomiting, excessive thirst, diminished excretion of urine, rapid emaciation and boat-shaped abdomen. The stomach was accompanied in its escape from the abdomen by the transverse colon, but this was not obviously obstructed. The patient was practically dehydrated, and the effect of saline infusion was such that operative treatment, although delayed, was made possible.

A Spaniard, aged 30, journalist, ✱ was admitted April 15, 1901. He was then very ill and emaciated, with sunken eyes and hollow cheeks. He complained of pain in the upper abdomen ; there was constant vomiting of thin fluid, and he had a feeble pulse. The abdomen was retracted and boat-shaped ; there was some tenderness in the epigastrium, especially to the left of the middle line. His thirst was great. On admission he was so ill that an intravenous saline solution to the extent of three pints was given. He did not look as if he could live through the night.[1]

The history of the case was as follows :—He had in the course of his professional duties in Spain, as a journalist, encountered successfully on some five occasions rivals in the political world, using a rapier as his weapon. When he again had a difference of opinion, which was referred to the arbitrament of the sword, his opponent thought it wiser to prevent an encounter which would very possibly have disastrous conse- quences to himself. He therefore hired a bravo who took an opportunity of stabbing our patient in the left side with a knife before the date of the duel. The doctor who treated him for this wound, which was received about six years before the man came under our care, said that " he saw the lining of the stomach." After recovery it was three years before any serious symptoms developed, and he then had an attack of

[1] *Lancet*, Vol. II., 1901, p. 1582.

vomiting, with severe pain in the region of the wound, from which he recovered in a few days. He had suffered occasionally from attacks of discomfort in the stomach and vomiting, from which he obtained relief by passing his fingers down his throat to make himself sick. A week before admission he crossed from France to England, and was violently sea-sick. The vomiting had continued and there had been complete constipation for six days. When seen the day after admission with Dr. Mackenzie, the vomiting and thirst continued, he was excited and restless, placed his fingers in his throat to make himself more sick, and asked for a large quantity of water to aid the vomiting. The reason why he did this was because he had found that in the less severe attacks of pain and sickness the use of the finger in this way with the effect produced would usually result in relief. The temperature was 96° and the pulse was hardly perceptible. There appeared to be some fulness under the left lower ribs, but no dulness. The chest was well formed and the ribs showed prominently owing to the great loss of flesh. There was a scar over the left hypochondrium in the left axillary line. The note on percussion was resonant all over and the breath sounds normal. There were a few crepitations at the base. The cardiac dulness began at the fourth rib and did not extend to the right beyond the left edge of the sternum. The apex beat was in the fifth intercostal space, 1 inch internal to the nipple line. The sounds were normal. The urine was scanty. The tongue was fairly clean, having a slight white coating. It was necessary to give another three pints of saline before we could operate, and this improved his pulse.

On opening the abdomen through an incision below the left costal margin, a quantity of collapsed gut was found. The descending colon was traced upwards to an oval aperture in the left side of the diaphragm about 2½ inches in greatest diameter. The stomach had also passed through this into the left pleura, and was gradually withdrawn by traction on parts as they presented. Some of the transverse colon and omentum were adherent and could not be withdrawn. The stomach was marked by the edge of the aperture and had evidently been tightly nipped.

Nothing could be done to repair the diaphragmatic opening ; he was too ill.

The effect of the operation was to relieve both pain and vomiting, but he still had much thirst. On the 18th it was necessary to put on a special nurse, he was so very excitable. During the day he frequently " practised dying," and during one of these practices he passed away. The temperature did not rise to normal at any time whilst under treatment.

At the *post-mortem* examination, which was made by Dr. J. J. Perkins, a large loop of transverse colon and omentum was still in the left chest and quite irreducible. There was no sac over the protrusion, but a spurious one had been formed by the omentum ; this was, however, very incomplete, but shut off the pleural cavity. The left lung was pushed up and there was pleurisy on both sides, chiefly on the left, and the lower lobe of the left lung was solid from septic pneumonia.

There was localised peritonitis, probably caused by the passage of organisms through the wall of the stomach at the point where it had been nipped after it had been freed at the operation. The opening in the diaphragm was in the muscular part 1 inch posterior to the limit of the pericardial sac, so that the hernia was in direct relation to the pericardium.

Mr. Lawford Knaggs, who has given an important contribution to this subject,[1] reminds us that protrusion of the stomach in these herniæ may be complete or partial, and therefore the signs will vary. The symptoms may be spread over a number of years dating from a sudden strain or injury :— (1) Attacks of dyspnœa, due to the tumour in the left chest. (2) Discomfort, pain, and vomiting after meals. (3) Obstruction and strangulation, as in the case described. (4) Tetany, as in a case under the care of the late Sir Russell Reynolds.

A woman of 29, in whom the hernia followed a stab inflicted seven years before death from tetany. The stomach, transverse colon, and omentum were found in a hernial swelling the size of two fists, in the left chest. There was no tight constriction.

The signs which are of importance in the diagnosis are the following : they assist very much when present, but they are not always present :—(1) Stomach or intestinal noises in the chest. (2) Intestinal or stomach peristalsis seen through a thin chest wall. (3) Displacement of the heart to the right. (4) A sound produced by the forcing of air from the thoracic part of the stomach into the abdominal part. Other signs of less importance are absence of breath sounds ; alterations in resonance ; changes in shape and deficient movements of the chest ; sinking in of the epigastric region ; inability to lie on the opposite side. Mr. Knaggs considers that in some instances the strangulation of the stomach may be the result of volvulus of the stomach or torsion of the small omentum. Few cases have been submitted to operation, but should operation be performed, and the condition of the case give opportunity, it may be possible to do something with the view of preventing recurrence of the hernia—(1) by suture ; (2) covering the opening by the liver (Berry) ; (3) " anchoring the stomach and omentum to the parietes in such a way as to prevent other abdominal contents finding their way into the opening " (Lawford Knaggs).

[1] *Lancet*, Vol. II., 1904, p. 358

INTESTINAL OBSTRUCTION.

In considering obstructions of the intestines, I have thought it best to present it from the clinical side and to avoid as much as possible the more purely pathological part. It is hoped that you may find what is essential in the diagnosis and so be able to cope with these cases although comparatively inexperienced and perhaps short-handed. It is at all events of the greatest importance that you should be able to " appreciate" a case when it comes before you, for the sufferer from acute intestinal obstruction requires prompt surgical assistance if his life is to be saved.

The arrangement which appears to me most practical is that of the comparative frequency of the various kinds of obstruction as met with in practice.

A. Acute obstructions other than intussusception.

B. Intussusception.

C. Acute supervening on chronic obstruction.

A. Acute intestinal obstruction is responsible for about 24 per cent. of all cases of the " acute abdomen," without including the cases of intussusception, which constitute about 16 per cent. The onset of the attack, with the symptoms of " peritonism "—abdominal pain, shock and vomiting—much resembles that in perforations of the hollow viscera ; and the same careful examination of the abdomen and analysis of symptoms will be required. The character of the pain is of little value, but it is much increased by percussion in peritonitis, more so than by palpation, whilst in obstruction percussion causes little or no pain, whilst palpation is less readily tolerated. The vomiting is severe, and changes its character as the case progresses, becoming very foul-smelling later. Shock may be profound, but varies greatly. The abdominal wall in obstruction is mobile and soft excepting during a paroxysm of pain, whilst in peritonitis it is rigid. Peristaltic movements are more commonly seen in obstruction, but may be found in peritonitis when the inflammation is localised, as I have shown in cases of perforated simple ulcer of the jejunum. In obstruction peristaltic waves can frequently be excited by friction of the abdominal wall. The bowels are confined, neither fæces nor flatus being passed.

In the severely toxic form, or the last stages of peritonitis, the abdominal wall, previously rigid, becomes soft and pliable again. As a rule, in the perforations leading to peritonitis the patient lies quiet, with flexed thighs ; in obstruction he moves about in bed, altering his position to that which appears for the moment to be most comfortable, and complains of almost intolerable griping pain, usually referred to the region of the umbilicus. In all a careful search should be made for any abnormal swelling, which in acute obstruction may be found in various parts of the abdomen. As the case progresses, general distension of the abdomen supervenes and increases, and any localised swelling will be gradually merged in the general enlargement. Septic absorption and inflammation are super-added and the case practically becomes one of peritonitis of the most grave nature. If seen for the first time at this stage a diagnosis of the exact cause of the inflammation is impossible, but prompt measures may yet prevent a fatal termination. Luckily patients do not often permit things to progress to this extent before applying for relief.

In those cases in which obstruction is not so acute in its onset you not infrequently find, before it becomes complete, complaints of griping pain and can see and feel local hardening and swelling of the abdominal wall, with gurgling as gas is forced past the obstruction.

An example of one of the most easily diagnosed (and remedied) forms of obstruction, both from its nature and the short time which elapsed before operation, may be given.

A married woman of 38 was admitted April 15, 1914, with a history that on the previous evening she had felt some stomach-ache, but it was not bad until she had gone to bed. It then became very severe and she had troublesome vomiting all night. At the time of operation (1.30 p.m.) she was still suffering from pain and was vomiting at intervals, the pain was paroxysmal and situated in the lower abdomen. The abdomen was somewhat distended, with shifting dulness in the flanks ; the pain was referred to the under surface of the lower end of the left rectus. Some of the coils of small intestine were very clearly outlined, and there was occasional peristaltic movement. Nothing abnormal was felt on vaginal examination. She had never had any previous illness. Altogether the evidence appeared to be in favour of volvulus of small intestine as a cause for the obstruction, although there was no tumour.

The right rectus was displaced outwards, and when the abdomen was opened a large quantity of clear fluid escaped. The small intestine was generally distended and the largest coil passed into the pelvis, from which a contracted ileum emerged. At the point where these met, about 2 feet from the ileo-cæcal valve, the dilated bowel was twisted and overlapping the contracted portion from left to right. When drawn to the surface, the end of the dilated bowel felt heavy and contained some irregular particles of undigested food. In view of the nearness of Easter Monday, it was suggested by one of the dressers that this might be part of an undigested cocoa-nut. The contents of the bowel were easily passed on, and the obstruction was relieved without any special manipulation. The wound was sutured in layers and the patient had

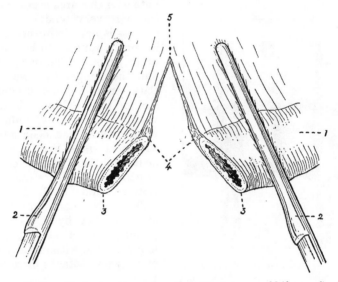

FIG. 31.—*End-to-End Anastomosis after Excision.* — Oblique Section of Bowel after application of Clamps : 1. Small intestine. 2. Clamps. 3. Oblique section of bowel. 4. Cut mesentery coming well beyond edge of section. 5. Wedge-shaped removal of mesentery of limited extent. The points of the clamps should be nearer to the cut edge of the mesentery.

an uninterrupted convalescence. Portions of cocoa-nut were passed with the first action of the bowels.

The obstruction was not complete, therefore there was an exudation of free fluid into the peritoneum. No localised swelling could be felt, partly because the twist was in the pelvis, and the coil affected was not distended with much gas. Early operation was all that was required to put things right.

As an example of volvulus producing a more severe form of obstruction in which early operation is most desirable the following case may be given :—

A.A.   R

G. D., aged 28, was admitted ✶ on November 7, 1904, with acute intestinal obstruction. At 4 p.m. on the day before admission he was suddenly seized with pain in the lower abdomen ; since that time his bowels had not been opened, neither had he passed flatus. There had been vomiting off and on since the onset. The pain had been continuous in character, with paroxysms. On admission it was stated : " The patient's face is drawn with pain, he continually moans and pants. He complains of pain in the abdomen, which does not move at all in its lower part during inspiration, and movement is poor in the upper part. There is a marked prominence in the hypogastric region in the middle line, looking like a much distended bladder. The percussion note over this area is resonant and the part very tender. The liver dulness is not diminished and the abdomen appears to be normal in other parts." The pulse was 120 and the temperature was 100·6°. Catheterism did not diminish the size of the swelling. When seen with Dr. C. R. Box, under whose care the man had been admitted, the local signs had become less acute and there was less complaint of pain. Acute intestinal obstruction was diagnosed, due to volvulus of small intestine, or strangulation by a band. The patient was a strong, healthy-looking man, without any history of previous attacks of abdominal pain.

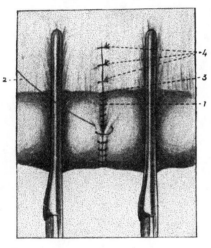

Fig. 32.—*End-to-end Anastcmosis of Small Intestine.*—The inner suture completed. 1. The outer suture continued. 2. On completion it will be tied to 3, which is the same thread left long for this purpose. 4. Sutures closing mesentery.

At 5.45 the abdomen was opened below the umbilicus to the right of the middle line, the rectus being displaced outwards. When the peritoneum was incised a very black coil of small intestine presented ; this was very tense and hard and could not be drawn up through the wound. It was therefore punctured with a trochar, and a quantity of fluid, which consisted almost entirely of venous blood, escaped ; this had a fæcal odour. This coil was then brought outside and found to be the ileum immediately before its junction with the cæcum. Another coil then presented itself and was also tapped and emptied of similar fluid contents and flatus ; it was now possible to lift the whole of the affected gut out of the abdomen. This was quite black, and when emptied of its contents without resiliency, although the peritoneal covering was not without polish. The twist which had occurred was one on the mesenteric axis from right to left, but when this had been reduced no improvement occurred in the circulation of the affected portion of small intestine ; it was necessary therefore to resect the whole of this, and to include an inch or two beyond. Altogether 43 inches of gut were removed from close to the ileo-cæcal valve upwards, Doyen's clamps being placed on the bowel above and below and the mesentery ligatured after the rapid application of artery forceps to each section before it was divided. The upper end was then joined to the part left at the ileo-cæcal opening with two rows of continuous sutures, an inner including all the coats, and a continuous "Lembert" outside that.[1] The upper part of the divided mesentery was also sutured. The pelvis contained dark blood-stained offensive fluid. There was no lymph present on any part of the peritoneum that came under observation. After washing out the pelvis and cleansing the parts involved in the operation with sterilised saline solution the wound was closed with deep and superficial sutures. Chloroform was administered, and during the operation two injections of 5 minims of liquor strychninæ were given hypodermically and, later, 15 oz. of saline solution *per rectum*. The operation was well borne.

Beyond the fact that a localised abscess, probably due to a *bacillus coli* infection, formed in the wound and discharged a fortnight after the operation, there was nothing of moment to record in the after-progress of the case. Rectal feeding was employed for three days. A good abdominal wall without hernial protrusion was obtained.

We had in this case a formidable complication—gangrene of the gut, one which required very prompt measures in dealing with it. Not many hours had elapsed since the onset of obstruction, but the strangulation of bowel had been absolute ; luckily it had not given way into the general peritoneal cavity.

Dr. C. L. Gibson, of New York, collected 1,000 cases of intestinal obstruction (including 354 cases of strangulated hernia), and amongst these there were 121 cases of volvulus. These were taken from various medical publications and included those affecting the large intestine, which are by far the most common, constituting practically the only form of acute obstruction of the large bowel. This variety of obstruction when affecting the large intestine has a mortality of 46 per cent. When affecting the small intestine the mortality is 70 per cent. This is accounted for by the fact that the small gut is of far greater importance, whilst the vitality of its walls is probably less. When the small intestine is the subject of volvulus the symptoms are more acute, manifestations of shock are more marked, and possibly its mobility allows of a tighter twist. Knowing the tendency there is to publish only successful cases, it is very probable that Dr. Gibson's statistics are more

[1] See Fig. 32.

favourable than they should be. He found only one record
of successful resection for gangrene due to volvulus of small
intestine, and this was performed by Riedel on the second day
of obstruction.

A somewhat similar clinical picture is presented by obstruction by Meckel's diverticulum, the symptoms of which are
practically those produced by any kind of band. There is
less frequently a history to guide you as to the actual cause of
the obstruction in these cases ; no account being given of a
previous inflammatory attack or of injury, although you may

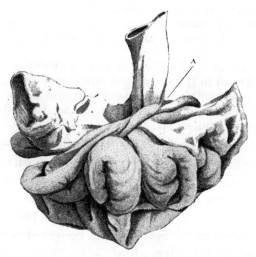

FIG. 33.—Obstruction produced by Meckel's Diverticulum, A.
(St. Thomas's Hospital Museum.)

at times hear of occasional " stomach-aches." Gibson gives
42 cases of obstruction by Meckel's diverticulum, as against
186 by bands of various other kinds. This seems to me to be
much too high a proportion as compared with actual practice ;
obstruction due to a Meckel's diverticulum is not often seen
in our hospitals.

The symptoms produced by the compression of small intestine by a band are practically the same as those described when
the cause is a twist—viz., " peritonism "—with the formation of
a localised swelling in the lower abdomen, which is resonant on
percussion. Any swelling of this kind should be regarded as of
importance and as an indication that nothing but operative

treatment is possible. The friends must be at once informed of this ; they will probably protest and the patient demand morphine for the relief of his pain, but you must be firm.

It is most important that abdominal operations should be performed before any general distension sets in ; operation is far more difficult in the face of distension, whilst the result is likely to be much less satisfactory.

In a stout man of 46 who had strangulation of gut by this diverticulum I found it necessary to excise some 46 inches of the small bowel, but the stitches gave way, because I probably placed them in damaged bowel. It is possible that a wider removal of the gangrenous gut would have had a better result, for I lost my patient.

In both these cases of gangrene the progress of events was rapid, the gut having become gangrenous in a few hours from the onset of symptoms. In dealing with volvulus it is only necessary to empty the involved intestine, and after drawing it from the abdomen twist it round in the required direction. In diverticulum, after the band has been found (not always an easy thing, if one may judge by recorded cases), it requires to be divided and the ends afterwards dealt with. Let me remind you of the necessity of examining carefully any band that may be divided during the progress of an operation for intestinal obstruction. I have known the careless division of a Meckel's diverticulum to allow of the escape of intestinal contents into the peritoneal cavity, which occurrence resulted in a rapidly fatal peritonitis.

In these cases we were met by a very formidable complication which requires special consideration. More or less extensive gangrene of the intestine may confront you in any acute abdominal case in which operation is performed, and you must be able to deal with it on the spot. It is of vital importance that the safe passage of the intestinal contents along the canal should be made possible. There will be no time to send a hurried messenger for button, bobbin, special forceps, or any one of the scores of suggested mechanical aids on which you may have decided to pin your faith ; in the presence of this complication you must immediately act, if you wish to save the life of the patient. The faith which was formerly placed in the special instrument should be put in an accurate method of suturing, after a judicious selection of the points of section of the gut, and in the precautions against sepsis, which are now a part of the usual technique.

There are many cases of localised gangrene in which it is found that a part of the gut does not look sound, but of which it is not possible to say that it will not recover if placed in favourable circumstances. When the portion of bowel affected is very localised, as when the pressure of a band has produced a transverse lesion, it may be possible to invert this by a row of Lembert sutures, as suggested by Professor Caird. I have done this with satisfactory results in early cases of strangulated hernia and pressure by band.

The treatment of gangrene of the small intestine when the entire circumference is affected will depend on the general condition of the patient, and the circumstances of the case, rather than on the extent of the gangrene, for the procedure will be much the same whether you resect 1 inch or 1 yard. In favourable circumstances excision should be the method adopted in the case of gangrenous intestine. Delivery of the affected part from the abdominal cavity, examination to define the extent, not only gangrenous but changed beyond this, cleansing of the part, careful packing off of the healthy area with sterilised gauze, covering of the gangrenous part with gauze to prevent possible contamination of the wound, resection, and subsequent joining of the ends.

In the resection of the gut in both cases which I have recorded Doyen's clamps were used and answered their purpose well. I used them because they were handy. In other cases of resection pieces of drainage tube passed through the mesentery and secured by tying or by forceps have answered equally well. Strips of gauze would answer in case you had no drainage tube available. The proximal and distal clamps should be placed 2 inches above or below the line of proposed section in a healthy part. I lay very special stress on this point, because in the case of obstruction by a Meckel's diverticulum it appeared that the suturing failed because the stitches could not hold in tissue which had been stretched and which underwent afterwards an inflammatory reaction and softening. The bowel seemed healthy, and one was naturally not anxious to excise more than was necessary. It is often advisable to cut the bowel a long distance away ; for instance, in January 1905, I resected 16 inches of small intestine with good result in a case of strangulated femoral hernia, although the part affected by gangrene was only about 1 inch in length. The bowel close to this was not in a healthy state. As each end of the bowel is separated it should be cleaned and wrapped in gauze until wanted. One or two vessels may require ligature. You need not excise a wedge-shaped portion of the mesentery, as in the removal of a new growth of the bowel (see Fig. 32).

The junction of the two ends should be made by careful suturing with a double row of silk sutures. These should be continuous, for they are more rapidly applied than the interrupted, and are equally efficient. According to the thickness of the intestinal wall should be the size of the suture material. As a rule, No. 1 is right for the adult. The first should include all the coats of the bowel ; the second will take only the two outer, as a rule. In applying this, you must see that the suture has a good hold. If you are satisfied on this point, it is not advisable to dip the needle more deeply, for if you pass your outer thread into the lumen of the bowel, in the endeavour to get a stronger hold, your patient will probably do badly. When applying the deeper stitch hold the two portions of bowel with forceps, one pair applied at the mesenteric point of attachment of each half, the other to a corresponding point opposite. If a pair of forceps is also placed half-way between these, closely applying the cut edges, the suture can be introduced still more rapidly. The mesentery should then be sutured, so as to present no raw surface to which adhesions can form ; the parts involved in the operation are cleansed, and the abdominal wound closed without drainage.

The amount of intestine resected in these cases appears large ; 43 inches in one case, and 46 inches in the other. But greater lengths have been excised. Mr. A. E. J. Barker, in a very instructive paper on the limitations of enterectomy, mentions a case in which Mr. Hayes, of Dublin, successfully excised 8 feet $4\frac{1}{2}$ inches of intestine for injury in a boy aged 10 years. Another paper by Mr. Barker will repay perusal. It is on enterectomy for gangrenous hernia. Many practical points are brought out. He also shows that the amount of shock is much less than is believed from such an extensive operation. I have mentioned these excisions of large pieces of intestine to show what can be done, so that you may not be intimidated should you meet with one of these extreme cases, remembering that if the gut at the point of union is sound, and you take proper precautions in following the various steps of the operation, you may gain a success, even in desperate circumstances.

The effect on the patient of the removal of a large portion of the small intestine is apparently very slight. In the former of the two cases of which I have just given details, there was, for a time, a tendency to looseness of the bowels ; but this passed off, and he regained good health, excepting for occasional "indigestion." The effect on the intestine has been recorded by Mr. Barker in two cases in which he had an opportunity of looking at the bowel during life some months (in one case five years) after operation. In both, the line of union was sound and without contraction, but the bowel on the proximal side was somewhat larger than that on the distal side, and showed smaller power of muscular contraction.

In the cases of volvulus the probable cause and position of the obstruction was known and the incision was made to give most direct access to it, due regard being paid to the anatomical arrangement of the muscles of the abdominal wall.

What is the best incision to use in cases where the cause of an acute obstruction is unknown, and what steps should be undertaken to find and remedy this when it is found ?

I think that an incision through the right rectus sheath to the inner side with displacement of muscle outwards is the best ; it should be of a size large enough to admit the hand, far too much time is lost in making a small incision and then enlarging it : you may make a small opening through the peritoneum at first, for it may be possible to quickly discover the cause of the symptoms. Anyway an extension of the incision in the peritoneum is very quickly effected. I have already pointed out the importance of operating before the onset of distension ; where the bowel is but slightly distended, manipulation within the abdomen is easy, for the hand can be passed from point to point without difficulty.

Where the small intestines are obstructed you should first examine the ileo-cæcal region, and if there is empty gut there follow it upwards to the obstruction ; but it is better to empty distended gut at more than one point where there is much distension rather than add to the danger of the case by bruising with your hand the already damaged wall of the gut. This not only enables you to explore the abdomen with greater rapidity and sureness, but gets rid of a large amount of toxic material, the absorption of which adds much to the dangers which the patient is facing. A loop of gut should be drawn out, placed over a sterilised vessel, and punctured opposite the mesentery with the point of a knife ; it is not needful that the opening be of large size. It is closed by means of a Lembert suture of silk (continuous), or by a purse-string stitch. The surface of the bowel is cleansed and the loop returned. It can be repeated with other coils. In examining the abdominal contents with the hand, search should be made for bands, which may be of various kinds, and these should be traced to their attachments if possible and cut short ; if there are adhesions which are too strong to be separated, it will be necessary to resect the bowel, do a short circuiting operation, or in a bad case open the bowel above after attaching it to the abdominal wall (enterostomy).

The operation of enterostomy must be regarded as a very unsatisfactory operation unless performed as a purely temporary measure for the relief of distension in advanced obstruction of the bowel or paralytic ileus. It is sometimes possible to save a life by this procedure when an injudiciously prolonged operation would cause a fatal ending. A local anæsthetic is required, and the opening should be made in the right iliac region, the cæcum or some presenting coil of small bowel being selected for the insertion of the tube. In an adult of ordinary size the incision should be about 3 inches in length. The part of the bowel to be opened is brought to the incision and sutured there by means of silk sutures placed in such a position that it will be possible to put a tube in the centre of the area brought up. A small-sized Paul's tube, or failing that a piece of rubber tubing with side openings near the extremity, or a Jacques catheter, will answer. A small fishgut suture should be passed through all the structures of the abdominal wall at the upper end of the wound, taking up the peritoneal and muscular layers of the bowel wall. Another should be passed in a similar

manner below.   Other sutures, of silk, should then be passed
on each side to fix the peritoneum and fascia of the abdominal
wall to the peritoneum and muscular layers of the intestine.
It is an advantage to the patient to have the tube put in at
once, and to facilitate this the loop should be pulled forward,
packed off with gauze, and the bowel partly emptied with a
trochar and canula.   Two pairs of forceps placed one above
and the other below the puncture will hold the gut in position
whilst an assistant compresses it behind to prevent further
escape of contents.   A purse-string suture is then placed round
the opening at a convenient distance and the tube inserted
through the enlarged puncture and secured by the suture.
The bowel and wound are washed with sterilised saline, and
the bowel now fixed to the abdominal wall with the silk sutures,
the parts again cleansed, a packing of thin gauze placed round
the junction, and the free end of the tube brought through the
dressings and put into a bottle.   To the Paul's tube there is a
wider and thinner tube already attached.   The tube comes
away in about four to five days.   After this the discharge
escapes on the skin, which rapidly becomes very excoriated
and painful.   Much may be done to mitigate the exceeding
discomfort of this by cleanliness and the application of oint-
ments.   The use of a solution of rubber may be useful, it should
be painted on after the skin has been cleansed and dried.

From the amount of misery which such an opening may
cause, and the tendency to rapid emaciation exhibited, if there
is reason to suspect that the fistula must become permanent
unless something more is done, the earliest opportunity must
be taken to explore the abdomen and do what the individual
case may require to restore the natural channel.

Another reason in favour of early operation for the re-
establishment of the normal track is the tendency to the
formation of iliac adhesions which such cases show.

Strangulation by bands is one of the most common of the
various forms of acute obstruction, and in its main features
differs very little from obstruction due to a volvulus.   I will
simply give cases which speak for themselves (see Fig. 1).

INTESTINAL OBSTRUCTION DUE TO A BAND.—On October 5, 1911,
C. P., a single woman, aged 75, was admitted.✶   She was an old woman
with sunken cheeks, and was lying propped up in bed complaining of

much pain in the abdomen which had commenced at 6 p.m. the previous day. This pain had been very severe, general throughout the abdomen, but extending under the ribs on both sides and shooting through to the shoulder blades. She had been vomiting all night and the morning of admission hiccough came on and continued at frequent intervals. The bowels, after having been constipated for four to five days, acted the morning before admission. The abdomen was well covered, lax, moving fairly well ; no distension, no abnormal dulness ; no tumour. There was tenderness chiefly above the umbilicus. Examination *per vaginam* showed nothing abnormal. Temperature, 98° : pulse, 92.

There was no history of any previous illness.

Operation, 6 p.m.—There was a large amount of blood-stained fluid in the peritoneum, but no spots of fat necrosis were visible anywhere, although the fluid suggested the possibility of acute pancreatitis. When the pelvis was examined a swelling like a top could be felt on the right side, which on fuller examination resembled a volvulus. A very firm band crossed this, running from the fundus of a sterile uterus to the posterior part of the pelvis. This was divided with scissors. The small gut affected was 2 feet in length, beginning 18 inches from the ileo-cæcal valve. It was of very dark colour, but resilient, and glossy. A drainage tube was inserted and much fluid drained away for four days, after which it was removed. There was nothing to show how the band originated.

The age of this patient did not prevent her recovery. The question of recovery depends more upon the stage of the illness than upon the age of the patient.

INTESTINAL OBSTRUCTION BY ADHESIONS (the result of old pelvic disease which had been treated by operation, a more common type).— M. M., a married woman, aged 25, was admitted October 31, 1911, ✳ with an illness of two days' duration.

She underwent an operation for double pyo-salpinx in January, and remained well afterwards until the 29th, when a sudden pain was felt in the epigastrium. This came on soon after 10 and was very severe. She vomited an hour later and had done so often since. The pain had remained constant in the same place. The bowels acted on the 30th.

The patient was pale and evidently suffering severe pain. Pulse 136 ; respirations, 32 ; temperature, 98·6°. The abdomen, which was well covered, moved poorly on respiration ; rather distended ; no visible peristalsis ; tympanitic all over. Abdominal wall soft and flaccid excepting in the epigastric region, where there was slight rigidity, and here she was very tender on palpation. The scar of former operation was visible in the mid-line below the umbilicus. The vomited material was bile-stained.

At the operation a coil of small intestine beneath the incision was adherent to the abdominal wall and to another coil. A large section of it was empty and collapsed. The distended coils were emptied by puncture and the obstructing adhesions divided. The surface of the gut was inflamed. There was some free fluid in the pelvis, which was removed with gauze swabs. The wound was closed. Suppuration in the wound ensued, but there was no other complication.

All the hernial apertures must be examined before operation, especially the femoral, in stout women.   I have myself operated for obstruction in two instances of this form of hernia.   The patients did perfectly well ; still I could but blame myself for imperfect examination.   It is not very unusual to find that digital examination of the rectum has not been carried out : this should always be done quite early, for very valuable help may be afforded by it—a rectal growth which was uusus- pected as it gave no symptoms ; a ballooned rectum ; an intussusception or gall-stone in the small intestine ; an impacted hydatid, or some other growth in the pelvis ; an inflammatory swelling about an appendix, or a suppurating tube. The surgeon should re-examine to confirm any statement. I have known the uterus when felt by rectum described as a tumour, and a distended ureter on the left side as an intussus- ception which could be easily felt.

In the case of married women a vaginal examination is also usually indicated.

There are certain varieties of acute obstruction which require special mention, because of their exceptional characters or special treatment required.   These are simple strictures ; various growths of the bowel, or affecting it secondarily ; gall- stones ; internal hernia ; and, in the large intestine, volvulus.

Simple stricture is not a very common cause of acute obstruc- tion, and is usually the result of injury from gut having been nipped in a hernial sac, sloughing of the part or the whole of an intussusception, tuberculous or dysenteric ulceration (not typhoid), a traumatic partial rupture of the intestine, or it may follow an acute appendicitis.

The congenital form is not only rare, but almost invariably fatal, the age of the infant rendering attempts to relieve the stricture almost hopeless.   In addition the presence of obstruc- tion cannot be promptly diagnosed in the majority.

In the acquired form the method of treatment will depend on the stage of the obstruction.   Should the stricture be a narrow one it may be possible to do an enteroplasty when the operation is undertaken early, but later nothing will be possible excepting (1) entero-anastomosis ; (2) excision of a sufficient length of intestine and an end-to-end, end-to-side or lateral anastomosis ; (3) enterostomy.

The history in acquired simple strictures is very much that of a growth invading or commencing in the small bowel, but has a longer course before the onset of complete obstruction. There is a complaint of attacks of colicky pain in the abdomen, often accompanied by sickness and a " rising in the stomach." Visible peristalsis is found if the abdomen is examined during one of these attacks. The attacks last for a variable time, but recur and increase in severity. In the case of growths [1] commencing in the wall of the small intestine the disease is usually far advanced when found, because the contents of the small intestine being fluid are able to pass through a small opening, and it is a long time before the growth contracts sufficiently to produce symptoms.

On Sunday, December 14, 1913, F. R. came to the ward in which she had previously been a patient to request permission to come for the ward festivities on Christmas Day. Whilst at the hospital she had an attack of abdominal pain and vomiting. The resident assistant-surgeon examined her and found some distension of the abdomen with peristalsis. A history of similar attacks for a period of three weeks was obtained. She was admitted and operation performed the same afternoon as it was evident some obstruction was present. The line of the previous incisions (see p. 267) was selected as the muscle fibres had not united well and there was a weak wall there. We could also feel a thickening about the size of a cherry under the upper extremity of the scar. This was adherent and placed at the angle of the loop which had been short-circuited before. There were one or two adhesions between the omentum and other parts, and when the pelvis was explored a tumour could be felt which was adherent to the summit of the bladder. It was some distance from the point of lateral anastomosis, encircled the small bowel, but did not quite occlude its lumen. The wall of the bowel above and below could be pressed into it, its shape, internally, resembling a dice-box. There was a tag of omentum adherent to it. The mesenteric glands were enlarged over a large area. After extension of the abdominal incision it was possible to cut away the growth from the summit of the bladder, the wall of which was sutured. The portion of small gut affected by the growth was excised (situated about 3 feet from the valve) with a few glands and an end-to-end anastomosis carried out. The glands were much too numerous for a complete operation. The small intestine above the growth was dilated and congested, that below somewhat

---

[1] An interesting paper by Dr. Speese on sarcoma of small intestine, will be found in the " Annals of Surgery," 1914, p. 727.

smaller than normal, but there had evidently been no complete obstruction.   There was a good deal of shock after the operation and the pulse
rose to 142 next day ; the bowels acted on the 17th, when the pulse
had fallen to 80.

Mr. Shattock reported that the growth was a round-celled sarcoma.
At one point the growth had become necrosed and here the omentum
was adherent externally so preventing perforation.   There had been no
bladder symptoms.

On January 20, 1914, exploration was again performed to see if the
glands would permit of removal
now that the patient was in
better health, but, although some
of them were smaller, they were
very extensively affected and one
or two nodules of growth could
be felt.   Ten days later the use
of Coley's fluid in increasing
doses was commenced.   She left
on February 12, 1914, for a convalescent home, from which Dr.
J. G. Duncanson reported a gain
of weight of about $\frac{3}{4}$ lb. a week
to the beginning of April, without
any signs of abdominal disease,
and she continued well when seen
in August.

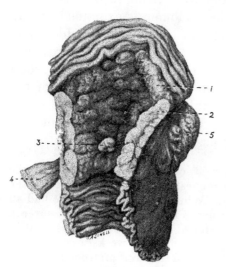

FIG. 34.—Sarcoma of Small Intestine
producing obstruction in a child.
1. Raised edge of growth, not hard
or everted.   2. Base going through
to the peritoneum.   3. Area which
had given way.   4. Omentum
attached and preventing general
peritonitis.   5. Situation of attachment to bladder.

When a sarcomatous growth
develops in the mesentery of
the small intestine it may
invade the intestinal wall and
fungate into its lumen, so
producing obstruction.

Mr. P., aged 50, was seen in
consultation with Dr. A. E.
Godfrey on May 12, 1911, for a swelling in the lower abdomen.   Two
years before he had had a swelling in the upper abdomen which disappeared.   There had been complaint of indigestion, but no vomiting.

The swelling of which he now complained was noticed at Christmas,
1910, and had increased slowly without pain.   The general appearance
of the patient was that of a healthy man.   In the lower abdomen was a
tumour the size and shape of a cocoa-nut ; it occupied the mid-line and
came forward above the pubes like an enlarged bladder.   It was quite
firm, feeling like a fibroid growth, and was fixed posteriorly to the
tissues at the back of the abdomen, but could be moved to some extent.
He complained of some loss of appetite, although this was never good,
and he had to take medicine to ensure an action of the bowels.

This tumour was removed on May 18 with the help of Dr. A. E. Godfrey, the anæsthetic being given by Dr. T. Godfrey.   Incision was made to the right of the middle line and the rectus displaced outwards.   The tumour was growing in the mesentery of the ileum,

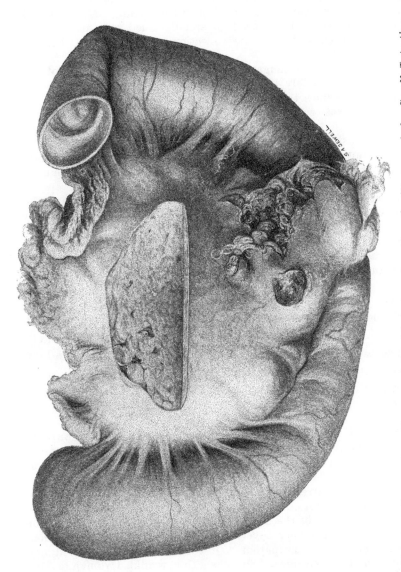

Fig. 35.—Sarcomatous Tumour of the Mesentery invading the Lumen of the Small Intestine. Removed successfully during life.   Dr. Godfrey's case.   The specimen is in the Museum of the Royal College of Surgeons.

and was difficult to lift out until an adhesion to the peritoneum on the right side of the pelvis had been divided.   It was crossed by a loop of small intestine (ileum), which was closely adherent.

The growth was very hard.   Clamps were applied to the small intestine involved and 18 to 20 inches of it were removed with the tumour and a large V-shaped portion of the mesentery, the vessels being secured as they presented themselves. End-to-end anastomosis with a double row of continuous sutures was performed and the mesentery sutured above and underneath, no raw surface being left. No glandular enlargement could be found. The wound was closed in layers. The recovery from this operation was uneventful. Mr. Shattock reported the nature of the growth as spindle-celled sarcoma, and the specimen has been added to the collection of the Royal College of Surgeons.

The specimen shows fungation of growth into the lumen of the intestine, not completely blocking the canal. Some peritoneum has been removed to show the rough section of the main growth.

This patient was seen again on March 4, 1912. During January and February he had two illnesses with night sweats, with some fever (102°—103°) lasting a week on each occasion. There had been no pain or bladder trouble, but he had constipation, and for ten to fourteen days had noticed renewed swelling in the lower abdomen. This was rounded in outline, tympanitic on percussion, and appeared fluctuating.

Exploration on the 9th showed an extensive growth with a broad base and infiltration of the mesentery. The peritoneum was very vascular with a quantity of large veins. The fluctuation was due to hæmorrhage into the growth. It was not considered operable and the incision was closed. The patient died in the following July. Coley's fluid produced no effect.

A hydatid cyst may press upon the intestine when it grows within the mesentery, or compress the large bowel when it develops within the pelvis. Uterine fibroids are very unlikely to cause acute obstruction, but it may arise as a secondary consequence owing to the formation of bands or adhesions when there has been inflammation of a fibroid possibly due to a twist.

OBSTRUCTION OF SMALL INTESTINE, DUE TO ADHESIONS SECONDARY TO A PEDUNCULATED FIBROID WHICH HAD UNDERGONE ROTATION. —A. M., a married woman, aged 48, was sent to me by Dr. Southey, of Colnbrook, on May 24 and left June 10, 1912. The catamenia had been more frequent and irregular for twelve months, and she had noticed increasing stoutness for six months, during which time she had suffered from occasional pain in the abdomen and backache. On May 12 she had been taken with very severe pain in the abdomen, which had continued since, with constipation. On the 22nd she had vomited, and this had occurred often since. She was a thin, wrinkled woman looking quite old, rather restless, and complaining of attacks of abdominal pain of varying severity. On examination of the abdomen, there was a hard centrally-placed tumour the size of a cocoa-nut, reaching above the umbilicus and going down into the pelvis, which it filled. It was slightly movable. On opening the abdomen we found the omentum adherent to a greyish-brown mass, and the transverse colon and small gut were also adherent round it. It was a pedunculated fibroid which had undergone one complete rotation on its pedicle, which was attached to the fundus uteri. Several bands were divided and a multilocular cyst of the right ovary removed. A groove was found in the wall of the ileum made by one of the larger bands. Above this the intestine was distended, below contracted. This groove was invaginated with a continuous Lembert suture.

Carcinoma is very rare as a primary growth in the small intestine.

I have only been called upon to operate for it once ; it was. in the jejunum high up. There was much glandular enlargement, and some secondary deposits in the peritoneum. A lateral anastomosis gave relief.

In obstruction from gall-stones there is a different clinical picture. A sudden attack of pain in the upper abdomen, with vomiting and shock, in a woman of advancing years. The vomiting is troublesome, and with the pain, which is paroxysmal, varies much according to the progress or arrest of the stone. The majority of stones are arrested in the ileum, because this part of the intestine is the narrowest, especially near the ileo-cæcal valve, but arrest is common in other parts as a result of muscular spasm. Absolute obstruction is temporary high up. During this time there is no action of the bowels. The pain moves to the neighbourhood of the umbilicus, and if the woman is thin the stone may be felt until a spasm of the bowels occurs, when peristalsis will be seen and tenderness complained of.

The stone which is shown in the illustration (Fig. 36) was removed at operation from a stout elderly woman, and before operation could be felt *per rectum* as a hard, very tender lump in Douglas's pouch. The mucous membrane was ulcerated over it and of a dark colour, making it probable that the stone had lodged there for some time. It could not be moved in either direction. The patient, who was very ill, did not recover.

These cases may go on for a long period if no operation is done.

I once saw an aged lady in consultation who had had symptoms for eighteen days, and as she was in bad health and unlikely to survive any operation the effect of local application of glycerine and belladonna was tried. On the twentieth day she passed a large non-facetted stone.

In another case the lady had been suffering with varying symptoms of obstruction, and was extremely ill. Her state was thought to be due to a gall-stone.

On March 26, 1913, a lady of 65 was seen with Dr. Spaull in consultation for intestinal obstruction. There was a history of an attack of gall-stones five years before, and the present illness began with rather severe epigastric pain on March 13. She had vomiting and was very ill for a day or two ; improvement ensued, but she kept her bed and her condition varied from day to day. The pain left the epigastric region and has varied in position since, being mostly in the umbilical region. On the 24th she had a severe attack of pain with vomiting and was very ill, with a rapid pulse. When seen on the 26th she was feeling much better, having passed wind, and at no time during the illness had she failed to have an action of the bowels, after enemata, for more than a day or two, excepting during the attacks of greater pain. The patient was rather stout, feeling ill, and not able to talk clearly about her condition. The abdomen was somewhat distended, without rigidity or particular tenderness anywhere, and without tumour. The tongue was furred and the bowels had acted after an enema. Pulse, 90 ; temperature, 99°. Suffers from hæmorrhoids.

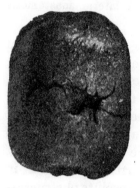

Fig. 36.—Gall Stone, natural size, removed from the Small Intestine during Life. It caused Acute Obstruction: St. Thomas's Hospital Museum.

She had an acute obstruction on the 28th and 29th and almost died, but this was relieved towards the evening of the 29th. On April 1 she probably passed the stone through the ileocæcal valve, as improvement began, and the stone was passed towards the end of the week, about twenty-three days from the commencement of symptoms : for a time it was fixed at the anal orifice. She regained her usual health.

The stone was not completely cylindrical, being compressed laterally, measuring about 1½ inches by 1¼ inches : one end was facetted, the other rounded.

In spite of such cases, early operation gives the best chance of success.

If you find a patient who is too ill, or who refuses operation, in whom you diagnose gall-stone obstruction, you are not justified in withholding all hope of recovery. You cannot estimate the exact size of the stone, and there is always a chance that it may be forced into the large gut at any moment should relaxation of local muscular spasm take place.

When you find a gall-stone in a coil of small intestine, the best treatment is to draw the loop outside, push the stone higher up the bowel (for you cannot estimate the amount of morbid change in the encircling mucous membrane), and cut down upon it from the ante-mesenteric border, suturing the incision through which it has been extracted with a double row of continuous sutures, the inner being passed through all the coats, the outer through peritoneum and muscular layers only.

Acute obstruction the result of passage of the small intestine through an aperture is not often seen, although several cases are on record. There is a specimen in the St. Thomas's Hospital Museum (Fig. 8), which shows an aperture of the kind, likely to snare intestine, in the mesentery. Apertures may be congenital or the result of injury to the abdomen. The symptoms are those produced by a band in a similar position. These obstructions are included under the heading Internal Hernia, which also comprises the cases where intestine becomes entangled in a retro-peritoneal pouch, the foramen of Winslow, or in an opening in the diaphragm. Pouches which have been found to ensnare intestine are found in both the upper and lower abdomen : of the former there are the duodenal (right and left) ; of the latter, the intersigmoid, the retrocæcal and the pouch of Douglas. As these pouches can mostly be demonstrated in the anatomical department and they rarely cause obstruction, it is probable that some abnormality exists when the intestine gets ensnared. As a rule the aperture can be dilated ; if incision is required, the possibility of the presence of vessels in the constricting fold must be remembered. After the intestine has been reduced, the opening of the pouch should be closed with a stitch. This statement does not apply to the foramen of Winslow, where the surgeon should not attempt to close the opening because of the very important vessels which surround it. In hernia into the lesser sac, in addition to acute symptoms there is a definite swelling in the epigastric region, with possibly retraction of the lower abdomen. It is possible that if the distended intestine which occupies the lesser sac and forms the tumour can be emptied, traction from outside the foramen will reduce it.

In duodenal herniæ it is possible to find a swelling in the region of the umbilicus, but in the series met with in the lower abdomen there is no special guide.

Diaphragmatic hernia is well illustrated by the dramatic case which has been related (p. 236).

The abdominal contents may pass into the chest and become strangulated through one of the natural openings of the diaphragm through a congenital deficiency in it, through a wound, or through the scar which follows a wound. This hernia is rarely recognised during life, but a consideration of the history with an examination of the chest may assist the surgeon in arriving at a correct solution of the case. The signs in the chest are often similar to those produced by a pneumo-thorax, with dyspnœa and palpitations. Before strangulation of the protrusion has taken place it may assist diagnosis if the patient is examined with the X-rays, but as the stomach is often implicated and vomiting frequent, when severe symptoms are developing, it is often too late (see " Strangulation of Stomach," p. 236 ; " Rupture of the Diaphragm," p. 15).

INTUSSUSCEPTION OR INVAGINATION OF THE BOWEL.

Under this heading is comprised a large group of the obstructions met with in practice ; in fact, it is so large and important that it requires a section to itself. There is hardly a week passes in which there is not some case admitted to the hospital, and as a rule they are brought at a comparatively early stage of the obstruction, because of the passage of blood from the bowel. This symptom is one which profoundly impresses the mother of the child, and she cannot pass it over, as it occurs in addition to pain of which the child gives evidence. She knows there is something wrong inside.

In this form of obstruction as met with in the living subject a varying amount of the bowel becomes invaginated into a section below. Thus a tumour of varying size is produced which consists of three layers—the entering, the returning, and the ensheathing. These layers, with possibly some omentum, form what is usually called the " sausage-shaped " tumour, which is so characteristic of the disease when it can be felt.

It is sometimes, especially in the chronic form, met with in adults, but is by far most commonly seen in children (male children) under one year old. A remarkable fact, which has been mentioned by many writers, is that the patient at the time of onset of the illness is often a very healthy and well-nourished child.

It is generally acknowledged that the cause of intussusception is an irregular peristalsis of the bowel, possibly due to intestinal irritation from within. The actual cause of this is, however, difficult to trace. There may be some swelling of a Peyer's patch, a hæmorrhage into the mucous membrane, or a polypus to start it. There is no clinical advantage to be derived from a minute division of the varieties of intussusception, and students only become confused if terms are multiplied. The divisions into enteric, colic, and entero-colic, as suggested by Mr. C. S. Wallace, are quite satisfactory ; more are superfluous. Practically, reducible and irreducible are recognised.

The symptoms are those of " peritonism," sudden abdominal pain, vomiting, and shock, followed by the passage of blood from the rectum and the formation of a tumour in the abdomen which can be felt.

There is a history given of a sudden screaming on the part of the child, which looks frightened, and becomes white-faced evidently from shock. Vomiting soon appears and the child rallies from the shock, but the attacks of pain and screaming continue at intervals. There is an action of the bowels, which contains little if any fæcal matter, but consists mostly of mucus and blood.

If the abdomen is examined between the attacks of pain it will be found flaccid and without distension. Sometimes the child is found kneeling in bed with his head buried in the pillow. Examination is not resisted as a rule until the swelling caused by the intussusception is touched, when there is a complaint of pain, the lump hardens, and the muscles over it become rigid. Sometimes rigidity is present when the child is examined and the tumour cannot be felt, examination being resisted by the frightened child, who instinctively hardens the abdominal wall until an anæsthetic has been given to relax the muscles ; but this anæsthetic should only be given when arrangements to operate have already been completed. The tumour varies in size and position, and is like a large sausage ; in the early stages it will be most frequently found on the right side below the liver. A rectal examination will often prevent the useless administration of an anæsthetic, for in cases where no blood has been passed some may be found on the finger when it is withdrawn after this examination.   In addition, the apex of the intussusception may be felt as a ring of mucous membrane within the rectum, into which the finger can be passed.   The tumour may also be felt bimanually, but not as a hard tumour, in the pelvis outside the bowel wall.   In cases where there is prolapse of the intussuscepted part this has been mistaken for a prolapse of the rectum, but examination shows in the latter that it is not possible to pass the finger up the bowel by the side of the protrusion owing to the attachment of the skin.

There may be no action of the bowels, but complete obstruction is very rare ; usually the intussusception permits the passage of intestinal contents through it, therefore distension may be regarded as a bad sign.   When it is present the case is a late one, and there is peritonitis as a complication.

One of the signs of intussusception which is not of great value is that known as the Signe de Dance.   It was first described by M. Dance, " Medicin de l'Hôpital Cochin," Paris, in 1824.[1]   It is applied to the condition of the right iliac fossa when the cæcum has been drawn away in an intussusception. This withdrawal of the usual contents is supposed to leave a comparative hollowness of the fossa when compared with the other side.

Adams and Cassidy (p. 182) say that they have known " abdominal section performed when the tumours were respectively the lower edge of the liver, Reidel's tongue-shaped projection from the right lobe of the liver, and the right kidney."

It is, however, obvious that a child with the passage of mucus and blood from the bowel and a tumour in the abdomen should be thoroughly examined, but the history given in these cases should prevent unnecessary opening of the abdomen. Henoch's purpura is sometimes associated with an intussusception and may require mechanical assistance to reduce the bowel to a condition more nearly approaching the normal.

Tuberculous affections of the glands, omentum, and peri-

[1] Repert. d'Anatomie, etc., 1824.

toneum are much more likely to cause difficulty in diagnosis in chronic rather than in acute intussusception. The position of these lesions, their shape and number, will help in the diagnosis.

When the intussusception has once commenced, the apex of the entering part remains constant and increases in size as a result of congestion from interference with the venous return. By peristaltic action of the sheath it is forced further along until it may protrude from the anus. Meanwhile the congestion of the entering layers has extended in amount and the difficulty in reduction increased. The mesentery enters with its section of bowel, and by its pull on the elongated swelling causes it to assume a curve with its convexity downwards. The compression of the mesentery increases, the venous return is more impeded, the bowel forming the intussusceptum becomes more engorged. There is an increased flow of mucus from the surface, the smaller veins yield to pressure, and as time passes there is an escape of blood-stained mucus from the anus, and hæmorrhage into the tissues from which it is escaping. Adhesions between the opposed peritoneal surfaces form early, and if relief is not afforded within a few hours gangrene of the intussusceptum ensues from complete stoppage of circulation, aided by bacterial invasion of the damaged tissues. Peritonitis is a frequent cause of a fatal ending, but the patient rarely dies from complete obstruction. If, however, the strangulation of invaginated bowel is complete from the first, blood and mucus will not be passed.

If no attempt is made to relieve the obstruction, death usually occurs before many days have passed, and although spontaneous reduction is spoken of, it is one of those rare occurrences which cannot be seriously considered. Some years ago Brinton made a collection of 500 fatal cases of obstruction and of these 215 were intussusceptions. Another way in which a patient may recover is by sloughing of the intussusceptum : of this there are many known instances.

A child under my care at the Royal Free Hospital was suffering from intussusception with prolapse for which the parents refused operation. The child was taken home to die, and was indeed very ill. About a fortnight afterwards the dresser of the case was walking through the street where the family resided and to her surprise saw the former patient playing with other children and sucking an orange. She made inquiries, and was told that a few days after leaving the hospital the portion of bowel which was prolapsed when she went home had come away and the child rapidly recovered health. It is not possible to say if stricture developed later.

It is interesting to see the various methods of treatment which have been tried in the past, many founded on a complete failure to understand the pathology of the disease. Fagge states that cases have been cured by the passage of bougies up the rectum.[1] Maydieu, of Argent,[2] used a mixture of No. 5 shot and olive oil, 7 oz. of the former to 4 oz. of the latter, and quoted twelve cases of supposed examples of the disease thus treated.[2] He has not found many imitators. Taliaferro relates the case of a prisoner who was cured by the use of effervescing powders in the rectum, but died of parotid bubo some weeks later; his gaoler acted as medical adviser. Iced injections have also been tried. The method of inflation which was in vogue some twenty years ago was introduced by Gorham[3] in 1838. This when combined with external manipulation and the use of chloroform in children not infrequently succeeded, but was uncertain and not without risk. Cheadle[4] wrote of this method : " The success of inflation in the cure of intussusception depends largely, no doubt, upon its early employment. Higginson's syringe proved of most use." Fagge[1] wrote of the same treatment : " It has now been frequently employed, and sometimes with the result of curing the disease. More often perhaps its success has been partial. The tumour has been reduced in size, or it has changed its position, returning towards the seat which it had occupied at an earlier period." Bryant wrote warningly : " Bowels have been ruptured by its use." The substitution of water pressure, by means of a funnel and tube introduced into the rectum, care being taken to prevent too much force being employed, has been similarly tried, and with varying success. The funnel should be elevated about 2 feet above the level of the rectum and warm saline solution allowed to flow quietly into the bowel whilst the child is under a general anæsthetic. Manipulation of the tumour

[1] Fagge, " System of Medicine," Vol. II., p. 413.
[2] Lancet, Vol. I., 1870, p. 737.
[3] Guy's Hospital Reports, Vol. III., p. 345.
[4] Lancet, Vol. I., 1888, p. 321.

through the abdominal wall should be carefully carried on as the injection enters. It is a method which I have used successfully in the past; it has been abandoned because of its uncertain effect, yet there may be occasions when it will appear to the attendant well worth a trial. To succeed the case should be an early one. The combination of this method with that of laparotomy has been found useful by some, but it is better in my opinion to trust entirely to opening the abdomen with manipulation of the intussusception. Incision on the

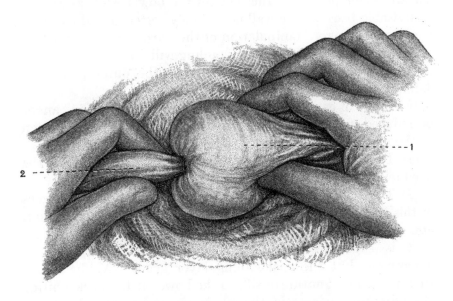

Fig. 37.—Reduction of an Intussusception by Manipulation outside the Abdomen. 1. Intussuscipiens, Intussusceptum. 2. The peritoneal cavity has been packed off with gauze.

right side over the rectus muscle, with opening of the sheath and displacement of the uninjured muscle outwards, is the best. You will not have a weak wound afterwards, as is often the case if the fibres of the muscle are separated. The upper limit should extend above the umbilicus. When the peritoneum is opened, the prolapse of small intestine is prevented by a gauze pad or plug and the position of the tumour defined. If two fingers are passed to the lower end of this and pressure is made over the end of the intussusception, it will quickly recede before the pressure until a variable amount is left, perhaps a firm sausage-like lump of 2 inches in length which is more resistant. This should be delivered out of the wound and complete reduction effected by firm but gentle pressure. As a rule some patience is required to reduce the part which has formed the apex of the intussusception, and sometimes when it has been reduced the operator has a doubt as to whether a thickening which is frequently felt inside the gut is a growth or only congested and œdematous mucous membrane. It is not wise to open the bowel in order to make certain ; growths are very rare in the acute variety and give some distinctive feature when present. Incision into a bowel such as this is inadvisable because the wall is probably softened and contains many organisms. Manipulation of the parts involved must be gentle but firm, violent or hasty pulling will do harm, and often cause a splitting of the peritoneum of the outer layer and damage which cannot be repaired.

If in spite of careful manipulation the intussusception cannot be reduced completely, there are practically two courses open to the operator in the case of children :—

(1) To perform a lateral anastomosis above and below the irreducible part when the bowel is healthy.

(2) To excise the intussusception by the method which goes in this country under different names : Maunsell, Jesset, Barker, etc.

It is especially indicated where the intussusception is gangrenous but the ensheathing layer good. Apply a continuous Lembert suture of silk to the bowel at the neck, uniting the adjacent surfaces in the whole circumference. With the usual precautions against the escape of bowel contents into the wound, make an incision in the ensheathing layer which shall fully expose the upper part of the intussusceptum. An incision is next made through this close to its upper end, by which the anterior two-thirds is divided into the central canal. Sutures are passed, four in number, through the entire thickness of this, one in front and one on each side. The fourth is passed in the following manner so that it may also act as a hæmostatic. The needle is made to penetrate the two parts of the intussusceptum from within outwards, is passed round the uncut part of this, which contains the mesentery with its vessels, and back again into the centre of the bowel. This is now tied, the complete division of the inner tubes (and mesentery) completed, and the opening in the sheath closed with a continuous Lembert suture, after the parts have been cleansed inside and out with warm saline.

If for some reason too much damage has been inflicted on the bowel during the manipulation for reduction to permit of its recovery, then it must be excised ; but the prognosis of this operation in the case of intussusception is very bad. If it has to be done, the peritoneum must be packed off with gauze moistened with warm saline and the operation done swiftly.

If the patient has stood the operation well, the wound in the abdominal wall may be sutured as usual ; if there is much shock, the best plan is to insert a number of interrupted sutures of thick salmon gut, which pass through all the layers.

It is unnecessary to give statistics : suffice it to say that prognosis depends very much on the ability of the surgeon to reduce the intussusception without resection of the intestine ; therefore every effort short of causing serious injury to the bowel must be made in order to effect that object. This is more likely to be successful if immediate operation is performed.

A CASE IN WHICH INTUSSUSCEPTION RECURRED, LATERAL ANASTO-MOSIS AT SECOND OPERATION.—F. R., a girl aged 8, was admitted ✳ on May 17, 1913. She was subject to constipation. For twenty-four hours she had suffered great pain in the abdomen with frequent vomiting. Nothing had passed by the bowel. She looked pinched and very ill, pulse 100 ; temperature, 100° ; respirations, 24. Examination showed a movable irregular mass in the right side ; the iliac fossa below felt empty and was tender on pressure, but the abdominal wall was everywhere soft. Examination *per rectum* normal. Operation was done through the right rectus (separation of fibres), and a large ileo-colic intussusception reduced with some difficulty after it had been brought outside. A hard button-shaped patch was left at the apex. She left on May 30, recovery having been uneventful.

On June 28 she returned from a convalescent home. Next day she had abdominal pain and vomiting ; the bowels acted twice, but there was no slime and no blood in the motions. She came in suffering from intermittent attacks of pain which caused her to roll about in bed and cry out. The abdomen was rather distended ; no visible peristalsis. On the 30th the bowels had not acted, although an enema of glycerine had been given. In the afternoon the old scar was reopened. The small gut was considerably distended, and there was some clear serous fluid in the peritoneum. The mesenteric glands were large. The intussusception was 2 to 3 feet above the ileo-cæcal valve and about 4 inches long. It was easily reduced in part ; the terminal piece, however, was much thickened and complete reduction impossible, firm adhesions extending between the peritoneal surfaces. The intestinal contents passed this section with difficulty. Lateral anastomosis above and below was performed. The mucous membrane of the lump looked rather sloughy examined through one of the incisions. There was no evidence of tubercle on examination and application of von Pirquet's test. She left the hospital well July 26.

Some months later this patient returned for symptoms of obstruction due to sarcoma of a different part of the small intestine (see p. 252).

A recurrence of the intussusception after complete reduction has been met with in more than one case, and to prevent this it has been recommended that the mesentery of the ileum near to the valve should be shortened by the insertion of a continuous stitch. It so seldom occurs that it is not advisable to adopt it as part of the routine treatment.

The separation of a slough of the mucous membrane may be seen some days later in consequence of strangulation from tight nipping. In the following case it came away about three weeks after operation, and, although there were some uneasy symptoms complained of about three years later, there has not been any proof of the formation of a stricture of the bowel, though such might be expected. The abdominal wall remained perfect.

The patient was a boy 3 years old, an only child, seen with Dr. Copeland on April 20, 1908. Vomiting had been present since the early morning and there had been complaint of abdominal pain. The bowels had acted, but no special attention had been paid to the character of the motion. There had been no blood or mucus passed. When seen earlier in the day by Dr. Copeland there had been nothing abnormal to be felt, and the temperature was about 100°, not over. In the evening when seen again there was a swelling in the iliac region. At 7 p.m. there was a flattened, sausage-shaped and somewhat tender swelling above the iliac fossa. The abdomen was generally flaccid elsewhere. Pulse, 80.

The abdomen was opened at 8.45 p.m. after displacement of the rectus ; and an ileo-cæcal intussusception reduced by manipulation. The terminal inch of ileum and early part of the cæcum were œdematous and thickened. He made a good recovery, but three weeks later passed a broad band-like circular slough of the mucous membrane from the lower ileum. The detachment of the slough was accompanied by some abdominal pain and a rise of temperature in the morning of the day on which it was passed.

With regard to the prognosis in cases where there is some sloughing of the intussusceptum a case recorded in

"Holmes' System of Surgery," Vol. II., p. 722, is very encouraging :—

A boy of 5 under the care of Dr. Buckley, of Sutton-on-Trent, passed 8 inches of the ileum, the cæcum with its appendix, and about 4 inches of the colon, after an illness of four months' duration, and recovered in six weeks' time. Sixteen years later he was reported as having had perfect health during the whole of the intervening time.

Chronic intussusception is mostly met with in adults, and is not infrequently due to a growth. These intussusceptions being mostly irreducible, are usually treated by excision of the affected portion of the bowel, the amount removed depending on the position and nature of any growth that may be present. A removal of a wedge-shaped piece of the mesentery will be necessary if the tumour is malignant. Under no circumstances should an attempt at a complete operation be made if acute has been superadded to chronic obstruction.

In those cases where a carcinomatous growth of the large bowel has been intussuscepted and prolapsed through the anus, I have on three occasions excised the growth with success so far as the immediate result of the operation was concerned, but one of them returned with general dissemination in the abdomen a few months later. The sphincter ani should be dilated and the growth drawn well into view. The bowel well above the growth, which is usually annular in shape, should be gradually divided with scissors completely round, forceps being put on the edges as they are cut. Silk sutures should then be passed through both layers and tied from before backwards. When the bowel is released it readily passes up into the upper part of the rectum. The objection to this operation is the fact that very few glands can be removed. The prolapse of itself indicates that there cannot be very much infiltration in the mesentery or great enlargement of the glands. There is usually some, but much of it may be secondary to a sloughy state of the growth, which is not uncommon, and often associated with hæmorrhage. The distress which it causes occasionally renders operative interference an urgent matter.

OBSTRUCTION OF THE LARGE INTESTINE.

In this section it is necessary to include a consideration of the forms of obstruction which are of a chronic nature, because the prevention of an acute and often fatal attack should be possible if the condition is recognised in time. It is far too common to find that for a long time the patient has had discomfort and troublesome constipation for which various forms of purgation have been tried, and succeeded, more or less imperfectly, in giving relief, then a complete obstruction has supervened which the most persevering and injudicious attempts at forcing a passage have failed to overcome. During the years 1903—12 inclusive, there were 121 cases under treatment in St. Thomas's Hospital in which a carcinomatous growth of the large bowel was present in acute obstruction, and of these 70 died and 51 recovered. Acute obstruction was produced in 14 others by the pressure of malignant growths, and of these nine died. A case of carcinoma of the jejunum also proved fatal.

The causes of death in the cases of malignant obstruction treated by colostomy are summed up as follows by Mr. Rouquette :—

Death due to operation, 21 per cent. : peritonitis, 9 per cent. ; pneumonia, 12 per cent.

Death due to prolonged obstruction, 79 per cent. : toxæmia, 67 per cent. ; perforation of growth or stercoral ulcer, 12 per cent.

This is a large percentage of fatal cases to be found in any series of diseases of the bowel at the present day which if recognised early are quite amenable to surgical treatment. It must be conceded that the subjects of malignant growth of the large bowel are often advanced in years, and may be suffering from bronchitis or some other complication ; but with the inevitable ending which awaits delay, it would often be the wisest course to take the smaller risk and submit to a palliative operation such as that of lateral anastomosis, if on exploration more curative procedures are not possible. It is very sad to find a patient suffering from an obstruction of some two to three weeks' duration, caused by a ring carcinoma of the colon which is quite operable, and have death follow a colostomy, because the patient is already poisoned by absorption from the distended bowel above the obstruction or exhausted by vomiting, pain and want of food. Even the causes of death which are put down to surgical interference are in most the result of changes in the bowel due to prolonged obstruction, and the pneumonia, a complication of the anæsthetic in an exhausted patient already suffering from hypostatic congestion of the lungs.

The majority of the cases of cancer of the intestine occur between 40 and 65 years of age, but it has been met with quite early in life. Nothnagel collected 61 cases the ages of which were between 20 and 30 years, and mentions others in which it was found at 3, $3\frac{1}{2}$, 11, 12, and 13 years of age. The youngest patient in my own series was a boy of 14, in whom it was necessary to perform colostomy for a fixed and extensive carcinoma of the pelvic colon. Maydl says that one-seventh of the cases are met with before 30 years of age.

Of the cases in our general series from the hospital the majority were males ; of a series of 151 in the London Hospital 65 were men and 86 women (Barnard).

The situation of the carcinoma is important and in a large series of cases was as follows, when it arose below the stomach:

	Duodenum.	Jejunum.	Ileum.	Small Intestine.	Appendix.	Cæcal, etc.	Ascending Colon.	Hepatic Flexure.	Transverse Colon.	Splenic Flexure.	Descending Colon.	Sigmoid Flexure.	Rectum.
Barnard : London Hospital, 1900—1905	5	3	2	5		41	6	3	17	12	6	103	278
Nothnagel : Vienna	7		10		2	23	6		80			53	162
St. Thomas's Hospital, 1903—1912 (incl.)			1			4		2	13	17	5	58	22*
Total..946.	12	3	13	5	2	68	12	5	110	29	11	214	462

* Producing acute obstruction only.

With reference to the malignancy of carcinoma of the large intestine, it is recognised that secondary deposits occur less frequently than in cancer elsewhere. The outlook in early excision is therefore more hopeful. When it does occur it is commonly in either glands or liver, but varies somewhat according to the exact nature of the growth.

A cancer of the large bowel may remain apparently without change for many months. A surgeon to one of our large hospitals told me of a case of carcinoma of the rectum for which he was consulted owing to an attack of obstruction which was relieved by castor oil.   Eight years later the patient was still alive and did not appear to suffer excepting from an occasional difficulty with the bowels which "his medicine" always relieved.   I can recollect the case of a woman of 40 who was treated for obstruction due to a ring carcinoma of the sigmoid. Lumbar colostomy was performed and gave relief for several years.   I saw her myself six years later, when the growth was assuming large dimensions.   This was in the days of lumbar colostomy, before excision was practised.

The early symptoms of the presence of a malignant growth of the large intestine are not very decided ; they may consist of a loss of strength, anorexia, lassitude, abdominal uneasiness, loss of flesh, and increasing pallor.

In the early stages pain varies very much, but it is not often a cause of much distress until obstruction has begun or peritonitis complicates the case.   In the small intestine, transverse colon, and sigmoid it is referred to the umbilicus ; when in the more fixed parts of the bowel it is at the point of fixation.   If there is an increase of pain when food is taken the growth may be in the lower ileum or cæcum.   Many parts are not accessible to palpation, and in fat people even a large growth may be difficult to find, whilst a contracted rectus may conceal it. There may be more than one tumour felt in the line of the colon, making the diagnosis difficult ; under these circumstances a purge will get rid of the scybala, and the growth can then be demonstrated.   In shape and size these cancerous growths vary very much ; if there is a large growth without any obstruction there may be a colloid change, a solid cylinder being formed without much, if any, contraction.

Blood, mucus, and pus may be found in the fæces if ulceration is present.

Occasionally a growth can be felt above the finger on examination *per rectum*, which from its mobility gives the impression that it is operable, but it is necessary to give a cautious opinion before examination from above has been done.   Quite recently two patients have been under my care ; in the male it was found at operation that the growth which had been felt was a carcinomatous deposit secondary to a stricture of the same nature higher up, and there were many secondary deposits in peritoneum and bowel wall without obstruction.   In the female, who had suffered from abdominal pain and irregularity of the bowels with some loss of flesh, the tumour was a small ovarian cyst which was adherent to the front of the rectum in Douglas's pouch.

Sometimes the X-rays give great assistance in the diagnosis of these conditions when the lumen of the bowel is narrowed but obstruction is not complete. A carcinomatous growth continues to contract and the symptoms associated with chronic obstruction appear sooner or later.

There is a complaint of increasing constipation which ordinary purgatives do not appear to relieve ; indeed, they cause pain. Enemata are then tried and fail after a time. There are attacks of diarrhœa which alternate with the constipation. Growths in the lower colon may cause almost continuous looseness of the bowels ; sometimes an alteration in the shape of the motions. Examination of the abdomen will often show a spasmodic contraction of the bowel above an obstruction, or abnormal thickening of its walls. This is found at or above the region to which the pain is referred. Later this becomes more extensive, and friction of the surface will excite painful peristalsis. Attacks of colic may come on with vomiting, rumbling of wind, and distension. In lead-colic and enteritis intestinal coils are not visible.

Continued distension of the abdomen follows when the obstruction is complete or almost so, and is greater the lower down the obstruction is placed ; it may increase until the whole abdomen is rounded and balloon-like, the distended intestine, both small and large, filling the peritoneal cavity and even pushing forward the ribs and ensiform cartilage. There will then be a general tympanitic note with perhaps a dulness in the flanks from the fluid fæces in the colon, whilst the superficial veins show up clearly in the stretched skin. I have seen some cases which had taken four to six weeks to get into this state and were still not much troubled by either vomiting or pain. Many of our hospital cases have been " worse " about three weeks : The first week, paroxysmal pain with wind and constipation ; second week, constipation, vomiting, distension, pain ; third week, increased pain, greater distension, with offensive vomiting, dry tongue, hiccough, thirst, and rapid emaciation.

Occasionally a patient who was " doing nicely " gets acute blocking of the carcinomatous stricture from a foreign body, a fæcal lump, or some other complication, and there is a rapid development of urgent symptoms. The pain is more severe and continuous with exacerbations, the vomiting is distressing and the vomit changes its character, becoming feculent. Nothing is passed by the bowel, and all enemata fail to bring away any fæcal matter or wind ; the distension increases rapidly, and at last the separate coils are indistinguishable. Should perforation now occur, or peritonitis arise from some other cause, tenderness and rigidity will be manifested, and there may be a temporary rise of temperature with a rapid failure in the strength of the pulse. The patient becomes collapsed, covered with cold sweat, the hands and feet are cold, pain ceases, the pulse dies away, and for some hours before death may cease altogether. The breath even gives a cold sensation to the hand, a quantity of foul fluid is perhaps poured from the mouth, and the end comes so suddenly that the friends, who are perhaps talking with the patient, are quite unprepared for it.

In the diagnosis of the cause of obstruction of the large intestine, besides cancerous growth there are various other conditions which must be considered, the chief of which are :—

(1) Fæcal impaction, distinguished from growth by the result of rectal examination and enemata.

(2) Ileo-cæcal tuberculosis ; can often only be told by a microscopical examination after removal.

(3) Foreign bodies, such as concretions and gall-stones, have been mistaken for growths until operation.

(4) Sigmoiditis, with thickening about the bowel secondary to the development of a pouch in the wall of the bowel, is more common than is generally believed.

(5) Tumours of neighbouring organs, such as—

A. The stomach.

On February 3, 1914, I operated for Dr. Mackenzie on a case of tumour of the abdomen which was regarded as one of growth of the descending colon. It was the size of a closed fist, on the left side below the level of the umbilicus, tender and adherent to the abdominal wall. There were no stomach symptoms, and free hydrochloric and free lactic acids were present in the gastric contents.

Cœliotomy and separation of the swelling from the parietal peritoneum enabled us to examine it thoroughly. It was lying to the outer side of the descending colon, but was in the stomach, having arisen in the greater curvature, and there were many enlarged and obviously malignant glands near.

B. Gall-bladder. A hard painful swelling in the right iliac fossa, the outline of which was not easily defined in an aged lady with constipation, proved to be a distended gall-bladder containing many stones.

C. Uterus and ovaries. Malignant growths having their origin in these organs may invade the bowel, and without operation it may not be possible to distinguish them. Palliative measures only would be possible.

In cases of obstruction due to a growth in the large intestine it is advisable to operate as soon as you can. Do not wait for the onset of vomiting and distension ; an early operation may give the patient a chance of cure. Unfortunately it is not possible to say, until the growth has been seen, if it will be possible to remove it. You will, however, have no reason for self-reproach if this is so, and may be able to save the patient much pain and suffering by performing a short-circuit operation. It cannot be too frequently repeated that anything like an attempt at immediate removal of the growth and the formation of an anastomosis when obstruction is present is certain to prove fatal. The patient's friends should be warned of the necessity of doing the operation in two stages. Many lives are still being lost in consequence of neglect of this rule.

When a patient comes for relief with a greatly distended abdomen, and the position of the obstructing cause is unknown, the best plan is to make an incision to one side of the middle line, open the rectus sheath, and displace the muscle outwards. A distended coil will present itself and should be drawn to the surface, precautions taken to prevent soiling of the wound or peritoneum, and the coil emptied through a puncture or small incision. After this coil is emptied of gas and fluid contents another should be taken and treated in a similar manner, and a third or fourth if necessary. Each puncture is closed with a purse-string suture, the coil cleansed and returned. By this means the distension is much diminished and the pressure on the diaphragm greatly relieved. It is now possible to pass the hand into the abdominal cavity and learn the position of the growth and its connections, also the presence or

T 2

absence of secondary growths in the liver, glands or peritoneum. This is important. On more than one occasion I have found an operable growth in the intestine with a short history of obstruction and a large secondary growth in the liver. If there is a fixed growth in the sigmoid or pelvic colon, and it is not possible to do a short circuiting operation, colostomy should be done on the left side in the usual position and a Paul's tube put in the bowel where it comes easily to the surface. A similar operation is required if there is a fixed growth in the rectum, but as a rule the rectal growths are found before operation and the exploratory incision is not needed. In the performance of colostomy for the relief of obstruction I am strongly in favour of the completion of the operation at the time. In this way relief is afforded at once, and experience convinces me that it is quite safe.

Many years ago I commenced a colostomy at the Royal Free Hospital for obstruction due to carcinoma in the pelvis. The patient was a woman in good condition and the obstruction did not appear very urgent. The colon was sutured to the wound ready for opening later. Two days afterwards the patient died suddenly and we found that the thickened but softened wall of the bowel had been ruptured above the sutured part by excessive muscular action. The obstruction was complete but the amount of distension not excessive.

Since that accident occurred I have always placed a tube in an opening in the bowel at once when operating under similar circumstances.

The operation is performed as follows :—An incision of 3 to 4 inches, according to the thickness of the abdominal wall, is made in the direction of the fibres of the external oblique— that is to say, at right angles to a line drawn from the left anterior superior spine to the umbilicus. The external oblique is divided in the same direction for the full length of the wound and the fibres retracted (Fig. 38). The internal oblique and transversalis are divided in the interval, which is in the centre of the wound and is shown by the line of fat deposit between the muscular fibres, which now extend at right angles to the incision. This part of the wound is also opened up with retractors and the subperitoneal tissue shown. Incision through this, the transversalis fascia, and the peritoneum should be of limited extent, according to the distension of the bowel to be brought outside. The bowel is recognised by its longitudinal muscular bands and appendices epiploicæ. To secure this in position, a loop of it is drawn up until the finger and thumb can be made to hold the mesentery beyond. A thick fishgut suture is then passed across from side to side of the wound so that the loop of the bowel is fixed well outside without tension. This suture should go through the meso-colon or meso-sigmoid about an inch from the posterior margin of the loop, and its passage is facilitated if forceps are placed on the peritoneum at the points near which it is to penetrate. These should be put below the middle of the opening, thus leaving the longer space for the proximal part of the loop (Fig. 39). Two silk sutures are passed above

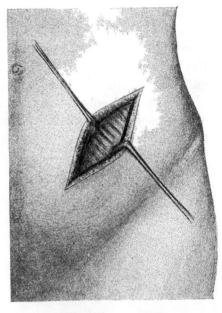

Fig. 38.—Left Iliac Colostomy. The line of incision, with retraction of divided external oblique. The arrangement of internal oblique fibres is shown.

and below the loop of bowel, which include muscle, peritoneum and the wall of the bowel itself. By these sutures the size of the opening through which the bowel passes is limited if necessary and no further protrusion is possible. They are also a safeguard against falling in of the gut should the stitch through the meso-colon give as a result of violent vomiting. I have never seen it do so. Other fishgut sutures are placed in the wound above and below as required. There is now

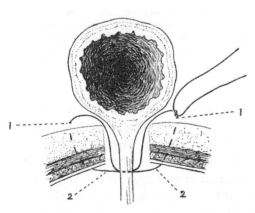

Fig. 39.—Colostomy. Diagram of cross-section of abdominal layers with fixation suture passed before tying externally. 1. Abdominal muscle, peritoneum and skin. 2. Meso-colon.

a good-sized loop of bowel protruding ; in order to open this at once and safely it is encircled with a strip of gauze, only the apex being left exposed.   An adequate incision is made in this for the insertion of the tube, the knife going into the lumen of the gut, any contents being wiped away.   Forceps are now placed at four equidistant points on the wall of this incision and a continuous stltch of No. 2 silk passed with a straight round-bodied needle.   A small-sized Paul's tube is inserted,

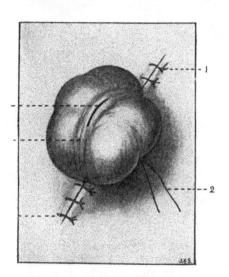

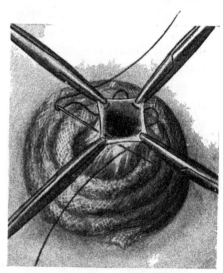

FIG. 40.—Colostomy. 1. The bowel has been brought outside and the wound closed. 2. Deep suture passing through abdominal wall and mesocolon.   3. Line of incision for tube. 4. Muscular band.

FIG. 41.—Colostomy.   Opening held by forceps to facilitate passing of running thread and introduction of tube.   The wound is protected by gauze, which is changed afterwards.

the suture tied, drawing the edges of the bowel incision round the tube beyond the flange.   The ends are passed round the peritoneal aspect outside and beyond the forceps, again tied, and cut off.   The bowel and surrounding parts are cleansed, and another strip of gauze drawn round and round the loop of bowel so that a thick layer protects the wound and at the same time supports not only the tube but also the loop into which it is inserted.   A dressing of sterilised gauze, reinforced with a thick layer of wool secured in position by a many-tailed bandage, supports the parts.   When the patient is in bed the thin rubber tube attached to the Paul's tube is placed in a convenient receptacle by his side. One effect of the circular stitch is to cause a slough to form, and the tube comes away in four to six days after the operation.

In all these cases it is advisable to empty the stomach with a tube before the operation and give saline afterwards by the rectum. These patients are often not only starved by their long abstinence from food, but dehydrated by the amount of fluid which they have vomited and been unable to replace. The results of this operation are very satisfactory.

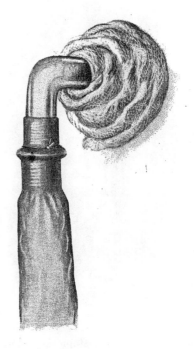

I recently saw (January, 1914) a woman for whom this operation was done for inoperable carcinoma of the rectum, and she spoke most enthusiastically of the benefit which she had derived from it, and the small discomfort which it caused. She had learned to manage her artificial anus excellently during the four years which had elapsed since it was made, and preferred the application of a pad and circular bandage to the more elaborate apparatus with which she had been supplied. She went about as usual both on foot and in public conveyances.

Fig. 42.—Colostomy. Completion of operation. The strip of gauze covers junction of tube and bowel; it also covers the wound in abdominal wall and the gut at its emergence.

Many surgeons are in favour of Paul's method of treatment of a malignant stricture of the bowel when it can be brought to the surface, whether there are secondary growths or not, and there is much to be said for it. By this operation the growth is brought outside, and either

(1) Fixed with the loop in which it is growing in the wound, a Paul's tube being put into the upper limb. Here the growth is removed later, or

(2) The growth is brought outside and cut away. A Paul's tube is then fixed in each end. These ends are sutured together

and fixed in the wound. Even if there are secondary growths, removal of the primary one will probably prolong life and make the future less liable to painful complications. No attempt is here made to restore the integrity of the canal, and there can be but inadequate removal of the glands in the second method. It is regarded as an operation rather more perfect than a simple colostomy.

The two-stage operation is often advisable when it is possible to perform a lateral anastomosis in cases where it is not good surgery to excise a growth. The wall of the bowel above, and often for some distance above, is so ill-fitted to hold sutures that they not infrequently give, and the patient dies from peritonitis.

In the same way ileo-colostomy may appear indicated in a case, but the condition of the distended small bowel with its softened wall will show how dangerous such a procedure would be until things have settled down.

Should, however, the obstruction be subacute after a more acute attack, the former operation may be done as follows :—

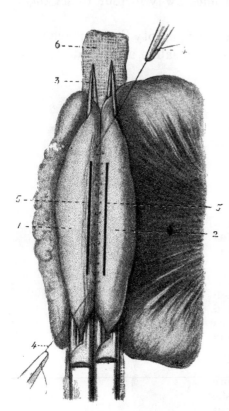

FIG. 43.—Lateral Anastomosis. 1. Large bowel. 2. Small bowel. These have been clamped and the clamps approximated. 3. The posterior continuous sero-muscular suture has been completed. 4. Incisions in back portions of bowel. 5. The ends of the sutures are held by artery forceps. 6. Gauze has been placed behind the parts engaged in the anastomosis, and structures around.

The portions of bowel to be united are brought outside and isolated by means of gauze strips. They are then placed side by side and clamps put upon them in such a way that there is a sufficiency of bowel isolated on each side to permit of a communication of about 3 inches being established. A continuous silk suture is then inserted commencing above and including the serous, muscular, and part of the submucous coats. The end of this suture is placed in artery forceps, and when it has been completed the needle is placed in gauze, or into one of the sterilised cloths, until again wanted. This line of suture should be about ¼ inch from the part of the bowel most distant from the mesentery. The intestine on each side in turn is now incised in a straight line in front of this suture (Fig. 43). The two incisions, being parallel, are carried down to the mucous membrane from which the outer coats have receded ; scissors are now used to open the bowel and cut away the ellipse of mucous membrane which is exposed. The parts of the bowel beyond the clamps are cleansed carefully with saline and gauze swabs held at the end of forceps. These forceps are again placed in the steriliser. A whipping suture including all the coats is then

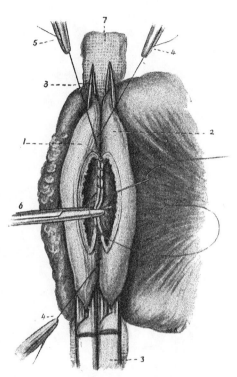

FIG. 44.—Lateral Anastomosis. The posterior part of outer suture completed, the bowel openings made, and the inner suture commenced. The needle passes through all the coats, which are held together with forceps. 1. Large bowel. 2. Small bowel. 3. Clamps. 4. Outer continuous suture. 5. Inner continuous suture. 6. Forceps holding the coats of both portions of bowel in position. 7. Gauze.

inserted, and it is a great help in doing this if the peritoneal surfaces are kept in apposition by forceps (Fig. 44). Much help is also afforded in the suturing if the needle, passed across the two opposed walls of the bowel, is grasped with forceps by the assistant, who holds it until you can take it, and keeps with his other hand the thread at the right degree of tension. This inner thread is passed through all the coats, at its commencement about ¼ inch from the end of the incisions and tied outside, the end being placed in forceps. It is continued circularly round the opening until the edges have been brought together, when it is tied to the end held by the pair of forceps. As the thread comes round to the front it is not difficult to continue it with the left hand. The clamps are now removed and the parts washed with sterilised saline. If the gloves are soiled they should be changed and fresh gauze packed round. Any bleeding point in the edge can be ligatured. The needle of the first thread is now taken and the outer suture continued in a manner similar to that which was done behind and at the same distance from the inner suture (Fig. 45). The ends are tied, cut short, and the junction is effected. If there is any doubt about the security of the suturing, extra sutures should be inserted at the ends to bring more of the peritoneum together in the long axis.

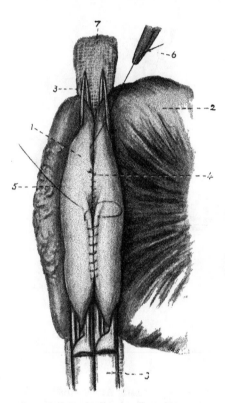

FIG. 45.—Lateral Anastomosis. The outer continuous suture almost completed. If there is any tension the clamps may be removed before this part of the suture is continued. 1. Large bowel. 2. Small bowel. 3. Clamp. 4. Inner suture. 5. Outer suture, to be tied to 6, which is left long for this purpose. 7. Gauze.

This anastomosis must not be too close to the growth, there must be no dragging on the line of sutures, and the two portions brought together should be isoperistaltic. Should it be considered best to make a short circuit between the ileum and large bowel, the same method by lateral anastomosis may be used or the end of the divided small intestine may be inserted into the large bowel, the distal end being closed with a double layer of sutures and dropped. The portion of large bowel selected is isolated with a clamp as it is in lateral anastomosis, and the free end of the ileum which projects beyond another intestinal clamp treated as follows :—

After thorough cleansing, the first outer suture is put in, taking up all the coats to the submucous layer ; this begins above about ¼ inch from the open mouth of the small bowel. An incision of length corresponding to the open mouth is made in the side of the large bowel and a running thread carried round to unite all the coats and act as a hæmostatic suture (Fig. 46). After removal of the clamp and cleansing of the parts the first suture is then continued round the line of anastomosis at the same distance from the completed inner suture. This union should also be without tension.

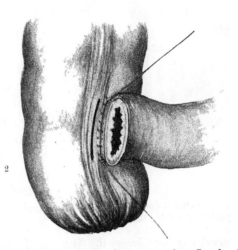

FIG. 46.—Ileo-colostomy. A. Implantation of the small intestine, end to side. The posterior part of the outer continuous suture, uniting the peritoneal and muscular layers, has been inserted and the incision made into the large bowel. The clamps are not shown. 1. Ileum. 2. Colon.

In order to give an aged patient relief for a distant journey when much distended I have punctured the transverse colon and given exit to enough gas to enable him to travel to his home in comparative comfort. He was a man who refused any other operative help.

Volvulus is the most common cause of acute obstruction of the large bowel, and is found in the sigmoid flexure, and at the ileo-cæcal junction. Of these the former is the more common and the patients mostly men.

The attack begins suddenly ; pain is severe and often

paroxysmal ; tenderness appears quite early. Vomiting is not usually a symptom which causes distress, and may even be absent. Distension of the abdomen comes on with considerable rapidity, and the respiration quickly becomes embarrassed in consequence of pressure on the diaphragm. The involved portion of the bowel tends to become gangrenous in a few hours, and peritonitis (as indicated by the marked tenderness) is an early complication. As a rule no separate coil of gut can be distinguished. When the ileo-cæcal region is affected the symptoms are of less urgency ; here there may be a resonant tumour of considerable size. Vomiting is present, but not usually of urgent character.

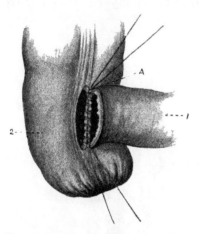

FIG. 47.—Ileo-colostomy. B. The posterior part of the inner suture encircling all the coats of the bowel has been inserted. The ends of both inner and outer sutures are left long, so that they may be continued and ultimately tied at A. 1. Ileum. 2. Colon.

Without early operation the prognosis is very grave. Very often the coil affected is gangrenous and resection is indicated. If the patient is very bad, the gangrenous bowel is drawn out of the abdomen and a Paul's tube put in. Later the gangrenous part is resected and the bowel restored by an end-to-end or lateral anastomosis.

RECURRENT VOLVULUS OF THE SIGMOID (Enterostomy : Recovery).—Mr. R., aged 76, was seen with Dr. A. E. Godfrey on March 22, 1914, for intestinal obstruction.

The present attack commenced with colicky abdominal pain and constipation ten days before. But having had some five or six similar attacks during the previous five years which had yielded to treatment, he had rather put off calling in medical aid. At first there had been a certain amount of relief from the use of remedies to act on the bowels, and enemata had been partly successful, but gradually the distension had become extreme and the pain paroxysmal, whilst little but coloured water could be washed from the bowel.

The abdomen was much distended, and the distension was most marked on the left side, where there was a large coil of the large intestine which contracted spasmodically during the examination. The abdomen was resonant all over (very tympanitic in front), but not tender. Rectal examination was negative. He was not sick, and was able to take fluid food. Pulse, 100 ; arteries rather hard ; tongue furred ; not emaciated.

Operation permitted on the 24th. An incision was made to the left of the middle line, the rectus displaced outwards, and the peritoneum opened. A very large coil of large intestine presented itself, so large that when outside the abdomen it measured 8 inches to 9 inches in diameter. This was emptied of a very large amount of gas by a stab wound with the point of a scalpel, there being only a few drops of fluid in the bowel. After closure of this opening with a stitch it was possible to examine the interior of the abdomen more fully and bring more of the sigmoid outside. It was then quite evident that the obstruction followed a volvulus of the sigmoid, there being a complete turn of a loop from left to right, the point of rotation being at the level of the promontory of the sacrum. The mesosigmoid was very long and the bowel wall thickened and hypertrophied. When this part of the gut had been emptied the upper abdomen looked quite concave, and although the small intestine was somewhat distended, it was quite remarkable how very little fæcal matter was seen and how little difference to the general distension had been contributed by the small bowel. A tube was placed in the sigmoid below the middle of the loop, and this was secured in the upper end of the wound. There was no evidence of growth which the recent history of the case had suggested before operation. The want of certainty made it advisable to explore before opening the large gut, as is usually done in the obstructed sigmoid when there is not a malignant stricture to be felt. He did well after the operation, and it was not long before the bowels acted naturally. The fæcal fistula was very useful for some days, and the attachment of the large bowel at that point will prevent a return of the volvulus.

PART VII

CONGENITAL DIVERTICULUM OF THE CYSTIC DUCT

IN considering fluctuating swellings in the subhepatic region, whether abscesses or suppurating hydatids, there is a condition to be referred to which, although very rare, closely resembles them. It is that of congenital diverticulum of the cystic duct. The remarkable characters which this disease may assume is shown by the case described.

F. G., a girl aged 14, was admitted ✳ on July 16 and died November 14, 1907.

She had been healthy until a month before, when she began to complain of pains in the right side with vomiting. For five days the pain had been continuous and more severe.

A fluctuating, prominent, rounded, very tender swelling was present on the right side below the liver, not moving well with respiration, and its outline towards the middle line was obscured by rigidity of the rectus muscle. The swelling passed backwards towards the lumbar region. Her pulse was 116; respiration 36; temperature, 103·2°. The tongue was furred and bowels confined. There was no jaundice.

An incision was first made in the loin and the peritoneum opened; the swelling was found to be covered with peritoneum and attached to the under surface of the liver. A second incision was made in front through the right rectus. Through this the cyst was tapped and 36 oz. of thick green bile drawn off. The wall of the cyst was very thick, especially the lining, which was white in colour. The gall-bladder was lying between the cyst and under surface of the liver, being flattened and empty, looking like a dog's tongue. The gall-bladder and cyst were removed and the cystic duct, which was a good deal elongated, secured in the wound. The cyst wall was composed of fibrous tissue and completely retroperitoneal. There were no calculi present, and there was no pus.

A tube was passed to the bottom of the wound and a gauze plug placed below it.

The patient improved quickly and bile came through the wound, all attempts later to make it flow in the normal direction being useless. At the end of October three attempts caused pain, and jaundice followed. On November 13 the cystic duct was inserted into the second part of the duodenum and sutured there with a double row of silk sutures. It was easily turned to the duodenum without tension, and no artery required ligature during the operation. It was thought best to place a tube and gauze plug down to the line of union. She became restless during the following night and died a few hours later.

Necropsy:—There had been extensive hæmorrhage into the right side of the abdomen, but Dr. Box could not find the source of the bleeding. The dilated bileduct had been anastomosed successfully to the duodenum immediately beyond the pylorus. The common duct terminated about an inch below the liver; beyond this it could not be traced downwards. Explored from the bile papilla in the duodenum, it ran up for an inch and then ended, but blindly. The intervening portion was missing. There was no peritonitis, but a certain amount of adhesions about the area of operation.

A case of diverticulum of the cystic duct is also found in the St. Thomas's Hospital Reports for 1907.

The case was that of a girl of 18 under the care of the late Mr. Clutton. She had complained of pain and swelling on the right side of the abdomen for a fortnight, and had vomited a day or two before admission. There was then a painless swelling in the right kidney region, extending slightly below the level of the umbilicus and almost to the middle line. The urine was normal; temperature, 98·2°. Eleven days after admission lumbar incision, paracentesis of an intraperitoneal cyst, withdrawal of two and a half pints of olive-green glistening fluid which did not contain bile, although fluid which flowed from the wound later did so. Cyst wall taken away; the colon was adherent to it, there was free venous hæmorrhage: arrested by plugs. There were numerous facetted calculi in it: a communication with cystic duct at a point where there was a small nipple-shaped projection. There was a discharge of bile after removal of the plugs, and she appeared to be progressing satisfactorily until twenty days after operation, when she died from hæmorrhage.

The internal opening was close to the neck of the gall-bladder in the cystic duct. The gall-bladder contained a few calculi; the common duct was normal. The hæmorrhage had probably come from a branch of the portal vein in the portal fissure.

Search has been made with the view of adding something to the somewhat bare records of these cases, but nothing has been found in surgical literature to give any help. It is very remarkable that both patients should have reached the ages attained before symptoms developed, and that there should have been no jaundice present in either of them at the time when they came to operation. It is also a curious fact that in each of them the fatal ending ensued after a hæmorrhage the origin of which was quite obscure.

APPENDIX

——◆——

THE OPERATION OF GASTROSTOMY

As gastrostomy may be required as an emergency operation in a neglected case of œsophageal obstruction, I have thought it advisable to add a few lines which may encourage its performance in a patient who appears almost at his last gasp. A man who has been taking even fluid nourishment with difficulty by the mouth, and is much emaciated, with a dry, harsh skin and sunken eyes, will improve marvellously as a result of the introduction of fluid through an opening into the stomach. There still appears to be a kind of prejudice against gastrostomy, firstly, because of the shock which it is supposed to cause; secondly, because of the inconvenience which leakage from the opening may produce.

If a local anæsthetic is used there is no shock, and the method of Senn prevents leakage of the stomach contents. The illustration (Fig. 48) shows the normal state of the skin in a patient who had gastrostomy performed two years ago for impermeable stricture of the œsophagus, the result of taking acid. There is not the slightest abrasion, whilst the girl is well nourished and looks healthy, although she is quite dependent for her food supply on the opening. The incision is made through the left rectus at its outer border, and should be from 2 to 3 inches in length, commencing just below the costal cartilage. The stomach is easily found, although usually retracted and small. Traction on the omentum will bring it down, and a point for the operation is selected. This should be about midway between the greater, and the lesser, curvatures, as far as possible from the pylorus. A rubber tube, or better, a Jacques catheter, No. 12—14, is introduced through an incision large enough to admit it, and fastened in position by means of a suture which includes all the coats of the stomach. A cone which projects into the stomach is made in the following

manner : A purse string suture is passed half an inch away from
the tube, completely encircling it, the tube is depressed by an

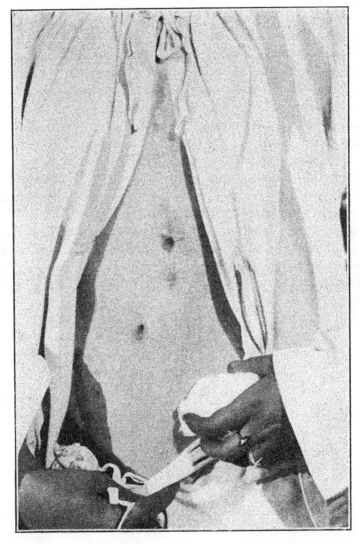

FIG. 48.—1. The opening two years after gastrostomy by Senn's
method, in a girl aged 16. 2. The scar of an operation for
acute appendicitis one year after the gastrostomy.

assistant whilst the suture is tied. Two similar sutures are
passed and tied, the tube being pushed in on each occasion.
The stomach is then fixed to the posterior rectal sheath and

A.A.   U

peritoneum of the wound, above and below, by sutures which
take good hold of it. Sutures are inserted on both sides,
shutting off the peritoneal cavity. The sheath of the rectus
above and below the opening is sutured and then the skin
incision.

The tube is brought through the dressing and secured outside
to the bandage with a safety-pin. A wooden plug is inserted
and prevents escape of fluid from the stomach. The stitch
through the tube rarely holds for more than ten days, but
unless the dressing is carelessly changed or the patient interferes
the tube will retain its position. No difficulty will be found in
changing the tube, but one of the original size should be retained
until the patient is used to feeding himself and has lost all
apprehension of hurting himself by passing it. It can then be
replaced by a gastrostomy plug, which is more easily managed
by a patient who wishes to get about.

Feeding should be commenced at once, a half a pint of milk
with an ounce of brandy being given on the table. Subsequent
feeds should be given through the tube, a small glass funnel
being used, and there should be no disturbance of the dressing.

INDEX.

CPSIA information can be obtained
at www.ICGtesting.com
Printed in the USA
BVHW04*1349210918
528174BV00011B/337/P